AF556798

Clinical Disorders in

PEDIATRIC GASTROENTEROLOGY AND NUTRITION

PEDIATRICS

Editor: **Charles Bauer**
Clinical Associate Professor of Pediatrics
Cornell University School of Medicine
New York, New York

Volume 1 CLINICAL DISORDERS IN PEDIATRIC GASTROENTEROLOGY AND NUTRITION, *edited by Fima Lifshitz*

Other volumes in preparation

Clinical Disorders in

PEDIATRIC GASTROENTEROLOGY AND NUTRITION

Edited by
FIMA LIFSHITZ
Cornell University Medical College
New York, New York
North Shore University Hospital
Manhasset, New York

MARCEL DEKKER, INC. New York and Basel

Library of Congress Cataloging in Publication Data

Main entry under title:

Clinical disorders in pediatric gastroenterology and nutrition.

(Pediatrics ; v. 1)
Includes bibliographical references and indexes.
1. Pediatric gastroenterology. 2. Nutrition disorders in children. I. Lifshitz, Fima, [Date] II. Series. [DNLM: 1. Gastrointestinal diseases--In infancy and childhood. 2. Nutrition disorders--In infancy and childhood. W1 PE191B v. 2 no. 1 / WS310 C641]
RJ446.C55 618.92'3 80-18516
ISBN 0-8247-6954-6

MARCEL DEKKER, INC.
270 Madison Avenue, New York, New York 10016

Current printing (last digit):
10 9 8 7 6 5 4 3 2 1

PRINTED IN THE UNITED STATES OF AMERICA

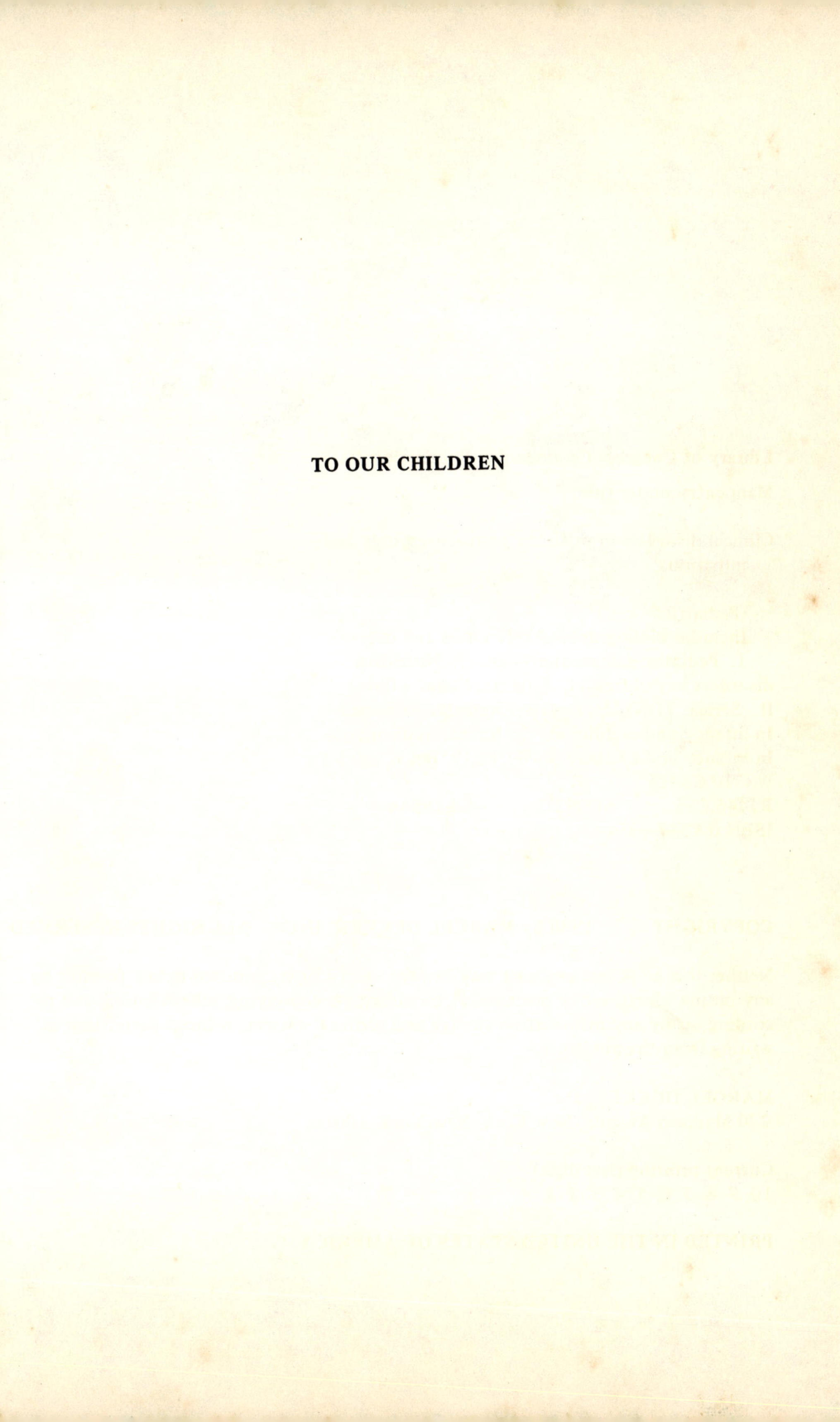

TO OUR CHILDREN

Contributors

Harvey W. Aiges, M.D. Assistant Professor, Department of Pediatrics, Cornell University Medical College, New York, New York; Associate Gastroenterologist, Department of Pediatrics, North Shore University Hospital, Manhasset, New York

R. Peter Altman, M.D. Professor, Department of Surgery, George Washington University School of Medicine, Washington, D.C.; Senior Attending Surgeon, Department of Surgery, Children's Hospital National Medical Center, Washington, D.C.

Jerrold M. Becker, M.D., F.A.C.S., F.A.A.P. Professor of Clinical Surgery, State University of New York at Stony Brook Health Science Center, Stony Brook, New York; Attending-in-Charge, Division of Pediatric Surgery, Long Island Jewish Hospital Medical Center, New Hyde Park, New York

Moshe Berant, M.D.* Visiting Research Scientist, Department of Pediatrics, Cornell University Medical College, New York, New York, and Visiting Research Scientist, Department of Pediatrics, North Shore University Hospital, Manhasset, New York

Sidney Cohen, M.D. T. Grier Miller Professor, Department of Medicine, University of Pennsylvania School of Medicine, Philadelphia, Pennsylvania; Chief, Gastrointestinal Section, Department of Medicine, Hospital of the University of Pennsylvania, Philadelphia, Pennsylvania

Fredric Daum, M.D. Associate Professor of Clinical Pediatrics, Department of Pediatrics, Cornell University Medical College, New York, New York; Chief, Division of Gastroenterology, Department of Pediatrics, North Shore University Hospital, Manhasset, New York

Sudhakar G. Ezhuthachan, M.D. (PED.), D.C.H., F.A.A.P.† Assistant Professor, Department of Pediatrics, Albert Einstein College of Medicine, Division of Neonatology, Bronx Municipal Hospital Center, Bronx, New York

Present Affiliation:

*Director, Department of Pediatrics B, Rambam Medical Center, Haifa, Israel.

†Assistant Professor, Department of Pediatrics, Albert Einstein College of Medicine, Bronx, New York; Associate Chief, Department of Neonatal-Perinatology, Bronx-Lebanon Hospital, Bronx, New York.

Ulysses Fagundes-Neto, M.D.* Research Fellow, Department of Pediatrics, Cornell University Medical College, New York, New York; Research Fellow, Division of Endocrinology, Metabolism and Nutrition, Department of Pediatrics, North Shore University Hospital, Manhasset, New York

D. Grant Gall, M.D., F.R.C.P. (C) Professor, Divisions of Pediatrics and Medicine, The University of Calgary, Calgary, Alberta, Canada

Lawrence M. Gartner, M.D.† Professor of Pediatrics, Department of Pediatrics, Albert Einstein College of Medicine, Bronx, New York; Director, Division of Neonatology, Bronx Municipal Hospital Center, Bronx, New York

Richard J. Grand, M.D. Associate Professor of Pediatrics, Harvard Medical School, Boston, Massachusetts; Senior Associate in Medicine and Chief, Division of Gastroenterology and Nutrition, Department of Medicine, Children's Hospital Medical Center, Boston, Massachusetts

Harold E. Harrison, M.D. Professor Emeritus, Department of Pediatrics, Johns Hopkins University School of Medicine, Baltimore, Maryland; Pediatrician, Children's Medical and Surgical Center, Baltimore, Maryland

Ellen I. Kahn, M.D. Assistant Professor, Department of Pathology, Cornell University Medical College, New York, New York; Attending Pathologist, Department of Laboratories, and Senior Assistant Attending, Department of Pediatrics, North Shore University Hospital, Manhasset, New York

Drew G. Kelts, M.D.‡ Research Fellow, Department of Pediatrics, Harvard Medical School, Boston, Massachusetts; Fellow, Division of Gastroenterology, Department of Medicine, The Children's Hospital Medical Center, Boston, Massachusetts

Gerald T. Keusch, M.D.§ Professor, Department of Medicine, Mount Sinai School of Medicine, New York, New York

Emanuel Lebenthal, M.D. Associate Professor, Department of Pediatrics, State University of New York at Buffalo School of Medicine, Buffalo, New York; Chief, Division of Gastroenterology and Nutrition, Department of Pediatrics, Children's Hospital of Buffalo, Buffalo, New York

Fima Lifshitz, M.D. Professor, Department of Pediatrics, Cornell University Medical College, New York, New York; Associate Director, Department of Pediatrics, Chief, Division of Endrocrinology, Metabolism and Nutrition, and Chief, Pediatric Research, Department of Pediatrics, North Shore University Hospital, Manhasset, New York

Present Affiliation:

*Assistant Professor, Division of Gastroenterology, Department of Pediatrics, Escola Paulista de Medicina, São Paulo, Brazil

†Chairman, Department of Pediatrics, Pritzker School of Medicine, University of Chicago, Chicago, Illinois

‡Assistant Professor, Department of Pediatrics, and Chief, Pediatric Gastroenterology, University of California at San Diego, California

§Chief, Division of Geographic Medicine, and Professor, Department of Medicine, Tufts University School of Medicine and New England Medical Center Hospitals, Boston, Massachusetts

Peter N. Perinchief, M.D. Fellow, Department of Pediatrics, Cornell University Medical College, New York, New York; Fellow, Division of Endocrinology, Metabolism and Nutrition, Department of Pediatrics, North Shore University Hospital, Manhasset, New York

Norton S. Rosensweig, M.D.* Associate Professor, Department of Medicine, Cornell University Medical College, New York, New York; Chief, Division of Gastroenterology and Nutrition, Department of Medicine, North Shore University Hospital, Manhasset, New York

Andrew Sass-Kortsak, M.D., F.R.C.P. (C) Professor, Department of Pediatrics, Faculty of Medicine, University of Toronto, Toronto, Ontario, Canada; Senior Scientist, The Research Institute, Senior Staff Physician, The Hospital for Sick Children, Toronto, Ontario, Canada

Keith M. Schneider, M.D., F.A.C.S., F.A.A.P. Clinical Professor of Surgery and Pediatrics, Albert Einstein College of Medicine, and Director, Pediatric Surgery, Hospital of Albert Einstein College of Medicine, Bronx, New York; Attending-in-Charge, Pediatric Surgery, North Shore University Hospital, Manhasset, New York

David L. Schwartz, M.D., F.A.C.S., F.A.A.P. Clinical Assistant Professor, Department of Surgery, Albert Einstein College of Medicine, Bronx, New York; Attending-in-Surgery, North Shore University Hospital, Manhasset, New York

Mervin Silverberg, M.D. Professor, Department of Pediatrics, Cornell University Medical College, New York, New York; Director, Department of Pediatrics, North Shore University Hospital, Manhasset, New York

Henry B. So, M.D., F.A.C.S., F.A.A.P. Clinical Instructor, Cornell University Medical College, New York, New York; Assistant Attending-in-Surgery, North Shore University Hospital, Manhasset, New York

Lani S. Stephenson, Ph.D. Research Associate in International Nutrition, Division of Nutritional Sciences, Cornell University, Ithaca, New York

Saul Teichberg, Ph.D. Assistant Professor, Department of Pediatrics, Cornell University Medical College, New York, New York; Chief, Electron Microscopy Section, Departments of Pediatrics and Laboratories, North Shore University Hospital, Manhasset, New York

Ramon B. Torres-Pinedo, M.D. Professor, Department of Pediatrics, University of Oklahoma Health Sciences Center, Oklahoma City, Oklahoma; Chief, Section of Pediatric Gastroenterology, Oklahoma Children's Memorial Hospital, Oklahoma City, Oklahoma

Present Affiliation:

*Medical Service, Department of Medicine, St. Luke's Hospital Center, New York, New York; Associate Professor, Department of Medicine, Columbia University College of Physicians and Surgeons, New York, New York

W. Allan Walker, M.D. Associate Professor, Department of Pediatrics, Harvard Medical School, Boston, Massachusetts; Pediatrician and Chief, Pediatric Gastrointestinal and Nutrition Unit, Massachusetts General Hospital, Boston, Massachusetts

Raul A. Wapnir, Ph.D., M.P.H. Professor of Biochemistry in Pediatrics, Cornell University Medical College, New York, New York; Head, Laboratory of the Child Development Center, and Chief Biochemistry Pediatric Research, Department of Pediatrics, North Shore University Hospital, Manhasset, New York

John B. Watkins, M.D. Associate Professor, University of Pennsylvania School of Medicine, Philadelphia, Pennsylvania; Division of Gastroenterology, Department of Medicine; Children's Hospital of Philadelphia, Philadelphia, Pennsylvania

Murray Wittner, M.D., Ph.D. Professor of Pathology and Parasitology, Department of Pathology, Albert Einstein College of Medicine, Bronx, New York; Director, Tropical Disease Clinic and Parasitology Laboratory, Bronx Municipal Hospital, Bronx, New York

Foreword

The present volume is based, in part, upon a postgraduate course for continuing medical education, designed for the practicing physician, which was held on April 24 and 25, 1978, in Manhasset, New York. The program was one of a series of educational modules offered by the Department of Pediatrics, North Shore University Hospital, Cornell University Medical College, and guest faculty. Over 120 pediatric practitioners and pediatric house officers participated in this postgraduate course, designed to bring to the audience the most current concepts in the pathophysiology and management of frequently encountered problems in children—as they relate to the rapidly changing fields of gastroenterology and nutrition. A distinguished faculty, both from Cornell's affiliated institution, North Shore University Hospital, and other major teaching centers, provided a stimulating program of major importance for today's pediatric practitioners, demonstrating thereby a significant contribution to Cornell's continuing medical education effort.

It is well recognized that even the best medical education program may not assure the continued competence and professional growth of the participating physicians; however, the wealth of knowledge, innovation, and creativity, available through the numerous programs around the nation, most certainly will have a positive effect on the implementation of medical care provided by physicians to the public. The publication of this volume is designed to contribute to this goal.

In our quest for knowledge we are reminded, as physicians, that eighty years ago, Sir William Osler, in a call to our profession, stated "no class of men need to call to mind more often the wise comment of Plato that education is a lifelong business." In this monograph it is hoped that you will find a valuable addition to your own education.

Lawrence Scherr, M.D.
Associate Dean
Cornell University Medical College

Preface

knowledge exists to be imparted
Ralph Waldo Emerson

This book reviews current information in the area of pediatric gastroenterology and nutrition. It is intended for those who want to acquire the most current knowledge in their battle against disease. The book focuses on current concepts in pathophysiology and management of frequently encountered gastroenterological and nutritional disorders in pediatrics. It is divided into five sections: (1) hepatobiliary disorders, (2) gastrointestinal disorders, (3) intestinal absorption disorders, (4) diarrheal disorders, and (5) consequences of gastrointestinal disorders. The subjects of each section are considered from the vantage point of experts in the field; the 31 contributors to this book have presented the most pertinent information for those who deal with these childhood disorders. Only this type of collaborative effort could appropriately cover this vast field. Each of the 27 chapters of the book denotes the "State of the Art" in the beginning of the new decade, and it presupposes no special competence or training in pediatrics, gastroenterology, or nutrition—only a wish to learn.

Fima Lifshitz, M.D.

Contents

Clinical Disorders in

PEDIATRIC GASTROENTEROLOGY AND NUTRITION

PART I

Hepatobiliary Disorders

1
Physiology of Bilirubin Metabolism

SUDHAKAR G. EZHUTHACHAN and LAWRENCE M. GARTNER* / Albert Einstein College of Medicine, Bronx, New York

I. Introduction

With each decade, investigators have come to a point in their knowledge of bilirubin metabolism at which they have believed they had a full understanding of the pathways of synthesis, transport, and conversion. Yet new questions emerge, and advances in knowledge are again made. This chapter attempts to summarize the current concepts in this area.

II. Synthesis of Bilirubin

Eighty-five percent of the total bilirubin load in adults is derived from senescent red cells. Studies in humans with radioisotope-labeled heme have demonstrated that peak production of bile pigment is derived from red cells formed 100-140 days prior to degradation [1]. This is known as the late peak of bilirubin synthesis. Two earlier peaks of bilirubin synthesis correspond to (1) hepatic heme turnover at 0-3½ hr and (2) ineffective erythropoiesis at 3-5 days after labeling of heme [2]. Bone marrow stimulation due to hypoxia [2], erythropoietin [2], or hemorrhage [2] increases the second early peak (3-5 days). Radiation-induced bone marrow aplasia results in suppression of this peak [3].

Other potential sources of bilirubin are the heme-containing proteins, the cytochromes, peroxidases, catalases, and myoglobin. Approximately 4 mg/kg of body weight of bilirubin is formed daily in the adult human. Heme is con-

*Present Affiliation:
Pritzker School of Medicine, University of Chicago, Chicago, Illinois

verted by alpha-heme oxygenase in the microsomes of the liver, spleen, and kidneys to biliverdin [4, 5], a water-soluble green pigment, which is further hydrogenated by biliverdin reuuctase, in the cytosol, to bilirubin [6], a fat-soluble yellow pigment. For each mole of heme degraded, one mole each of carbon monoxide (CO), ferric iron, and bilirubin is formed [7, 8]. The rate of CO production, once considered a reliable measure of heme degradation, has been questioned recently because of evidence that the peroxidation of microsomal lipids may also result in the formation of CO [9].

Data from experimental animals suggest that alpha-heme oxygenase is far more active in immature animals than in the adult of the species. The activity of alpha-heme oxygenase can be induced by hemoglobin. Hemolysis is associated with a three- to fivefold increase in activity [7], as is splenectomy [7].

Red cell sensitization, fasting, glucagon, and epinephrine are also known to induce heme oxygenase activity. It has been suggested that several cofactors, including ascorbate and O_2, are required for the conversion of hemoglobin or heme to bilirubin. In the reticuloendothelial system, heme is degraded to bilirubin IXα, the major isomer. Small amounts of other isomers are also found.

Unconjugated bilirubin (UCB) is highly insoluble in an aqueous medium having a pK of 7.95 and a true water solubility of the order of 0.0056-0.0058 mg/dl. The methyl, vinyl, and propionic side chains have specific positions on each of the four pyrrole rings, determining the water solubility of the molecule [5]. Bilirubin IXα is extremely insoluble in water at pH 7.4, despite the presence of apparently ionizable hydroxyl and carboxyl groups, because of intramolecular hydrogen bonding [10], which sequesters the polar groups. Rearrangement of the side chains, as found in the isomeric forms, prevents intramolecular hydrogen bonding, resulting in markedly increased water solubility.

III. Plasma Transport of Bilirubin

The albumin molecule has been shown to possess at least two binding sites for bilirubin. A third site and possibly other, weaker sites have also been suggested. The first or "tight" site has an affinity constant variously reported as from 10^7 to 10^8 M. Globulins, lipoproteins, and red cells are other circulating blood constituents that are capable of binding bilirubin. At bilirubin-to-albumin molar ratios of less than 1, bilirubin is all firmly bound to albumin in the normal individual. At a molar ratio of 1, each gram of albumin can bind 8.4 mg bilirubin. Thus, for an albumin concentration of 3.5 g/dl, up to 30 mg/dl of bilirubin can be tightly bound. Saturation of both major sites will occur at 60 mg/dl. By means of a variety of methods for estimation of bilirubin binding, some newborn infants have been shown to have deficient capacity and/or affinity [10a]. The explanation for such deficiency is unknown, but competing anions, a structural abnormality of albumin, and the effects of altered physical states have been suggested.

IV. Uptake of Bilirubin

Despite the tight binding of bilirubin to albumin, bilirubin is transferred readily into the hepatocyte by a mechanism not as yet fully defined. No active transport system has been demonstrated; simple diffusion and carrier-mediated or facilitated diffusion have been suggested. Albumin and bilirubin dissociate prior to the entrance of bilirubin into the liver cell [11]. The "Y protein," also known as ligandin [12], an intracellular cytoplasmic protein capable of binding bilirubin, transports the bile pigment from the sinusoidal membrane to the smooth endoplasmic reticulum and may also permit storage of unconjugated bilirubin within the liver cell [13]. Ligandin is an anion-binding protein not only for bilirubin but also for other substances such as azo carcinogens and cortisol [12].

The rate of entry of bilirubin into the circulation and the rate of uptake of bilirubin by the liver determine the serum bilirubin concentration. An imbalance in this relationship, as in the hepatic uptake deficiency found in Gilbert's syndrome in humans, results in an increased serum unconjugated bilirubin concentration.

Tracer studies with UCB in rats suggest that 70% of hepatic bilirubin is in the cytosol, the remainder being distributed among the microsomes, lysosomes, mitochondria, and cell-membrane nuclear fractions [14, 15]. Only 50% of injected bilirubin enters the hepatic pool, however. In the hepatic parenchymal cell cytosol are the two major anion-binding proteins: ligandin (Y protein) and Z protein [13]. Ligandin is also found in the kidney, brain, and gut—and in liver consitutes 5% of all the protein in the hepatic cytosol [12]. The Z protein has a lower affinity for the anions than ligandin, but has a greater potential binding capacity and appears to be identical with fatty acid-binding protein (FABP) [13]. Hepatic Y protein content can be augmented by administration of phenobarbital and DDT.* Ligandin is the more important of the two proteins with regard to bilirubin transport, whereas Z protein seems to play a greater role in fatty acid transport. It remains unsettled at this time whether ligandin has a higher affinity for bilirubin than albumin, and thereby enhances uptake by stripping bilirubin off albumin, or has a lower affinity than albumin and facilitates bilirubin movement into the liver cell by preventing reflux of bilirubin back into plasma.

*1,1,1-Trichloro-2,2-bis(*p*-chlorophenyl)ethane (DDT).

V. Conjugation of Bilirubin

Bilirubin is conjugated in the hepatocyte, converting the fat-soluble pigment into a water-soluble compound. The major conjugate of bilirubin is the glucuronide [16], with uridine diphosphoglucuronic acid (UDPGA) acting as the donor. Xylosyl and glucoside conjugates are also formed [17]. Thin-layer chromatography of azo dye derivatives of bile pigments demonstrates that approximately 85% of bilirubin bile in normal adults is in the form of bilirubin diglucuronide [18]. Only small amounts of bilirubin monoglucuronide and nonglucuronide conjugates are found [19]. In patients with Gilbert's syndrome, a marked increase in the proportion of bilirubin monoglucuronide in bile is found. How this relates to the development of unconjugated hyperbilirubinemia in these individuals is unknown.

The conjugation of bilirubin with glucuronic acid takes place in two separate steps, with formation of the monoglucuronide occurring in the microsomal fraction of liver, while the conversion from monoglucuronide to diglucuronide takes place at the hepatic cell canalicular membrane. The reactions are summarized in the following sections.

A. The First-Step Process

In the cytosol:

Glucose-1-phosphate + uridine triphosphate $\xrightarrow{\text{uridine diphosphoglucose pyrophosphorylase}}$ uridine diphosphoglucose + pyrophosphate

Uridine diphosphoglucose + $2NAD^+$ + H_2O $\xrightarrow{\text{Uridine diphosphoglucose dehydrogenase}}$ UDPGA + $2H^+$ + 2NADH

In the microsome:

Bilirubin + UDPGA $\xrightarrow{\text{UDPGA glucuronyl transferase}}$ bilirubin monoglucuronide + UDP

This monoglucuronide formation can be saturated if 100 times the normal load of bilirubin is presented to the hepatocyte. Unconjugated hyperbilirubinemia would be expected to occur only when enzyme activity has been reduced to 1% of normal or less, as observed in patients with the recessively inherited (type I, Crigler-Najjar syndrome) [20] and dominantly inherited (type II, Arias's syndrome) forms of conjugating deficiency [20a].

B. The Second-Step Process

Uridine diphosphoglucuronate glucuronyl transferase is the enzyme catalyzing the conversion of bilirubin monoglucuronide to bilirubin diglucuronide. In this reaction at the site of the canalicular membrane, the glucuronic acid of one bilirubin monoglucuronide is shifted to a second molecule of bilirubin monoglucuronide, resulting in the formation of one molecule of bilirubin diglucuronide and one molecule of unconjugated bilirubin, which then is returned to the endoplasmic reticulum for subsequent reconjugation. The necessity for the second step is not known with certainty since bilirubin monoglucuronide is water-soluble and can be excreted into bile. The second-step enzyme, better known as transglucuronidase, may, because of its proximity to the canaliculus, bear a close relationship to excretory function. In severe chronic hemolysis increased serum concentrations have been found, suggesting that transglucuronidation operates at a lower rate than monoglucuronidation.

The significance of xylose, glucose, polysaccharide, and even sulfate conjugation of bilirubin for the human is uncertain. Drugs, natural and synthetic steroids, may also be conjugated in the liver with glucuronic acid to render them metabolically inactive. Most of these nonbilirubin conjugations are believed to be catalyzed by a different set (or different sets) of enzymes from those used for bilirubin conjugation, but the process is not entirely clarified at this time.

VI. Excretion of Bilirubin

Bilirubin excretion from the liver cell into bile is believed to be an active, secretory process [21] at the canalicular membrane, with generation of a 100-fold concentration gradient from liver cell cytoplasm to bile [21]. Linked to bile salt excretion, bilirubin competes with other substances for excretion, including bromsulphthalein (BSP), indocyanine green (ICG), and Rose Bengal [22]. Excretion is the rate-limiting step in the overall transfer of bilirubin from blood to bile. Maximum bilirubin excretory capacity in monkeys ranges from 17 to 24 μg/100g body weight per minute. Maximum rates for uptake and conjugation are at least twice that of the excretory rate, an indication that neither of these earlier steps is normally rate limiting.

Disease affecting the excretory function of bilirubin, including hepatitis, cause retention of both bile salts and conjugated (direct-reacting) bilirubin, designated as cholestasis. In contrast, in both the Dubin-Johnson and Rotor syndromes, conjugated hyperbilirubinemia results from an isolated reduction in bilirubin excretion without bile salt excretory failure.

VII. Enterohepatic Circulation of Bilirubin

One additional factor which influences serum bilirubin concentration is the enterophepatic circulation of bile pigment [23, 24]. Although bilirubin excreted from the liver cell is all in the form of conjugated pigment and is water-soluble

[25, 26], it is readily hydrolyzed to unconjugated bilirubin by the alkaline pH of the duodenum and mucosal β-glucuronidase [24]. Both unconjugated and conjugated bilirubin can be reduced to urobilinogens and stercobilins by the intestinal bacteria, particularly the *Escherichia coli* and clostridial organisms, this change taking place mainly in the distal small bowel and colon. Unconjugated bilirubin (but not conjugated bilirubin) can be absorbed across the intestinal mucosa, returning to the portal circulation for reexcretion by the liver after reconjugation. Although the proportion of intestinal bilirubin reabsorbed is not clearly known in the human, it has been estimated that 25% returns to the portal circulation. Nonabsorbable substances that bind bilirubin, including activated charcoal and agar, may reduce intestinal bilirubin reabsorption.

A portion of the urobilinogens formed are reabsorbed as well, to be excreted in bile and urine. The absence of urobilinogens in the stool and urine, in the presence of conjugated hyperbilirubinemia, implies obstruction of bile flow into the bowel.

VIII. Fetal Bilirubin Metabolism

Despite severe reductions in hepatic bilirubin transport and metabolism in fetal life, unconjugated hyperbilirubinemia does not develop. Cord bilirubin concentrations are normally less than 1.5 mg/dl. Even in the case of severe hemolysis in utero, bilirubin concentrations rarely exceed 6 or 7 mg/dl unless the conjugated fraction is also elevated. The placenta efficiently permits transfer of unconjugated bilirubin into the maternal circulation, but does not permit significant transfer of conjugated bilirubin. Thus, diseases affecting fetal liver excretory function, such as neonatal hepatitis, causing an elevation of conjugated bilirubin, will manifest as significant jaundice in the fetus and in the newborn at birth, since the placenta cannot excrete conjugated bilirubin, and this remains in fetal circulation. The process of placental transfer of unconjugated bilirubin is believed to be one of passive diffusion in both directions. It is possible that an elevated maternal serum unconjugated bilirubin level will be reflected in the fetus as well.

The presence of unconjugated bilirubin has been noted in amniotic fluid from the 12th through 37th week of gestation in association with fetal hemolytic disease. Its possible sources include diffusion across the fetal membranes, umbilical cord, and fetal skin–and from pulmonary and tracheobronchial secretions.

IX. Bilirubin Metabolism in the Neonate

Virtually all newborns develop serum unconjugated bilirubin elevations (greater than 2 mg/dl) in the first week of life. The normal newborn, in comparison with the older child and adult, produces approximately twice the amount of unconjugated bilirubin per day (8.5 mg/kg body weight)–due to a greater red cell volume, shortened red cell life-span (even shorter in prematures), and an increased quantity of early-labeled fraction bilirubin.

The unconjugated hyperbilirubinemia of the newborn referred to as physiologic jaundice has been characterized as occurring in two distinct phases [27]. The first phase (phase I) starts at birth and peaks at around 3-4 days in full-term infants and at 5-7 days in prematures. This peak is followed by a rapid decline over the next 2 days and is followed immediately by phase II, which is characterized by a sustained UCB level of 2-3 mg/dl until the end of the second week of life, when adult levels of less than 1 mg/dl are achieved. In the premature, phase I is exaggerated in concentration, and phase II is prolonged for up to 4-5 weeks; in postterm infants, phase I is much lower in concentration than in term infants, while phase II is the same as in term infants [27, 28].

In newborn rhesus monkeys the total load of bilirubin which the liver must excrete is about 5-6 times greater for the first 3-6 weeks of life than it is in older monkeys [27, 28]. With diversion of bile from the gut in monkeys more than 3 days old, it has been observed that almost all of the markedly increased serum bilirubin is derived from exaggerated intestinal reabsorption of uncongugated bilirubin, and not from de novo synthesis, after the first week of life [27]. Considering differences in rates of maturation, this would suggest that human newborns may have increased intestinal bilirubin absorption for up to 18 weeks of life.

Hepatic glucuronyl transferase, the enzyme involved in the first step of conjugation, is markedly deficient in the immediate newborn period [27]. The activity of the enzyme in the full-term rhesus monkey at birth is 5% that of adult monkeys [28]. This reduction in activity, coupled with the sixfold increase in bilirubin load, produces phase I physiologic jaundice. The increase in enzyme activity after the first 24 hr in the rhesus monkey newborn, and after 72 hr in the human, coincides with the decline in serum bilirubin concentration.

The administration of phenobarbital to the rhesus monkey mother during the last weeks of pregnancy increases the enzyme activity by about twofold and significantly reduces phase I hyperbilirubinemia [29]. This has also been confirmed in humans, following administration of 30-60 mg per day of phenobarbital to near-term pregnant women for 2 weeks prior to delivery. In the *premature* monkey and human, little or no effect is observed from the administration of phenobarbital to the mothers. Thus far, evidence exists only that the first-step enzyme is deficient in activity in the neonate; developmental studies of the transglucuronidase enzyme have not yet been reported.

The second phase of physiological jaundice (phase II) also is the result of a combination of at least two factors: i.e., increased bilirubin load and delayed hepatic bilirubin uptake. The former is derived from exaggerated enterohepatic circulation of bilirubin [30]. Reduced hepatic bilirubin uptake results, in part at least, from developmentally deficient ligandin synthesis.

X. Summary

Bilirubin is derived from a variety of heme sources. Its structural peculiarity, specifically intramolecular hydrogen bonding, necessitates its conjugation to render it water-soluble and therefore excretable in bile. The process of conjugation has now been shown to be a two-step process, the second step involving the enzyme transglucuronidase.

In the newborn, the developmental process responsible for physiologic jaundice has been shown most recently to resolve into two distinct clinical and functional periods, in which conjugation and uptake deficiency interact with exaggerated enteric bilirubin absorption.

References

1. C. H. Gray, A. Neuberger, and P. H. A. Sneath. Studies in congenital porphyria. II. Incorporation of ^{15}N in the stercobilin in the normal and in the porphyric. *Biochem. J. 47,* 97-92 (1950).
2. S. H. Robinson, M. Tsong, B. W. Brown, and R. Schmid. The sources of bile pigment in the rat: Studies of the "early labelled" fraction. *J. Clin. Invest. 45,* 1569-1586 (1966).
3. L. G. Israels. The bilirubin shunt and shunt hyperbilirubinemia. In *Progress in Liver Diseases* (H. Popper and F. Schaffner, Eds.), Vol. 3. Grune & Stratton, New York, 1970, pp. 1-12.
4. F. H. Jansen and M. S. Stoll. Separation and structural analysis of vinyl and isovinyl-azobilirubin derivatives. *Biochem. J. 125,* 585-597 (1971).
5. P. O'Carra. Heme-Cleavage: Biological systems and chemical analogs. In *Porphyrins and Metalloporphyrins* (K. M. Smith, Ed.), Elsevier Scientific, Amsterdam, 1975, pp. 123-153.
6. C. D. Wise and D. L. Drabkin. Degradation of hemoglobin and heme to biliverdin by a new cell-free enzyme system obtained from the hemophagous organ of the dog placenta. *Fed. Proc. 23, 223* (1964).
7. R. Telhunen, H. S. Marver, and R. Schmid. Microsomal heme oxygenase: Characterization of the enzyme. *J. Biol. Chem. 224,* 6388-6394 (1969).
8. C. D. Wise and D. L. Drabkin. Enzymatic degradation of hemoglobin and hemin to biliverdin and carbon monoxide. *Fed. Proc. 24,* 222 (1965).
9. D. G. Wolff and W. R. Bidlack. The formation of carbon monoxide during peroxidation of microsomal lipids. *Biochem. Biophys. Res. Commun. 73,* 850-857 (1976).

10. R. Bonnett. Recent advances in tetrapyrrole chemistry. *Ann. N.Y. Acad. Sci. 206,* 722-733, 1973.
10a. J. Kapitulnik, R. Horner-Mibashan, S. H. Blondheim, N. A. Kauffmann, and A. Russell. Increase in bilirubin binding affinity of serum with age of infant. *J. Pediatr. 86*:442-445 (1975).
11. E. A. Jones, R. Shnager, J. R. Bloomer, P. D. Berk, R. B. Howe, and N. I. Berlin. Quantitation studies of the delivery of hepatic synthesized bilirubin to plasma, utilizing amino levulinic acid-4-^{14}C and bilirubin-^{3}H in man. *J. Clin. Invest. 51,* 2450-2458 (1972).
12. G. Fleischner, J. Robbins, and I. M. Arias. Immunological studies of Y protein. A major cytoplasmic organic anion-binding protein in rat liver. *J. Clin. Invest. 51,* 677-684 (1972).
13. A. J. Levi, Z. Gatmaitan, and I. M. Arias. Two hepatic cytoplasmic protein fractions, Y and Z, and their possible role in the hepatic uptake of bilirubin, sulfobromophthalein and other anions. *J. Clin. Invest. 48,* 2156-2167 (1969).
14. L. H. Bernstein, J. Ben-Ezzer, L. M. Gartner, and I. M. Arias. Hepatic intracellular distribution of tritium labelled unconjugated and conjugated bilirubin in normal and Gunn rats. *J. Clin. Invest. 45,* 1194-1201 (1966).
15. W. R. Brown, G. M. Gradsky, and J. V. Larbone. Intracellular distribution of tritiated bilirubin during hepatic uptake and excretion. *Am. J. Physiol. 207,* 1237-1241 (1965).
16. B. H. Billing and G. H. Lathe. Bilirubin metabolism in jaundice. *Am. J. Med. 24,* 111-121 (1958).
17. L. J. Schoenfield and J. L. Bollman. Further studies on the nature and source of the conjugated bile pigments. *Proc. Soc. Exp. Biol. Med. 112,* 929-932 (1963).
18. P. G. Cole, G. H. Lathe, and B. H. Billing. The diazo reacting pigments of serum, urine and bile. *Biochem. J. 57,* 514-518 (1954).
19. E. W. Callahan, Jr., and R. Schmid. Excretion of unconjugated bilirubin in the bile of Gunn rats. *Gastroenterology 57,* 134-137 (1969).
20. S. H. Robinson, C. Yannoni, and S. Nagasawa. Bilirubin excretion in rats with normal and impaired bilirubin conjugation: Effect of phenobarbital. *J. Clin. Invest. 50,* 2606-2613 (1971).
20a. I. M. Arias, L. M. Gartner, M. Cohen, J. Ben Ezzer, and A. J. Levi. Chronic non-hemolytic unconjugated hyperbilirubinemia with glucuronyl transferase deficiency: clinical, biochemical, pharmacologic and genetic evidence for heterogeneity. *Am. J. Med. 47*:395-409 (1969).
21. L. M. Gartner, D. L. Lane, and C. E. Cornelius. Bilirubin transport by liver in adult *Macaca mulatta*. *Am. J. Physiol. 220,* 1528-1535 (1971).
22. I. M. Arias, L. Johnson, and S. Wolfson. Biliary excretion of injected conjugated and unconjugated bilirubin by normal and Gunn rats. *Am. J. Physiol. 200,* 1091-1094 (1961).
23. R. Brodersen and L. S. Hermann. Intestinal reabsorption of unconjugated bilirubin: A possible contributing factor in neonatal jaundice. *Lancet 1,* 1242 (1963).

24. R. D. Poland and G. B. Odell. Physiologic jaundice: The enterohepatic circulation of bilirubin. *N. Engl. J. Med. 284,* 1-6 (1971).
25. J. Jacobsen. A chromatographic separation of bilirubin glucuronides from human bile. *Acta Chem. Scand. 23,* 3023-3025 (1970).
26. F. H. Jansen and B. H. Billing. The identification of monoconjugates of bilirubin in bile as amide derivatives. *Biochem. J. 125,* 917-919 (1971).
27. L. M. Gartner, K. S. Lee, S. Vaisman, D. Lane, and I. Zarafu. Development of bilirubin transport and metabolism in the newborn rhesus monkey. *J. Pediatr. 90,* 513-531 (1977).
28. L. M. Gartner and D. Lane. Hepatic metabolism and transport of bilirubin during physiologic jaundice in the newborn rhesus monkey. *Pediatr. Res. 5,* 413 (1971).
29. S. L. Vaisman and L. M. Gartner. Pharmacologic treatment of neonatal hyperbilirubinemia. *Clin. Perinatol. 2,* 37-58 (1975).
30. R. A. Ulstrom and E. Eisenklam. The enterohepatic shunting of bilirubin in the newborn infant. I. Use of oral activated charcoal to reduce normal serum bilirubin values. *J. Pediatr. 65,* 27-37 (1964).

2

Bile Acid Pathophysiology in the Neonate

HARVEY W. AIGES and RAUL A. WAPNIR / Cornell University Medical College, New York, New York, and North Shore University Hospital, Manhasset, New York

I. Background

Perhaps in the nineteenth century and for most of the twentieth century the axiom "no jaundice, no liver disease" was a useful one simply because there were no other techniques or methods of detecting liver disease. As we approach the twenty-first century, a new interest has developed in anicteric liver disease. The interest lies not so much in identifying the infant who clearly has a problem at birth because he is jaundiced, but in recognizing those types of cryptogenic diseases which do not become apparent until the child has reached the age of 8 or 9 years. These children often present with hematemesis and are found to have portal hypertension, cirrhosis, and frequently a vague neonatal history, such as jaundice which cleared after an evaluation revealed no etiology for the icterus.

The problems of these patients are not common in pediatrics. Indeed, liver disease is uncommon as compared with diseases of all the other major organs. Statistically, the liver disorders we are discussing occur in 1 of every 25,000 to 1 of every 40,000 births. However, it is a goal to devise methods of screening for liver defects in the neonate—comparable to the method of screening for phenylketonuria (PKU)—so that we can detect these problems early in life and perhaps alter the natural history.

Dr. Wilbur C. Davidson, in his book *The Complete Pediatrician,* pointed out in its preface that the book was not written to cover the field of pediatrics and all its problems, but really to go into the problems without making any pretext of covering them. In the area of bile acid metabolism, so much has developed in the last 20 years that—rather than write a comprehensive paper—it is better to confine this discussion to the problems of the neonatal period. This may allow a more detailed review without an attempt to skim the whole area of bile acid metabolism.

II. Bile Acid Synthesis

Bergström, with his associates at the Karolinska, has made outstanding contributions since 1955 regarding the synthesis of bile acids from cholesterol. This group's original observations remain substantially correct for the adult, and perhaps even for the neonate. They found that the synthesis of bile acids may begin with the addition of a second hydroxyl group into the cholesterol molecule to form 7α-hydroxycholesterol, the first intermediate in the pathway of bile acid synthesis [1]. However, there are now reasons to believe that bile acids can also be synthesized by side chain oxidation with 26-hydroxycholesterol as the initial intermediate (Fig. 1). At present, there is good evidence to suggest that this alternate pathway may be very important in newborn and fetal life [2].

The classic Bergström experiment considered the cholesterol molecule as made up of two separate parts: the sterol ring and the hydrocarbon side chain. Bergström's group postulated that bile acids are built either by first changing the ring or by first changing the side chain. Had they had access to 7α-hydroxycholesterol or 26-hydroxycholesterol, which would be the first theoretical intermediates, they probably would have used them; but these were not yet available in the 1950s. So the group approached the problem by using a compound in which the side chain had been converted to that of a bile acid. Thus, they started with 3β-hydroxy-5-cholenoic acid, a model compound of transformation of the side chain, with a sterol ring essentially like that of cholesterol (Fig. 1). The other model compound they were able to synthesize was just the opposite; that is, they tranformed the sterol ring into that of a bile acid and left the side chain like that of cholesterol: 3α-7α-trihydroxy-5β-cholestane. After they injected each of these compounds into a rat with a bile fistula, they found that these compounds were excreted into the bile as cholic acid (a primary bile acid).

Recently, both labeled 26-hydroxycholesterol and 7α-hydroxycholesterol of very high specific activity were prepared and injected into a man with a bile fistula [3]. Evidence was obtained by gas-liquid chromatography of chenodeoxycholic acid and cholic acid synthesis. After intravenous injection of the 26-hydroxycholesterol and 7α-hydroxycholesterol, the labeled peaks obtained duplicated exactly the peaks of the standards of chenodeoxycholic acid and cholic acid. So it appears that there are two pathways for bile acid synthesis: one going directly via the side chain, one initiated via the sterol ring.

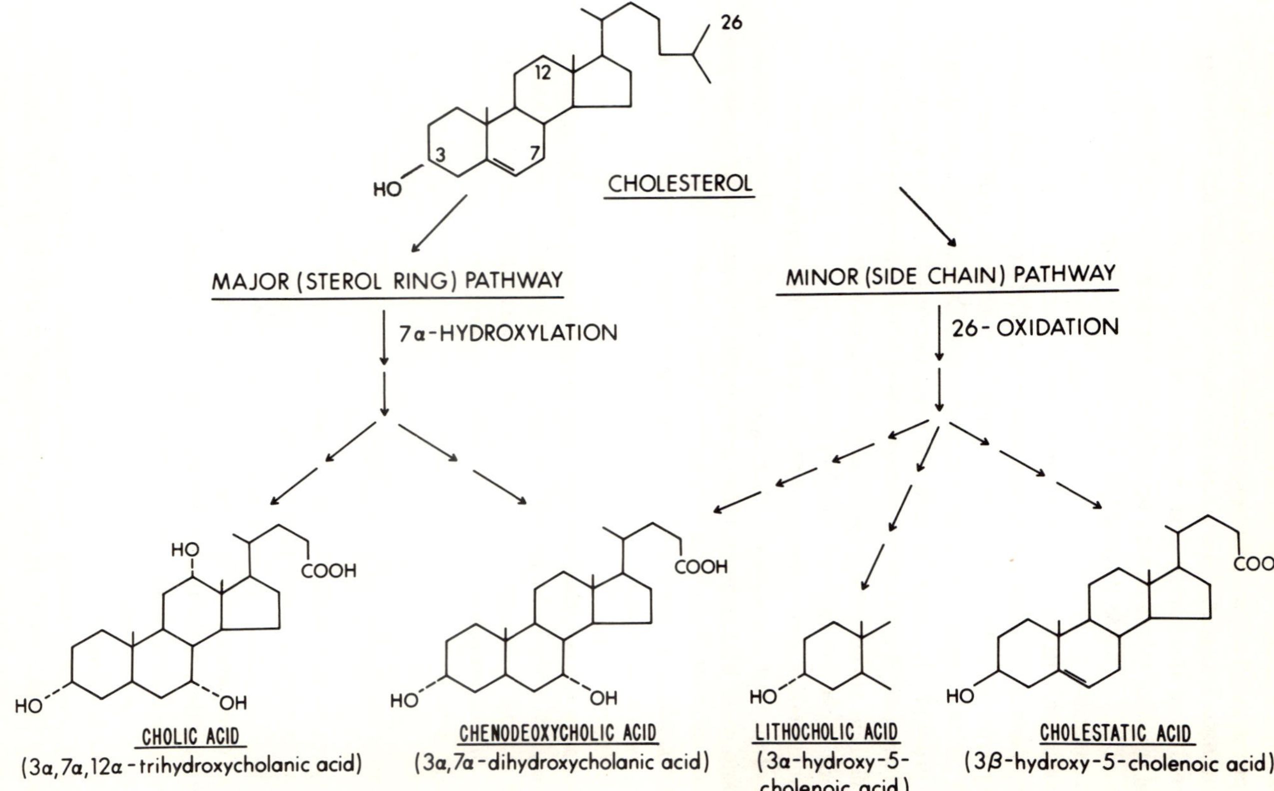

Figure 1 Biosynthesis of bile acids. The two possible pathways may be initiated either by the sterol ring hydroxylation (7α-hydroxylation) or the side chain oxidation. The side chain oxidation occurs in both cases, and chenodeoxycholic acid is a common end product.

However, the injection of an intermediate and its subsequent metabolism does not prove that such a compound actually existed in the liver, or that it was really a natural intermediate. Actually, very few intermediates have ever been isolated from the human liver, because reactions go so quickly from cholesterol on, that bile acid may be synthesized in a matter of seconds. Therefore, obtaining these intermediates as the native compound is extremely difficult technically.

It is now known that the normal human infant has a large amount of 26-hydroxycholesterol in its meconium, but it is not clear where this compound originates [4]. One thing we do know is that this cannot be an artifactual product, since it is clear that 26-hydroxycholesterol is not an auto-oxidation product. It has to be made by some enzymatic system and is probably derived directly from cholesterol. While 7α-hydroxycholesterol is probably derived enzymatically by cholesterol 7α-hydroxylase, it may be an artifact since it can be an auto-oxidation product.

Atheromata taken from adults after extraction of the cholesterol yield the sterol of greatest abundance: 26-hydroxycholesterol. As previously stated, it is also known to be the major sterol component of meconium. In the past several years substantial evidence has accumulated to suggest that this is a normal intermediate, metabolized in several ways. There are recent data showing that there is a cholesterol 26-hydroxylase in mitochondria that uses cholesterol as a substrate [5]. Thus, bile acid synthesis may begin in the mitochondria by oxidation of the side chain of cholesterol, and by sterol ring hydroxylation via 7α-hydroxycholesterol. It is presently known that in humans, rats, hamsters, and every other species investigated, the two primary bile acids chenodeoxycholic acid and cholic acid—can be derived from either intermediate [6].

III. Bile Acid Metabolism in the Neonate

Bile acid synthesis starting by the side chain pathway may yield monohydroxy bile acids as an end product. However, in the late 1960s it was found that monohydroxy bile acids can completely stop bile flow, with potentially deleterious consequences [7, 8]. Therefore, it is of particular interest to evaluate what is happening to this substance in fetal and neonatal life. We know that an end product of 26-hydroxycholesterol would be coprostanic acid. Recent reports have shown that coprostanic acid, which is normally found only in trace amounts in newborn infants, may be found in at least two pathologic conditions: (1) there is a form of familial cholestasis, described by Eyssen et al. [9] and Hanson et al. [10], in which there is trihydroxycoprostanic acid in large amounts—suggesting that there is a block in the normal oxidation of cholenoic acid; (2) more recently, coprostanic acid has been implicated in

Zellwegger's syndrome (cerebrohepatorenal syndrome). At present it is known that the finding of coprostanic acid indicates a marked derangement of bile acid metabolism, with alterations in side chain oxidation. In health, when the side chain of the normal cholenoic acid is oxidized, a new, interesting compound is obtained: 3β-hydroxy-5-cholenoic acid, the compound Bergström originally used.

Research on bile acid metabolism in the newborn is very new and exciting. As mentioned earlier, abnormal conditions unfortunately can go for a long time without being recognized. In the neonate, the step where cholenoic acid can actually be metabolized to di- and trihydroxy bile acids is unknown. If this metabolism is not operative in the neonate, an excess of monohydroxy bile acids will occur, which may be cholestatic. Investigators have shown that indeed, in the normal meconium, there are monohydroxy bile acids, and, in fact, more of them in the premature than in the mature neonate [11, 12]. Since these monohydroxy bile acids are constantly present in the developing healthy neonates, they must have some important, but as yet undefined role.

Recently, Paumgartner et al. showed that in the amniotic fluid, lithocholic acid is found, reaching a peak at about the sixth month of pregnancy [13]. This finding has attracted a lot of attention since this monohydroxy bile acid may be hazardous in excessive amounts. In fact, it is known that lithocholic acid can produce severe hepatic inflammation and biliary ductular proliferation [14]. Cholestatic acid, which has also been found in neonates, is a compound that may be of concern in fetal and neonatal life, since it has a potential for severe cholestasis because it is very insoluble.

With an appropriate supply of di- and trihydroxy bile acids, bile flow increases, and the insoluble monohydroxy bile acids will be incorporated within the micelle structure of the di- and trihydroxy bile acids. However, if the proportion of the monohydroxy from being excreted exceeds the tolerable concentrations, then precipitation can occur within the biliary tree—which can then cause a reduction in bile flow.

It is becoming clear that the neonate, in a way, is normally rather well protected. Although neonates may produce 26-hydroxycholesterol and 3β-hydroxy-5-cholenoic acid, they have a very competent sulfation mechanism, solubilizing both of these compounds and accounting for their excretion in the meconium and the urine [15]. Probably 26-hydroxycholesterol can also be metabolized to chenodeoxycholic and cholic acids, which are then excreted in bile. As long as there is an active sulfation mechanism, the infant remains well even with a limited bile flow; so, even though normal neonates have traces of 3β-hydroxy-5-cholenoate, it does not cause problems.

IV. Pathologic States

One of the major problems that can occur could be related to abnormal sulfation. In situations where the capacity to sulfate is impaired, the monohydroxy bile acids are not solubilized; they are excreted into the biliary canaliculi and begin to obstruct the biliary tree. Alternately, other cholestatic mechanisms can occur, such as a primary defect in the capacity to transport bile acids [16]; or, as previously mentioned, there are situations where there is a block in normal oxidation. These are all problem areas that have not been fully elucidated.

However, even if cholestasis occurs in the neonate, it can be very mild, and the child may be able to recover without deleterious effects. This can happen because chenodeoxycholic acid will increase in the serum in cholestasis, but, if the sulfation mechanism is operative, this primary bile acid will be sulfated and therefore safely excreted into the urine. This may very well be the major mechanism of compensation in neonatal cholestasis.

Therefore, we can conceive of a system called *compensated cholestasis,* a defect of bile acid excretion balanced by the sulfation step used in the alternate pathway (side chain oxidation). A child with this condition could really go undetected, since jaundice may be absent, and the problem could probably resolve spontaneously.

One can also envision an *uncompensated cholestasis,* where the capacity to sulfate is lost, resulting in an inefficiency of bile acid excretion, with these metabolites accumulating in the serum. A vicious cycle can develop, where an inability to sulfate 3β-hydroxy-5-cholenoic acid causes more cholestasis, and that blocks the excretion of chenodeoxycholic acid. However, with the sulfation mechanism lost, the primary bile acid accumulates rather than being safely excreted. There is good evidence that, as serum concentrations of bile acid increase, liver cell levels also increase, with consequent deterioration of liver cell function and progression to cirrhosis. Fortunately this situation is infrequent [17-19].

V. Summary

The synthesis of bile acids in the fetal liver may, in addition to the usually accepted sterol ring pathway, occur via a side chain pathway which has lithocholic and cholestatic acids as intermediates. These monohydroxy bile salts do not usually have deleterious effects, because they can be metabolized to the primary bile acids; moreover, even in cholestasis, they can be sulfated, increasing their solubilization and markedly increasing their excretion.

There can be significant pathology produced when: (1) there are abnormlities of side chain oxidation leading to trihydroxycoprostanic acid; (2) there is a defect in 7α-hydroxylation alone, with a defect in sulfation, and resultant loss of this alternate pathway.

Fortunately, the two pathways of bile acid metabolism are a beautifully complementary system and infrequently fail to compensate for each other.

Acknowledgment

This article includes concepts presented by Dr. N. B. Javitt at the Symposium on Clinical Disorders in Pediatric Gastroenterology and Nutrition, held in Manhasset and New York City, on April 24 and 25, 1978.

References

1. S. Bergström and H. Danielsson. Formation and metabolism of bile acids. In *Handbook of Physiology,* Sect. 6, The Alimentary Canal, Vol. 5. The American Physiological Society, Washington, D.C., 1968, pp. 2391-2407.
2. Mitropoulous, K. A. and N. B. Myant. The formation of lithocholic acid, chenodeoxycholic acid and α- and β-murocholic acids from cholesterol. *Biochem. J. 103,* 472-479 (1967).
3. K. Anderson, E. Koh, and N. B. Javitt. Bile acid synthesis in man: Metabolism of 7-hydroxycholesterol-^{14}C and 26-hydroxycholesterol-^{3}H. *J. Clin. Invest. 51,* 112-117 (1972).
4. P. Eneroth and J. A. Gustafsson. Hydroxylated cholesterol derivatives in the steroid monosulfate fraction from meconium. *FEBS Lett. 3,* 129-131 (1969).
5. I. Bjorkhem, J. Gustafsson, G. Johansson, and B. Persson. Biosynthesis of bile acids in man: Hydroxylation of the C_{27} steroid side chain. *J. Clin. Invest. 55,* 478-481 (1975).
6. T. Masui and E. Staple. The formation of bile acids from cholesterol. The conversion of 5-beta-cholestane-3-alpha,7-alpha-triol-26-oic acid to cholic acid via 5-beta-cholestane-3-alpha,7-alpha,12-alpha, 24-xitetrol-26-oic acid. *J. Biol. Chem. 241,* 3889-3893 (1966).
7. Javvitt, N. B. Cholestasis in rats induced by taurolithocholate. *Nature 210,* 1262-1263 (1966).
8. N. B. Javitt and S. Emerson. Effect of sodium taurolithocholate in bile flow and bile acid excretion. *J. Clin. Invest. 47,* 1002-1014 (1968).
9. H. Eyssen, G. Parmentier, F. Compernolle, J. Boon, and E. Eggermont. Trihydroxycoprostanic acid in the duodenal fluid of two children with intrahepatic bile duct anomalies. *Biochim. Biophys. Acta 273,* 212-221 (1972).
10. R. G. Hanson, J. N. Isenberg, G. C. Williams, D. Hachey, B. Sczepknik, P. Klein, and H. L. Sharp. The metabolism of 3α,7α,12α-trihydroxy-5β-cholestan-26-oil acid in two siblings with cholestasis due to intrahepatic bile duct anomalies. *J. Clin. Invest. 56,* 577-578 (1975).
11. P. Back and K. Ross. Identification of 3 beta-hydroxy-5-cholenoic acid in human meconium. *Hoppe Seylers Z. Physiol. Chem. 354,* 83-89 (1973).

12. H. L. Sharp, J. Peller, J. B. Carey, and W. Krivit. Primary and secondary bile acids in meconium. *Pediatr. Res. 5,* 274-279 (1971).
13. G. Paumgartner, G. Deleze, and G. Karlaganis. Nachweis von 3-beta-hydroxy-5-cholensaure im Menschlichen. *Fruchtwasser Schweiz. Med. Wochenschr. 107,* 529-531 (1977).
14. R. H. Palmer and Z. Hruban. Production of bile duct hyperplasia and gallstones by lithocholic acid. *J. Clin. Invest. 45,* 1255-1267 (1966).
15. A. Stiehl. Bile salt sulphates in cholestasis. *Eu. J. Clin. Invest. 4,* 59-63 (1974).
16. J. Makino, J. Sjövall, A. Norman, and B. Strandvik. Excretions of 3-beta-hydroxy-5-cholenoic acid and 3-alpha-hydroxy-5-alpha-cholenoic acids in urine of infants with biliary atresia. *FEBS Lett. 15,* 161-164 (1971).
17. A. Norman and B. Strandrik. Excretion of bile acids in extrahepatic biliary atresia. *Acta Paediatr. Scand. 63,* 97-102 (1974).
18. A. Norman, B. Strandvik, and O. Ojamae. Urinary bile acid conjugates in extrahepatic biliary atresia. *Acta Paediatr. Scand. 63,* 97-102 (1974).
19. I. Makino, H. Hashimoto, K. Shinozaki, Y. Koichi, and S. Nakagawa. Sulfated and nonsulfated bile acids in urine, serum and bile in patients with hepatobiliary diseases. *Gastroenterology 68,* 545-553 (1975).

3
Chronic Liver Disease in Children

MERVIN SILVERBERG and ELLEN I. KAHN / Cornell University Medical College, New York, New York, and North Shore University Hospital, Manhasset, New York

I. Introduction

Chronic liver disorders in children involve a wide variety of diseases, the majority of them occurring with relative infrequency. The authors have randomly selected a few of these conditions from a clinical-pathological point of view, excluding the general category of cirrhosis and those topics which are well covered elsewhere: e.g., genetic-metabolic disorders (Chapter 4).

II. Chronic Hepatitis

Acute viral hepatitis in children is generally a benign disease with more than 90% of patients returning to a normal or near-normal status within 3 months of the onset of the illness. According to the purists, chronic hepatitis requires a 6-month observation period before the diagnosis can be made. However, the majority of children with significant physical and biochemical abnormalities 3 months after onset, particularly those with icterus, are at high risk to develop chronic hepatitis. Other known risk factors are found in immunocompromised patients (due to primary illness or drugs), those who are chronically exposed to blood or blood products, and those patients with persistent surface hepatitis B antigenemia (HB_SAg) or circulating DNA polymerase. The adolescent female and the newborn also appear to be more vulnerable to chronicity. Most cases of chronic hepatitis in children are believed to be due to hepatitis A, hepatitis B, or hepatitis non-A, non-B. Chronic persistent hepatitis and chronic active hepatitis are the two most common varieties of chronic hepatitis (Table 1).

Table 1 Manifestations of Chronic Hepatitis

Manifestation	Chronic persistent hepatitis	Chronic active hepatitis
Relative incidence in children	Uncommon	Common
Male-female ratio[a]	2:1	1:2
Extrahepatic manifestations	Rare	Common
Severity of symptoms	Mild	Mild to severe
Jaundice	Rare	Common
Response to steroid Rx	Not indicated	Good to fair
Cirrhosis	Never	Common
Disturbances of T- or/and B-cell function	Common	More common
Prognosis	Good	Usually poor

[a]Approximate.
Source: From M. Silverberg. *Pediatr. Ann. 6,* 312 (May 1977).

A. Chronic Persistent Hepatitis

Chronic persistent hepatitis (CPH) occurs predominantly in patients who are exposed to blood and blood products. In the pediatric age group, most of the cases appear in adolescent drug abusers and in the offspring of mothers who are drug addicted or are carriers of HB_sAg for other reasons. It is a relatively mild, self-limited disease with distinct clinical-pathologic features.

1. Case History. A. G. is a 17-year-old male who denied taking parenteral drugs, but admitted that many of his friends indulged. He developed anorexia and nausea with mild jaundice over a 2-week period. His liver was minimally enlarged and slightly tender, and no spleen was palpable. The initial SGOT/ SGPT* ratio was 1100/1210; IgG was 1620 mg%. Six months later he was well, with normal immunoglobulins but the SGOT/SGPT ratio was 68/76. Initially and at 6 months HB_sAg was positive; anti-HB_s was detected 4 months after the onset of his illness. A percutaneous liver biopsy was performed.

2. Microscopic Features. (Fig. 1) The parenchymatous changes are minimal and consist of nodular proliferation of Kupffer cells (Spaetknoetchen), at times

*Serum glutamic oxaloacetic transaminase (SGOT); serum glutamic pyruvic transaminase (SGPT).

surrounding isolated degenerated hepatocytes. Diastase-resistant, PAS-positive* material is present in Kupffer cells. The portal areas show round cell infiltration, which is predominantly lymphocytic, diffuse, or nodular, at times with germinal centers. This infiltration is restricted to the portal spaces, without spilling over into the region of adjacent hepatocytes.

3. Comments. The above features share the common characteristics of any chronic hepatitis: i.e., predominance of portal over parenchymatous changes and variability from field to field. The latter characteristic is important, inasmuch as it may lead to an erroneous interpretation due to sampling. Evidence of chronic active hepatitis may be present elsewhere, although it is rare for the bonafide CPH patient to convert to the more serious chronic active form. Clinical correlation is, therefore, important.

Spaetknoetchen formation and Kupffer cells containing diastase-resistant, PAS-positive material are hallmarks of chronicity. The absence of destruction of the limiting plate by inflammatory cells, i.e., *piecemeal necrosis,* distinguishes histologically chronic persistent from chronic active hepatitis.

B. Chronic Active Hepatitis

Chronic active hepatitis (CAH) is a more virulent form of chronic hepatitis and in children usually occurs without evidence of hepatitis B infection [1]. The marked female-adolescent preponderance is noteworthy. Multiple-system involvement is common, and occasionally the extraintestinal manifestations, such as glomerulonephritis, may overshadow the hepatic disease. The biochemical diagnostic hallmarks are serum aminotransferases at least two to five times normal, in addition to the elevation of IgG, which is usually in excess of 2.0 g%.

The clinical and histologic features may be simulated in Wilson's disease, as well as by drugs such as the laxative, oxyphenisatin acetate, and the antihypertensive, α-methyldopa.

1. Case History 1. S. K. was a 14-year-old girl who was seen 2 months after the onset of a "typical" case of hepatitis. She continued to show signs of cholestasis (D/T† bilirubin, 4.5/6.8), IgG level was 2.6g%, and there was significant hepatosplenomegaly. A percutaneous liver biopsy was performed 1 month later, since there was no change in her clinical status.

*Periodic acid-Schiff (PAS).

†Ratio of "direct" to "total" (D/T) measurements.

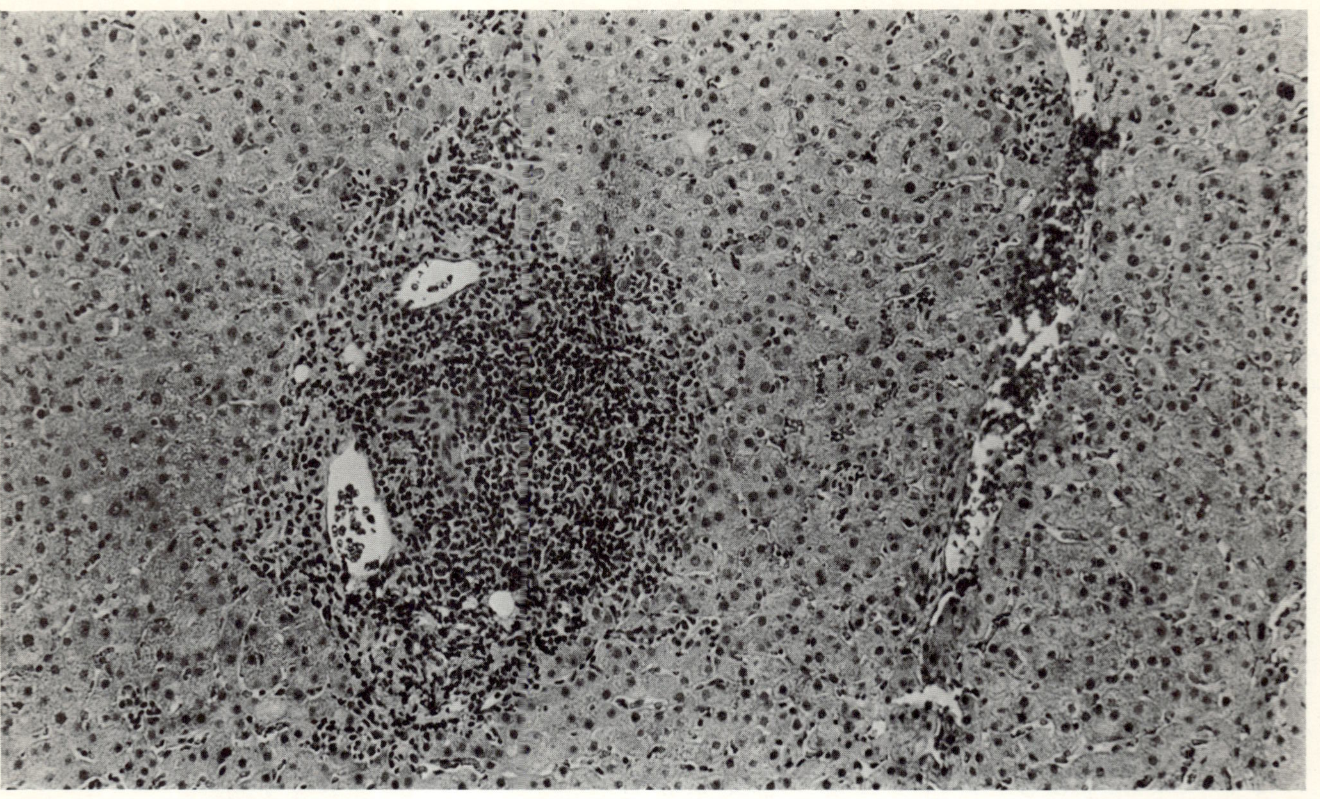

Figure 1 Chronic persistent hepatitis. Well-defined nodular lymphoid infiltration of portal space with preservation of limiting plate, i.e., hepatocytes at the interphase with the portal space. H&E. × 102.5.

2. *Microscopic Features* (Fig. 2). Portal spaces show varying degrees of mononuclear infiltration extending into adjacent hepatocytes of the limiting plate, with degeneration and necrosis of the cells (*piecemeal necrosis*). The portal infiltration at times links adjacent portal areas (porto-portal bridging). The lobular architecture is lost, due to bands of fibrous connective tissue which surround small regenerative nodules. Three types of lobular changes are noted: nodular proliferation of Kupffer cells; diastase-resistant, PAS-positive material in Kupffer cells; and giant cell transformation of hepatocytes characterized by large cells with pale-staining cytoplasm associated with several nuclei. Cell plates, two cells thick, and pseudoacinar formation are noted.

A follow-up biopsy after 6 months of steroid therapy showed similar changes, although the portal infiltration was less severe. Giant cell transformation was still noted.

3. *Comments.* The features are those of chronic active hepatitis with cirrhosis. The diagnosis of chronic active hepatitis is based on the presence of piecemeal necrosis. Evidence of regeneration, such as two-cell-thick cell plates, pseudo-acinar formation, and the presence of fibrous connective tissue strands sub-dividing the hepatic lobules into micronodules, characterizes a pattern of cirrhosis.

Giant cell hepatitis is the usual reaction of an infantile liver to various nosologic factors. It represents a regenerative phenomenon in young cells, and its presence in older children is rare. Giant cell transformation in adults has been described in chronic active hepatitis [2], in viral hepatitis, and in toxic hepatitis associated with toxins such as methotrexate, aminosalicylic acid, vinyl chloride, chlorpromazine, and 6-mercaptopurine. The prognostic implication of this cellular reaction is unknown.

4. *Case History 2.* M. L. was a 12-year-old male who presented with acute thyrotoxicosis and unexplained mild splenomegaly. He developed transient abnormalities of serum aminotransferases, which were thought to be secondary to antithyroid drugs. A liver biopsy was performed (Fig. 3). One year later, he became hyperthyroid again, in association with an attempt to withdraw propylthiouracil. Concurrently, the liver function tests showed deterioration, and his spleen enlarged progressively. A second liver biopsy was performed (Fig. 4). He responded dramatically to corticosteroid therapy, and liver function tests and immunoglobulins were normal after 1 year. After 2 years on prednisone he had a third liver biopsy, and the prednisone was discontinued, since the biopsy specimen was normal.

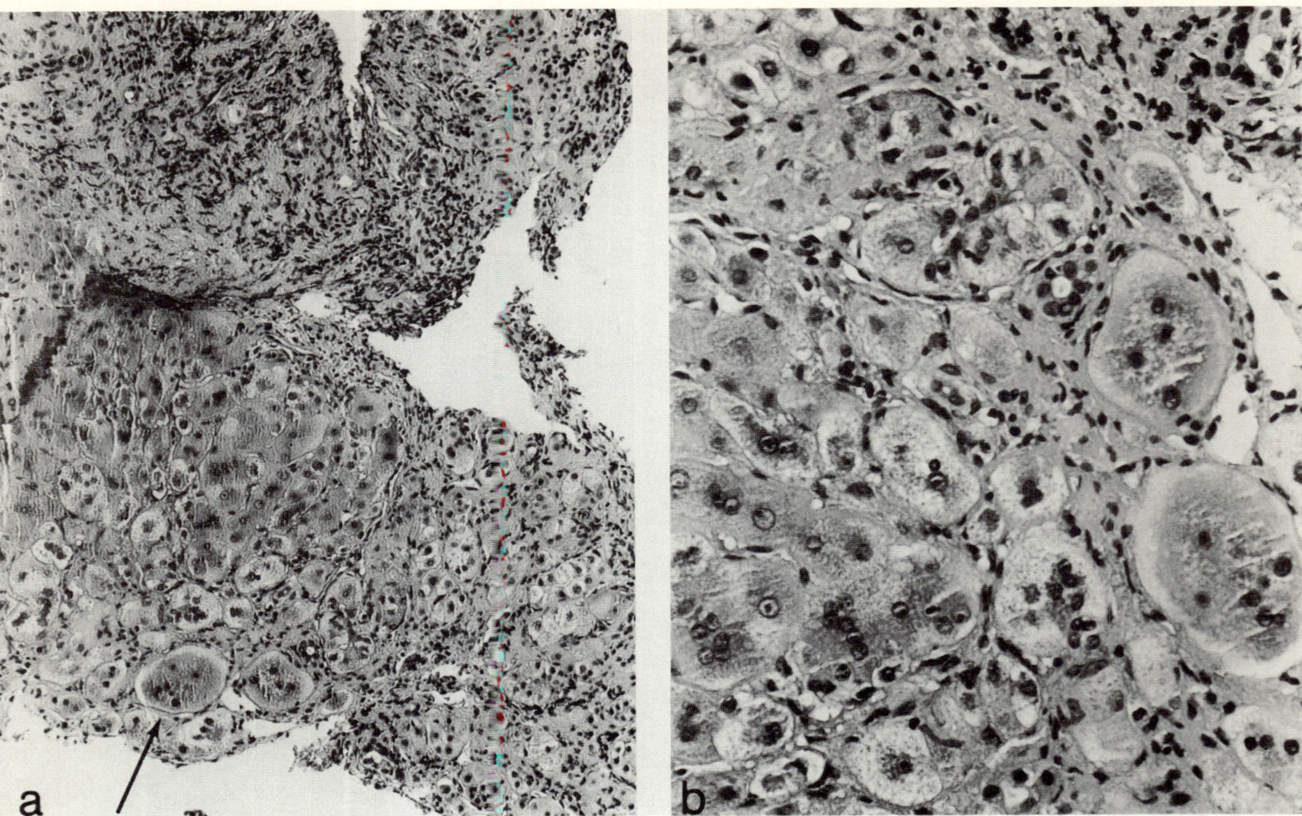

Figure 2 (a) Chronic active hepatitis with cirrhosis and giant cell transformation. Giant cell indicated by arrow within a regenerative nodule. H&E. × 102.5. (b) Details of giant cell transformation. H&E. × 280.

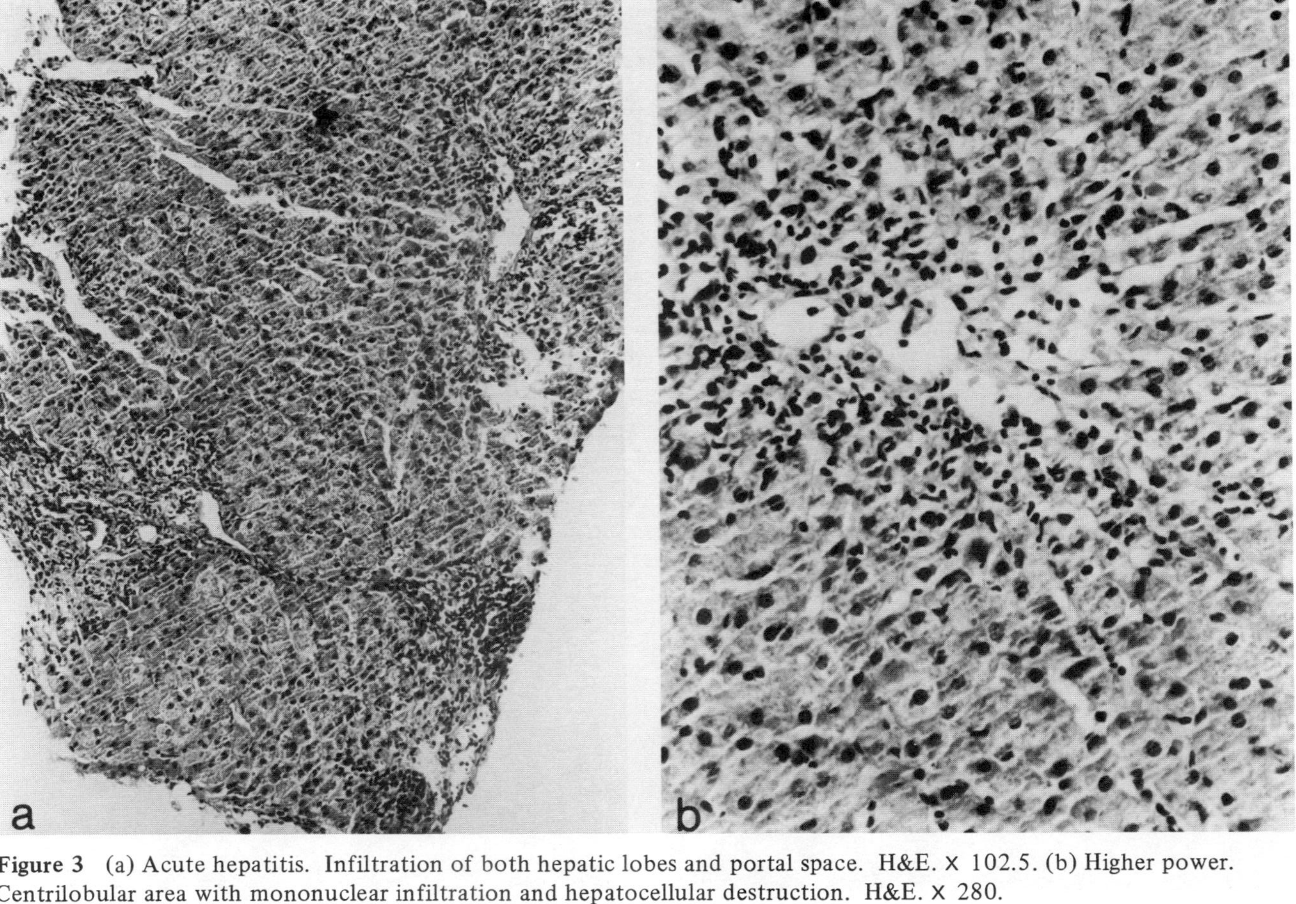

Figure 3 (a) Acute hepatitis. Infiltration of both hepatic lobes and portal space. H&E. × 102.5. (b) Higher power. Centrilobular area with mononuclear infiltration and hepatocellular destruction. H&E. × 280.

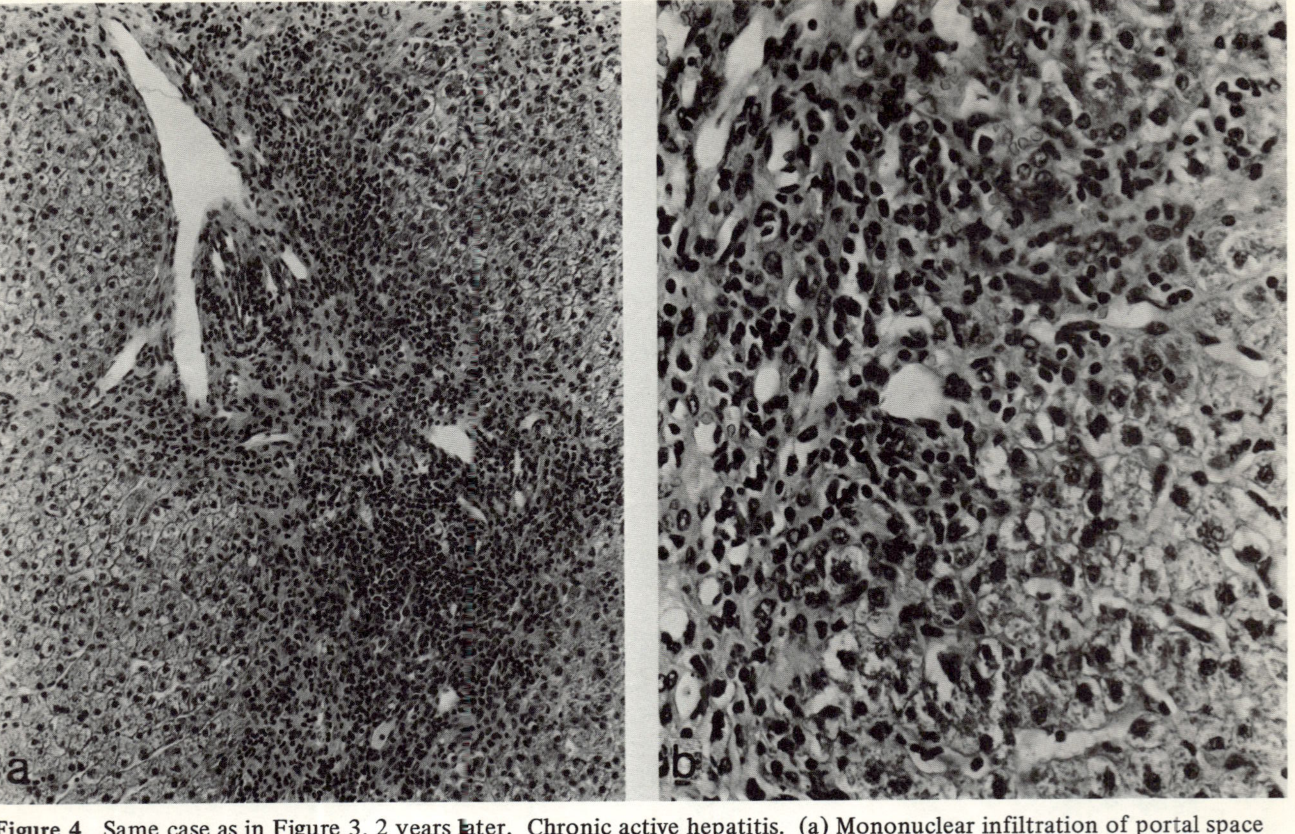

Figure 4 Same case as in Figure 3, 2 years later. Chronic active hepatitis. (a) Mononuclear infiltration of portal space with destruction of limiting plate and extension into adjacent hepatic parenchyma–piecemeal necrosis. H&E. × 102.5. (b) Higher power, portal space (left of center) with piecemeal necrosis. H&E . × 280.

5. *Microscopic Features.* In Figure 3, the changes are uniform and diffuse, involving both hepatic lobules and portal spaces. Hepatocytes show degenerative changes with ballooning–swollen, clear cytoplasm–and acidophilic body formation, round hepatocytes with dark eosinophilic cytoplasm and pyknotic nuclei. These changes are associated with moderate lymphocytic infiltration. Centrilobular areas are more severely involved, at times with linking of these areas with the portal spaces (porto-central bridging). The portal areas are widened by mononuclear infiltration, predominantly lymphocytic, extending into adjacent hepatocytes.

In Figure 4 the portal spaces are expanded by mononuclear infiltration associated with piecemeal necrosis. Nodular Kupffer cell proliferation is present, as well as diastase-resistant, PAS-positive material in Kupffer cells.

6. *Comments.* The pattern in Figure 3 is characteristic of an acute hepatitis with a diffuse, uniform type of change and predominance of parenchymatous over portal lesions. Acidophilic bodies suggest a viral origin. Spilling over of the portal infiltrate does not have the same prognostic meaning as in chronic hepatitis. The severity of the changes in the centrilobular areas is more pronounced than usual and is prognostically somewhat worrisome. In the present case, it may be explained by the association with hyperthyroidism.

Note that the pattern in Figure 4 is that of a chronic active hepatitis, impossible to predict from the antecedent biopsy. The absence of porto-central bridging constitutes a favorable prognostic point.

III. Fibropolycystic Disease

Fibropolycystic disease of the liver refers to a variety of disorders characterized by hepatic fibrosis and a spectrum of intrahepatic bile ductular abnormalities. They all share the features of minimal parenchymal involvement, genetic patterns of inheritance, and in more than 50% of patients, renal "cystic" changes are also noted.

The three basic subtypes are congenital hepatic fibrosis, childhood fibropolycystic disease, and adult fibropolycystic disease [3]. Congenital hepatic fibrosis is most frequently diagnosed in the pediatric age group, and a variant is reported with ectatic intrahepatic bile ducts, i.e., Caroli's syndrome.

A. Congenital Hepatic Fibrosis

Congenital hepatic fibrosis is usually diagnosed in the first decade of life, with the presenting features associated with portal hypertension, hepatosplenomegaly, or pyelonephritis, in decreasing order of frequency. The portal hypertension is presinusoidal in origin, and there are only mild abnormalities of liver function tests. The renal manifestations are usually due to renal tubular ectasia, renal dysplasia, or cysts. There is increased susceptibility to renal infection, however glomerular function is generally intact. The condition is believed to be inherited as an autosomal recessive disorder.

1. Case History. K. B. is a 2-year-old-girl who presented with persistent hematemesis, 20 hr in duration. She had had a recent fever with an upper respiratory infection, which had been treated with aspirin. She was extremely pale and had a hematocrit of 24%. The liver was very firm and extended 4 cm below the right costal margin. Liver function tests were normal. Intravenous pyelogram revealed tubular ectasia, but normal renal function. Liver and kidney biopsies were performed when the patient was stabilized. A cousin had a similar disorder, and both sets of parents were related to each other.

2. Microscopic Features. The liver biopsy (Fig. 5a) shows portal triads which are expanded and reveal three changes involving fibrous connective tissue, biliary ducts, and vessels. Portal fibrosis with dense, fibrous connective tissue, not associated with inflammatory reaction, is responsible for the widening and incomplete porto-portal bridging. The histologic picture may be confused with micronodular cirrhosis. Ductal proliferation is prominent, especially at the periphery of the portal areas, and at times the ducts appear irregular and slightly dilated. The lining cells are cuboidal (Fib. 5b). These changes are an exaggerated replica of the *von Meyenburg complex.* The walls of the hepatic artery branches are thickened, and the number of portal vein branches is reduced. The lobular architecture is preserved. The limiting plate is intact, without evidence of regeneration.

In the kidney biopsy (Fig. 6) most of the glomeruli are intact, although some are small and immature. A small number of renal tubules having a cystic appearance are lined by cuboidal cells. A few dysplastic tubules lined by cuboidal cells and surrounded by smooth muscle are noted. There is focal interstitial fibrosis associated with lymphocytic infiltration.

3. Comments. Congenital hepatic fibrosis is explained by some as persistent von Meyenburg complexes, with overproduction of the mesenchyme-inducing ductal proliferation. The associated portal hypertension is explained by portal fibrosis with hypoplasia of portal vein branches.

Congenital hepatic fibrosis can remain stationary or subclinical—or can progress to more severe states of hepatic fibrosis. An association with

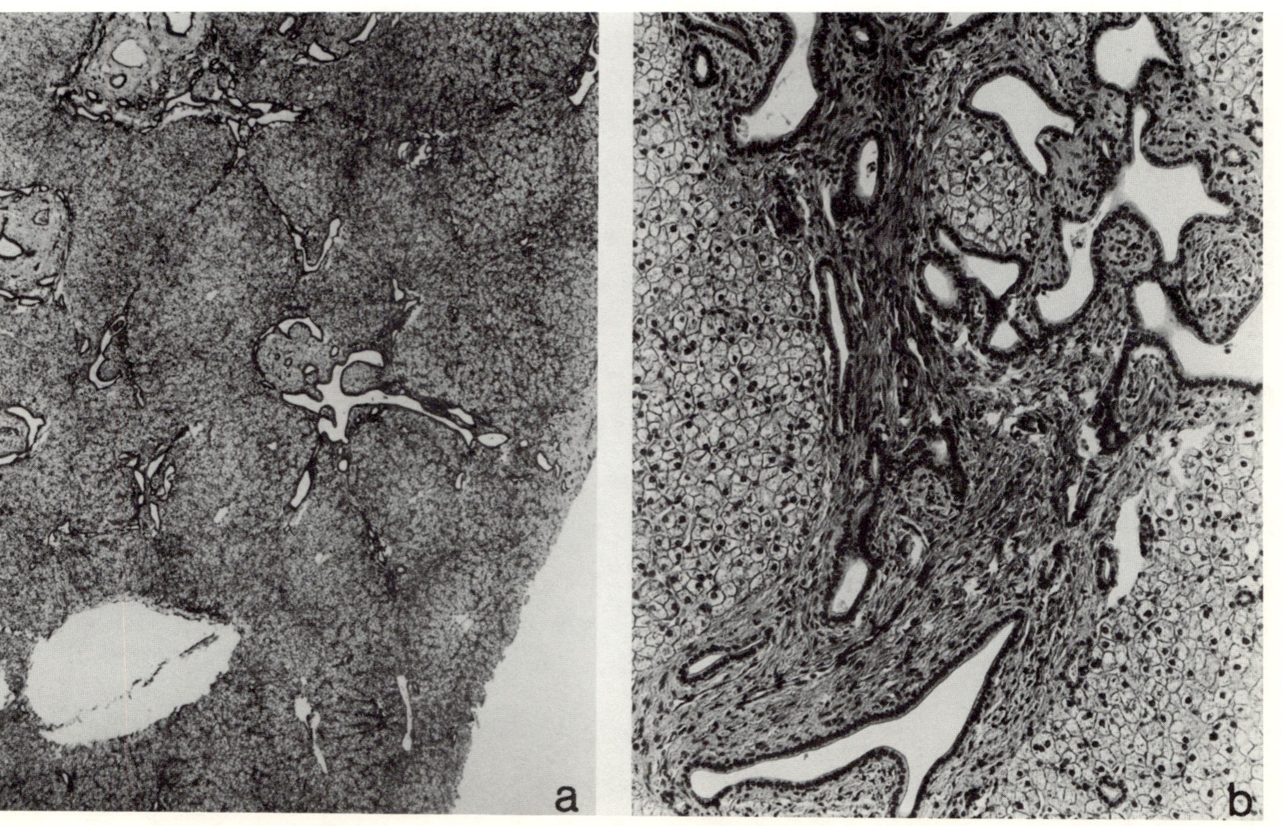

Figure 5 (a) Congenital hepatic fibrosis. Widening of portal spaces with hyperplasia and dilatation of bile ducts. Trichrome. × 102.5. (b) High power, portal space. Note dilated bile ducts, absence of inflammation, intact limiting plate. Trichrome. × 280.

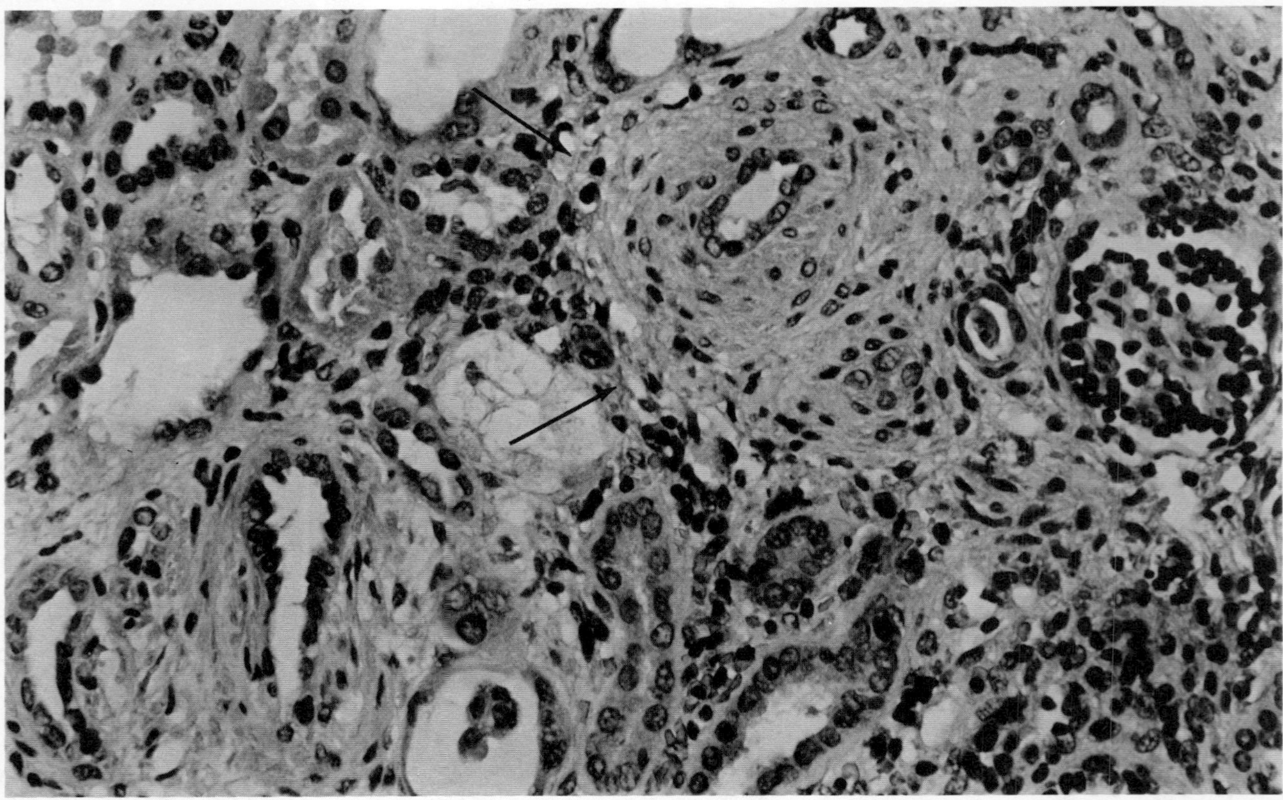

Figure 6 Renal dysplasia. Renal biopsy specimen from same case as in Figure 5, with dilated, and at times dysplastic, tubules surrounded by smooth muscle (arrows). H&E. × 280.

cholangiocarcinoma [4] and hepatoma has been described. There are no histologic clues to predict any of these evolutions.

B. Caroli's Syndrome

In rare cases of congenital hepatic fibrosis, an associated cystic dilation of the intrahepatic bile ducts is reported. Caroli's original paper did not mention this association [5], but it has been found in the majority of all subsequent reports [6]. As a result of segmental or diffuse dilatation of the intrahepatic biliary tree, cholangitis is a common complication and presenting problem. Intrahepatic cholelithiasis, sepsis, amyloidosis, and cholangiocarcinoma [7] have also been reported. The diagnosis is usually made by transhepatic cholangiography, sonography, or computerized axial tomography.

1. Case History. J. S. had intermittent diarrhea and thrived poorly from age 2-6 years. At the age of 7 years he was noted to develop progressive hepatosplenomegaly without jaundice or significant abnormalities of liver function tests. A liver biopsy was performed (Fig. 7). Two years later, he began to spike recurrent fevers and developed progressive cholestasis. A transhepatic cholangiogram demonstrated generalized dilatation of the intrahepatic bile ducts. Another liver biopsy and a modified Longmire operation were performed.

2. Microscopic Features. In Figure 7 there is marked fibrosis with hepatic lobules partially or completely surrounded by dense, fibrous connective tissue. The number of bile ducts is slightly increased. No inflammation is noted. The hepatocytes are unremarkable.

3. Comments. The pattern suggests, at first glance, the diagnosis of hepatic cirrhosis. Closer examination should lead the observer to the diagnosis of congenital hepatic fibrosis. There is no evidence of hepatic regeneration. The central veins are preserved. The portal fibrosis is not associated with inflammation or ductular proliferation. The number of bile ducts is increased.

The second liver biopsy shows two additional changes: fibrous obliteration and the collapse of large bile ducts, surrounded by a concentric rim of fibrous connective tissue; and portal fibrosis with porto-portal bridging as a prominent feature.

The pattern of congenital hepatic fibrosis is complicated in this case by features of healing cholangitis in a large intrahepatic ductal structure. This last finding suggests the clinical diagnosis of Caroli's syndrome. This entity may manifest itself as an isolated finding or, more commonly, is associated

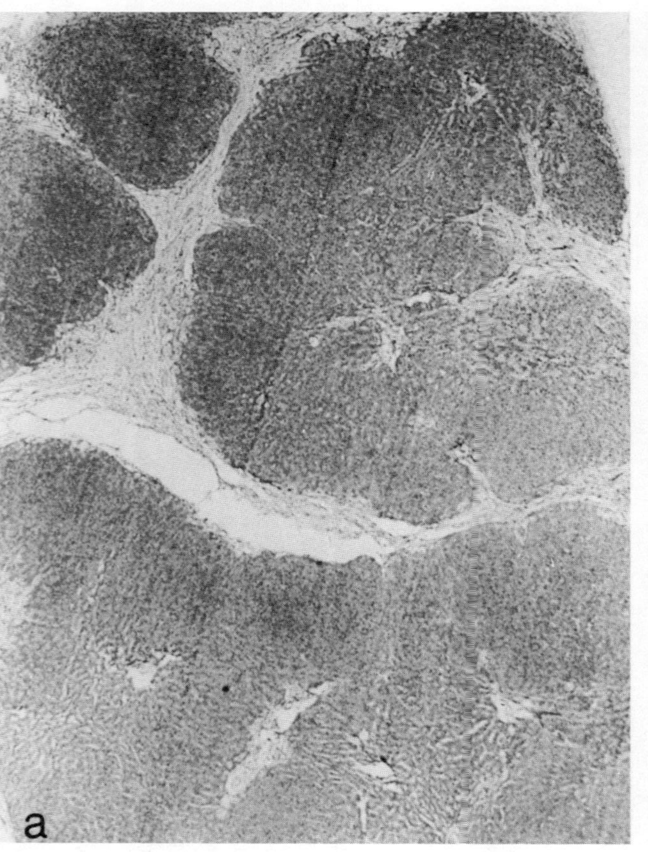

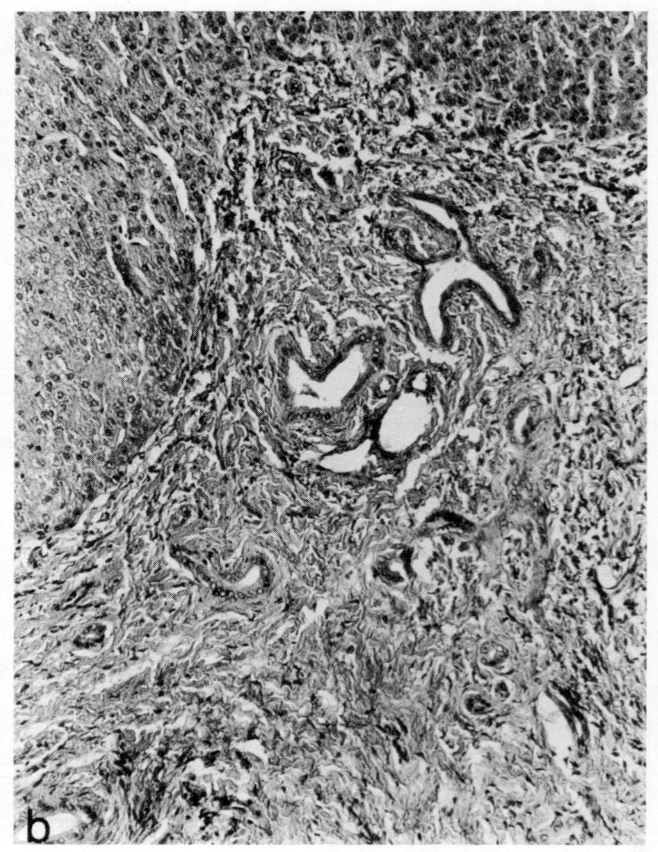

Figure 7 (a) Congenital hepatic fibrosis with Caroli's syndrome. Periportal fibrosis simulating pattern of cirrhosis. Trichrome. × 25.9. (b) High power, portal space with features of congenital hepatic fibrosis. Trichrome. × 87.5.

with congenital hepatic fibrosis, as this case exemplifies. Renal tubular ectosia or seldom adult cystic disease of kidneys and pancreas may also be noted. The pathogenesis of Caroli's syndrome is unknown.

IV. Chronic Intrahepatic Cholestatic Syndromes

Chronic intrahepatic cholestatic syndromes refer to a group of disorders with cholestasis and a normal extrahepatic biliary system. Many are heredofamilial and are associated with disturbances of bile acid metabolism. Morphologically, the intrahepatic bile ducts may be normal, hypoplastic, or markedly reduced in number (Table 2).

In terms of severity of illness, children with *benign recurrent cholestasis* have an excellent prognosis. At the other end of the spectrum, children with *Byler's disease* [9] and those with retention of unusual bile acids (e.g., lithocholic acid [10] and trihydroxycoprostanic acid [11]) invariably end up with hepatic failure before they reach adolescence.

Clinically, these patients are characterized by poor growth and development, pruritis, jaundice, steatorrhea, and retention of bile acids and lipids in the blood.

A. Arteriohepatic Dysplasia Syndrome

Of the numerous cholestatic syndromes which have been described, one of the most unusual includes a typical facies and multiple congenital anomalies. The

Table 2 Chronic Intrahepatic Cholestatic Syndromes

Normal intrahepatic bile ducts
Benign recurrent
Familial progressive—e.g., Byler's disease; associated with elevated lithocholic acid
Associated with lymphatic anomalies—e.g., in Norwegian kindreds [8]
Paucity or dysplasia of intrahepatic bile ducts
Arteriohepatic dysplasia
Defect in bile acid metabolism—e.g., trihydroxycoprostanic acid
Miscellaneous- acquired abnormal intrahepatic bile ducts
Fibropolycystic disease and cholangitis—e.g., Caroli's syndrome
$Alpha_1$-antitrypsin deficiency

descriptive name "arteriohepatic dysplasia" seems appropriate, since the most common manifestations are hepatic and cardiovascular abnormalities [12]. The syndrome appears to be inherited in a dominant fashion with varying penetrance.

1. Hepatic Features. A number of hepatic phenotypes have been described: (1) asymptomatic liver disease; (2) transient cholestasis of early infancy; (3) cholestasis of early infancy, progressing to periportal fibrosis and/or cirrhosis; and (4) late-onset cholestasis.

In addition to a familial pattern of the paucity of intrahepatic bile ducts, rare instances of familial coexistence of neonatal hepatitis and extrahepatic biliary atresia have been described.

2. Cardiovascular Abnormalities. Peripheral pulmonary artery stenosis is the most common lesion, occurring in more than 50% of the cases. Additionally, pulmonary valve stenosis, aortic valve stenosis, and coarctation of the aorta or other major arterial vessels have been reported.

3. Miscellaneous Findings. Other features occurring in decreasing order of frequency are:

1. Facies: Most patients resemble each other, with a prominent forehead, deep-set eyes, and mild hypertelorism. The nose is straight, and the chin is small and pointed.
2. Skeletal abnormalities: Vertebral arch defects are most common, due primarily to failure of fusion of the anterior arches of the vertebrae. Although this defect may be noted early in infancy, it is more evident with increasing age. Other skeletal abnormalities include decreased medullary-cortical ratios, densification of the metaphyseal plate, osteoporosis, and dilated metacarpal and phalangeal medullary cavities.
3. Growth retardation, with normal growth hormone studies.
4. Mental retardation, usually of a mild degree.
5. Hypogonadism, associated with a small testicular volume and occasional interstitial fibrous tissue proliferation or abnormal spermatogenesis.

1. Case History 1. K. H. had a relatively uneventful infancy except for the persistence of a significant heart murmur from the fourth day of life. At the age of 1 year he was diagnosed as having a mild aortic stenosis. Two years later he developed prolonged recurrent episodes of itchiness, which were originally attributed to a generalized keratosis pilaris. At the age of 9 years he was noted to have chemical evidence of cholestasis. He had experienced a few mild episodes of unexplained rectal bleeding during the preceding year. Six months later (age 9½) a liver biopsy was performed. The pruritis has been well controlled with the use of cholestyramine. At present, he is 15 years old, with a typical facies (i.e., deep-set eyes, frontal bossing, and a pointed chin), and has evidence of short stature, mild sexual infantilism, minimal thoracic and lumbar scoliosis, and biochemical evidence of bile acid and triglyceride retention. At all times he has had only minimal hepatomegaly.

2. *Microscopic Features* (Fig. 8). The lobular architecture is preserved. The portal triads are mostly delicate, the majority not associated with bile ducts. A total of five portal triads are encountered in each section; only one contains a bile duct. Patchy portal fibrosis is noted, with porto-portal bridging or extension into adjacent parenchyma.

3. *Comments.* The biopsy shows a decrease in the number of bile ducts, if one considers as normal a ratio of 1:2 in the number of portal spaces to the number of bile ducts. Caution is necessary to interpret this finding; an adequate number of portal spaces must be present in the biopsy sample.

4. *Case History 2.* N. P. was a small-for-date baby with obvious right coronal suture craniosynostosis, but was otherwise normal. She developed progressive cholestasis, and at 11 weeks of age a laparotomy was performed. Normal extrahepatic bile ducts were found, and a liver biopsy was done (Fig. 9). At the age of 7 months she had a typical facies, and cardiac catheterization demonstrated the presence of peripheral pulmonary stenosis; a second liver biopsy was done (Fig. 10). At 24 months of age a third biopsy was performed because of persistent, severe cholestasis and hepatosplenomegaly (Fig. 11).

5. *Microscopic Features.* The section (Fig. 9) is characterized by predominantly periportal cholestasis with feathery degeneration of periportal hepatocytes and minimal giant cell transformation. There are foci of extramedullary hematopoiesis. Iron is present in macrophages of portal spaces and in Kupffer cells. Regeneration of hepatocytes, with pale-staining cytoplasm and at times pseudoacinar formation, is noted in the outer two-thirds of the hepatic lobules. Some portal spaces without bile ducts are completely devoid of inflammatory reactions. Others are associated with diffuse or patchy mononuclear infiltration, at times with segmented leukocytes, associated with collapse of bile ducts. The epithelium of the bile ducts is flattened, occasionally pyknotic; and in some areas no bile ducts can be identified. Ductular proliferation can be noted with inflammatory infiltrate spilling over to adjacent parenchyma. Reticulum stain demonstrates porto-portal fibrosis and intralobular fibrosis.

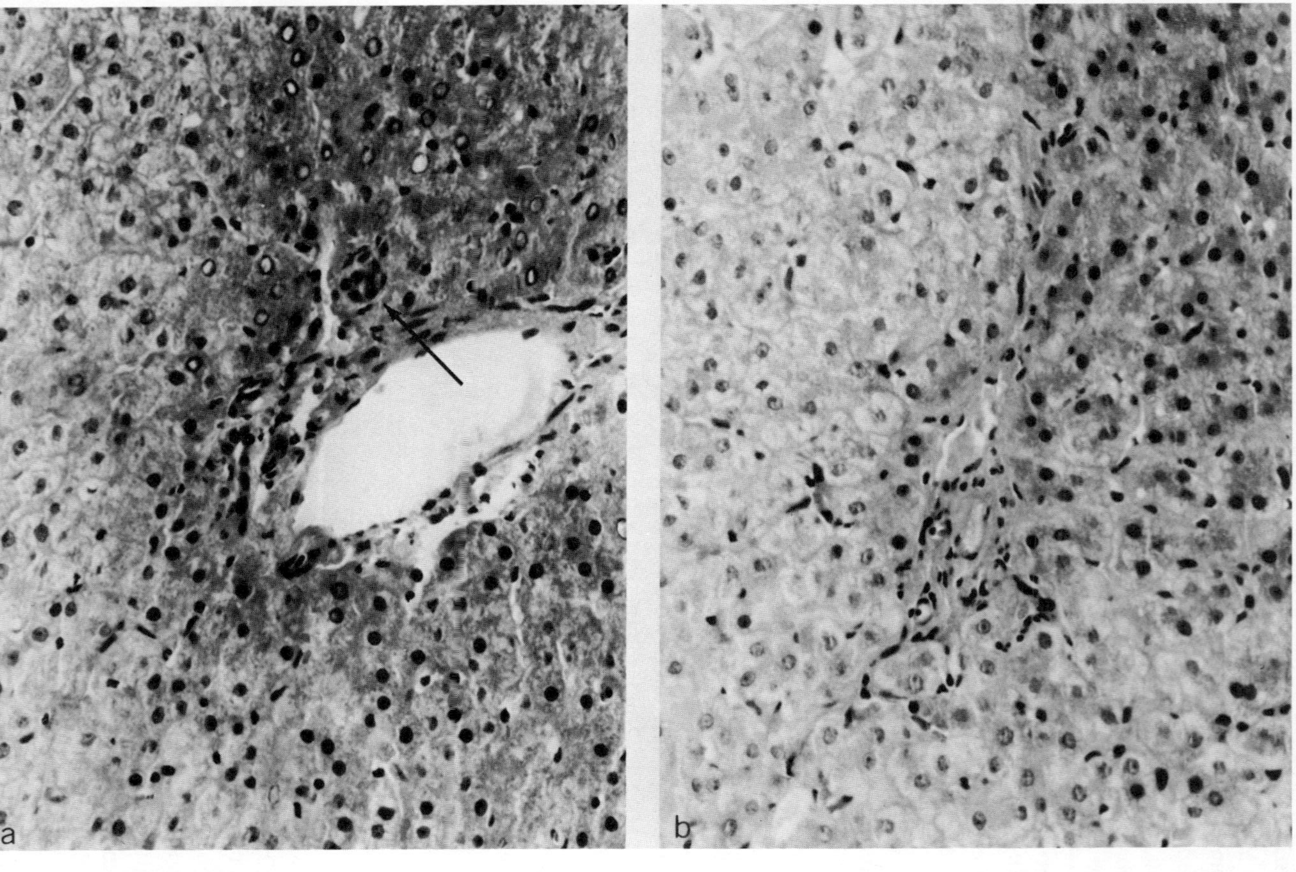

Figure 8 (a) Paucity of intrahepatic bile ducts. Isolated portal space with bile ducts (arrow). H&E. × 280. (b) Same patient–portal space without bile ducts (arrows). H&E. × 280.

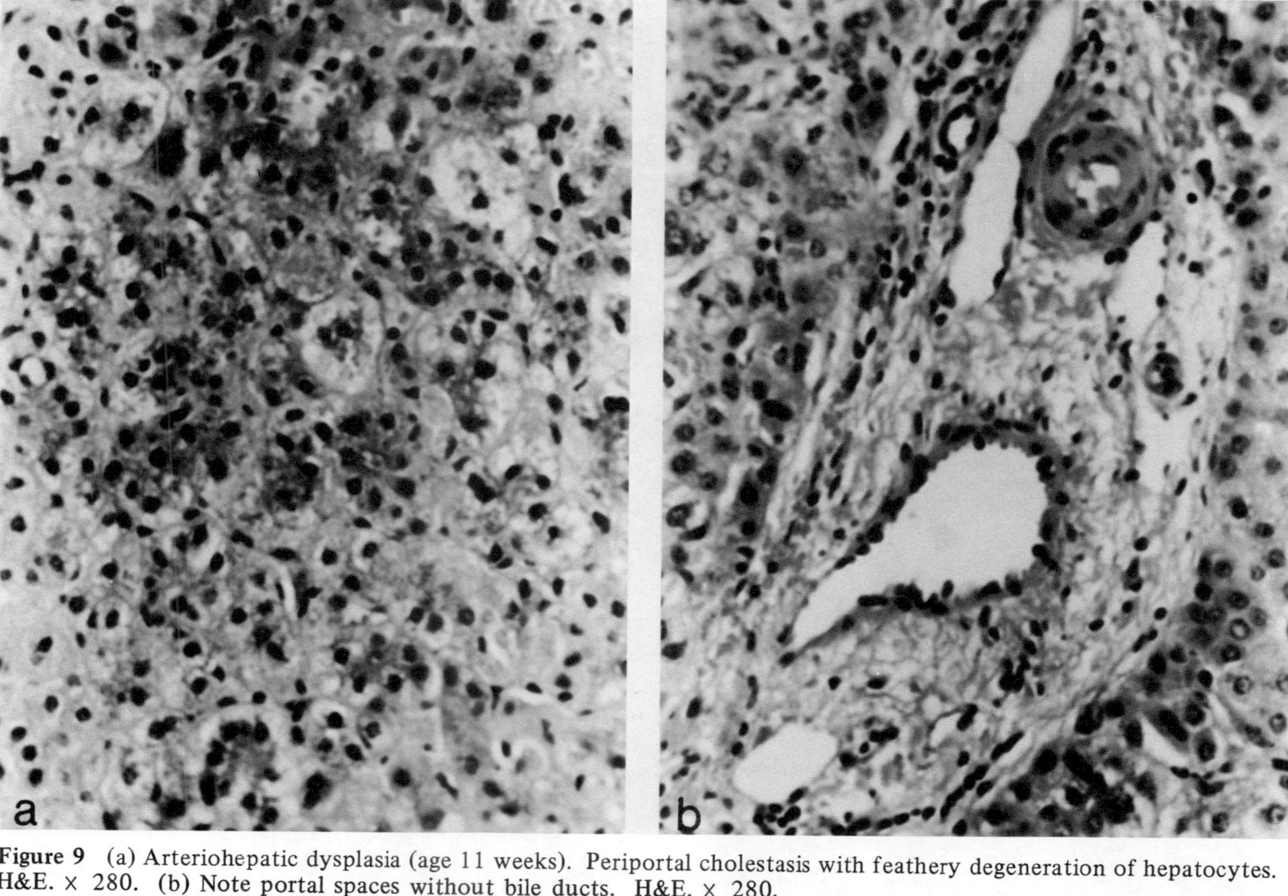

Figure 9 (a) Arteriohepatic dysplasia (age 11 weeks). Periportal cholestasis with feathery degeneration of hepatocytes. H&E. × 280. (b) Note portal spaces without bile ducts. H&E. × 280.

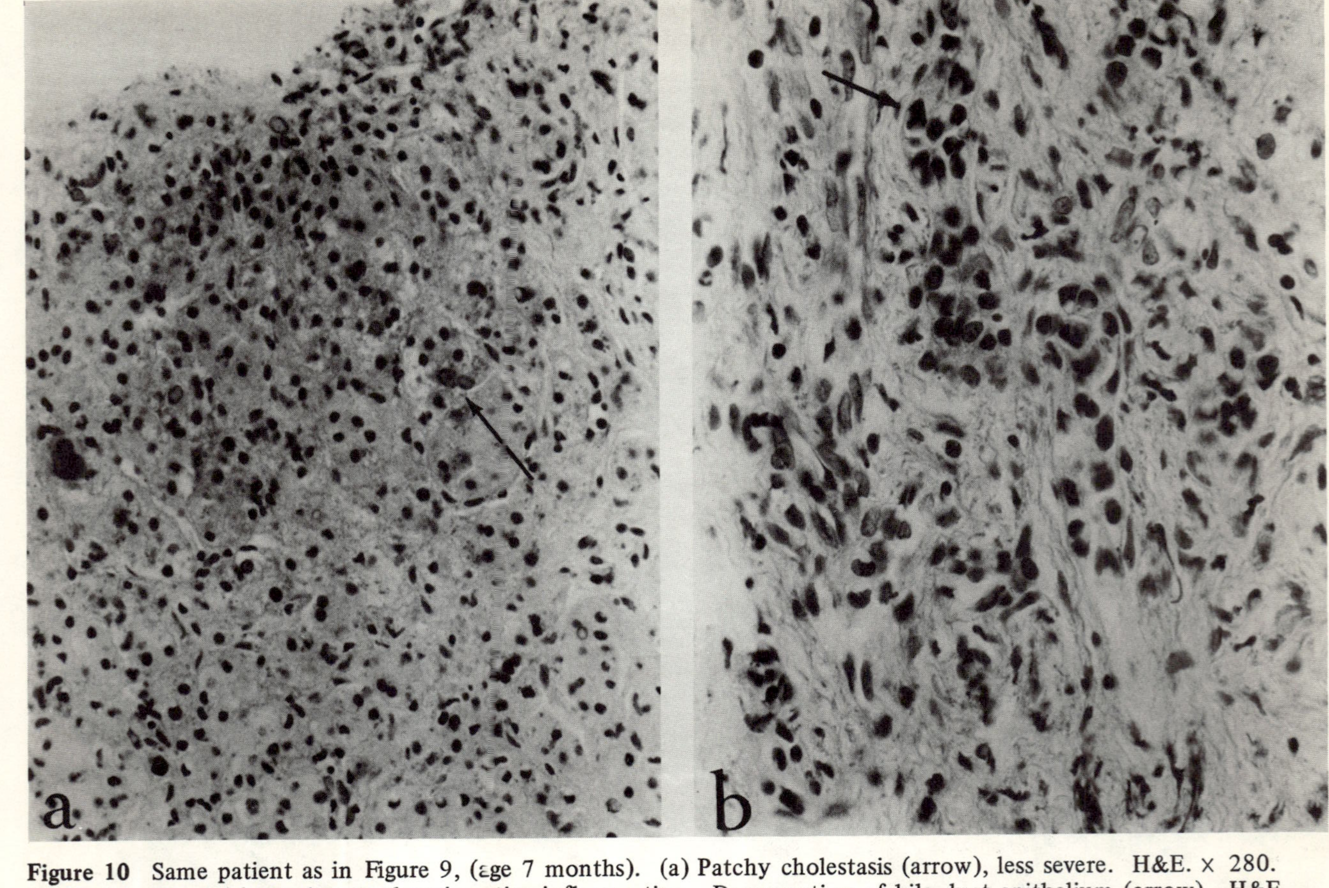

Figure 10 Same patient as in Figure 9, (age 7 months). (a) Patchy cholestasis (arrow), less severe. H&E. × 280. (b) Portal space with persistent, chronic active inflammation. Degeneration of bile duct epithelium (arrow). H&E. × 280.

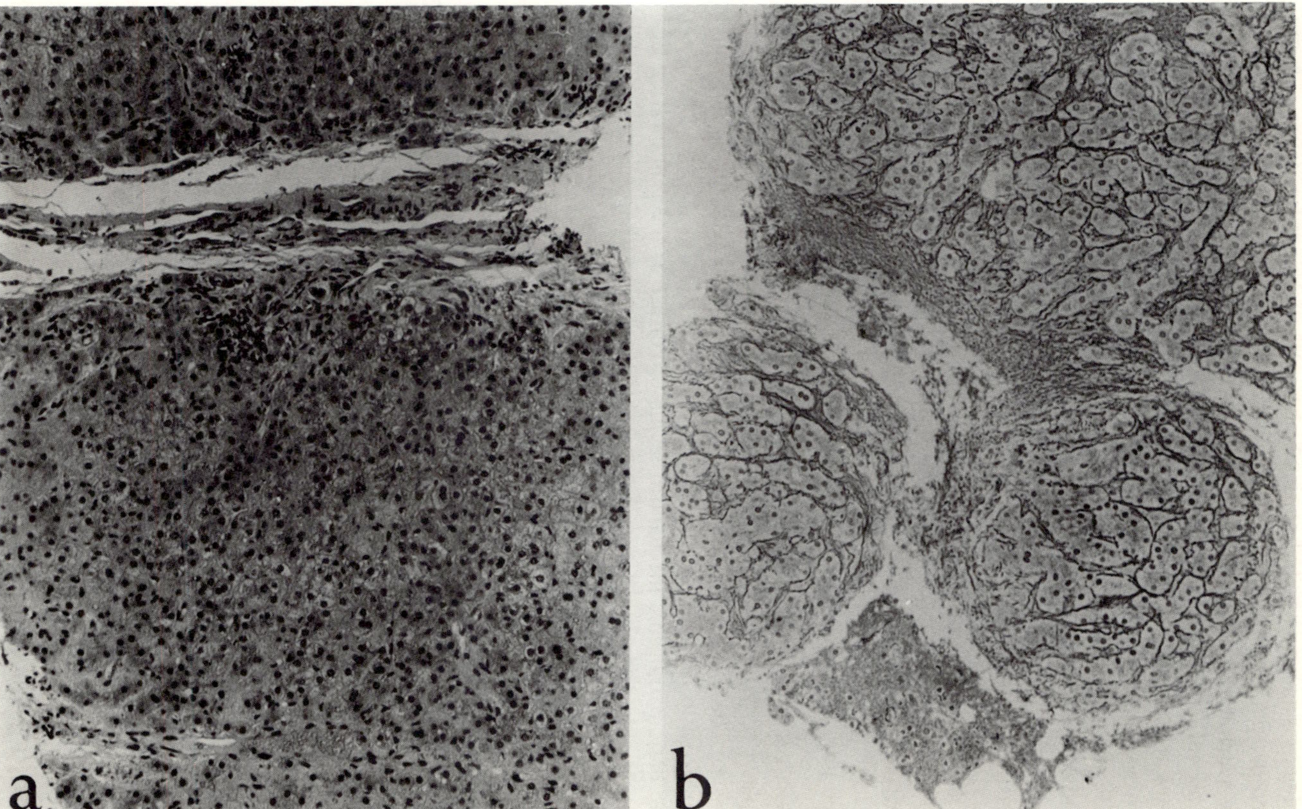

Figure 11 Same patient as in Figures 9 and 10, at age 2 years. (a) Portal space without bile ducts. Note absence of inflammation and longitudinally cut artery. H&E. × 102.5. (b) Progression to micronodular cirrhosis. Reticulum stain. × 102.5.

In Figure 10a, patchy cholestasis persists, although it is less severe. A generalized regenerative pattern of the hepatocytes is noted. In this needle biopsy specimen, most of the portal spaces are associated with bile ducts and show the inflammatory changes described above (Fig. 10b). As a new feature, incipient concentric fibrosis around isolated bile ducts is noted. Portal fibrosis is more severe, with the presence of collagen fibers.

In Figure 11a, cholestasis is still present. A large portal space (cut longitudinally) does not show bile ducts. Inflammatory reaction is absent. Portal fibrosis with subdivision of the hepatic parenchyma into small regenerative nodules is noted (Fig. 11b).

6. *Comments.* This case illustrates the progression of the fundamental process from a pattern simulating patchy giant cell hepatitis with a decreased number of intrahepatic bile ducts at 3 months, with progressive destruction of bile ducts at 7 months, terminating at the age of 2 years with a well-defined pattern of paucity of intrahepatic bile ducts and hepatic cirrhosis.

7. *Discussion.* These two cases exemplify different types of intrahepatic hypoplasia or paucity of intrahepatic ducts, associated with arteriohepatic dysplasia. The process is usually limited to the intrahepatic ducts, but can also progress to involve the extrahepatic biliary system.

The basic pathogenic mechanism seems to consist of the proliferation of smaller bile ducts around larger ones, with fibrosis and disappearance of the latter. A reduction in the number of portal spaces has been described, suggesting that there is also injury to the vascular anlage.

B. Cerebrohepatorenal Syndrome (Zellweger's Syndrome)

The cerebrohepatorenal syndrome [13] is an autosomal recessive hereditary complex with the main features of: (1) generalized hypotonia, often associated with seizures; (2) abnormal craniofacial development, including a high forehead, hypertelorism, and shallow orbital ridges—the facies may be confused with that of Down's syndrome; (3) liver disease, varying from mild periportal fibrosis to micronodular cirrhosis, often associated with gastrointestinal bleeding; (4) asymptomatic renal cortical cysts; and (5) minor skeletal anomalies, including chondral calcification and hand and foot deformities.

Most of these infants do not thrive, and they die within the first 6 months of life. Excessive amounts of urinary pipecolic acid has been noted in many cases in Australia [14]. Hepatic acatalasia, absent peroxisomes and abnormal-looking mitochondria, which have been described [15], may be related to the underlying defect.

1. *Case History.* The infant was the product of a normal full-term pregnancy and delivery. At birth she was noted to be unusually flaccid and had a facies suggestive of Down's syndrome. She failed to thrive and at 1 month developed

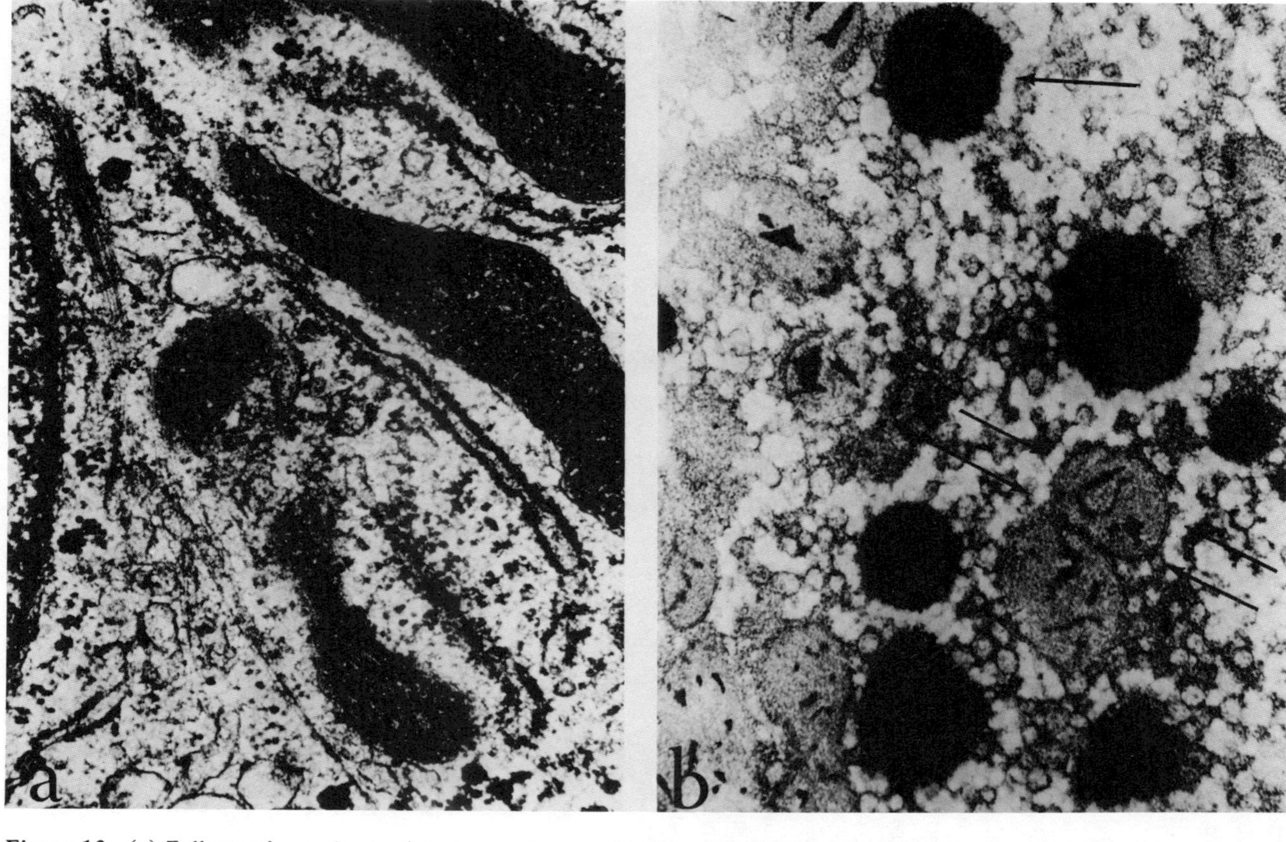

Figure 12 (a) Zellweger's syndrome (electron micrograph). Hepatocyte from Zellweger's syndrome. Absent peroxisome; deformed mitochondria. (b) For comparison, normal hepatocyte with peroxisome (arrow) and normal mitochrondria (double arrows). (Courtesy Dr. S. Goldfischer). X 30,000.

generalized seizures. At 2 months of age she presented with cholestasis and hepatosplenomegaly. The liver disease progressed rapidly, and the patient died at 4½ months of age, with hepatic failure and portal hypertension.

2. *Microscopic Features.* Electron microscopic abnormalities (Fig. 12a) in the liver consist of changes involving mitochondria and peroxisomes. The shapes of the mitochondria are distorted, they have a dense appearance, and the cristae are indistinct. Peroxisomes are absent. (Fig. 12b shows a normal hepatocyte for comparison.)

3. *Comments.* The routine histologic pattern of the liver and brain is nonspecific, whereas the electron microscopic appearance is very suggestive of Zellweger's syndrome. The syndrome is characterized histologically by an increase of iron in the liver, spleen, kidney, skin, and brain. There is also an increase of lipids in kidney and brain. The brain shows signs of macrogyria or polymicrogyria. An increase of neutral lipids is noted in astrocytes of the white matter (sudanophilic leukodystrophy).

The mitochondrial changes have been described in the liver and might be the morphological representation of the basic defect in iron metabolism. The absence of peroxisomes has been noted in hepatocytes and in the renal tubular epithelium. It is not certain that their absence is related to an increase of neutral fat.

References

1. R. S. Dubois and A. Silverman. Treatment of chronic active hepatitis in children. *Postgrad. Med. J. 50,* 386-391 (1974).
2. J. Richey, S. Rogers, D. von Thiel, and R. Lester. Giant multinucleated hepatocytes in an adult with chronic active hepatitis. *Gastroenterology 73,* 570-574 (1977).
3. S. Sherlock. The liver in infancy and childhood. In *Diseases of the Liver and Biliary System.* Blackwell, Oxford, 1975, pp. 553-556.
4. P. J. Daroca, R. Tuthill, and R. J. Reed. Cholangiocarcinoma arising in hepatic fibrosis. *Arch. Pathol. 99,* 592-595 (1975).
5. J. Caroli and V. Corcos. La dilatation congenitale des voies biliairies intrahepatiques. *Rev. Medicochir. Mal. Foie 39,* 1-70 (1964).
6. J. Caroli. Diseases of intrahepatic bile ducts. *Isr. J. Med. Sci. 4,* 421-425 (1968).
7. A. W. Jones and D. R. Shreeve. Congenital dilation of intrahepatic biliary ducts with cholangiocarcinoma. *Br. Med. J. 2,* 277-278 (1970).
8. O. Aagenaes, C. B. Van der Hagen, and S. Refsum. Hereditary recurrent intrahepatic cholestasis from birth. *Arch. Dis. Child. 43,* 646-657 (1968).
9. R. J. Clayton, S. L. Iber, B. H. Ruebner, and V. A. McCusick. Byler's disease; fatal familial intrahepatic cholestasis in an Amish kindred. *J. Pediatr. 67,* 1025-1028 (1965).

10. C. N. Williams, R. Kaye, L. Baker, R. Hurwitz, and J. R. Senior. Progressive familial cholestatic cirrhosis and bile acid metabolism. *J. Pediatr. 81,* 493-500 (1972).
11. J. N. Isenberg, R. M. Hanson, G. Williams, P. Sczepanik, B. D. Klein, and H. L. Sharp. A clinical experience with familial paucity of intrahepatic bile ducts associated with defective metabolism of trihydroxycoprostanic acid to cholic acid. In *Liver Diseases in Children* (D. Alagille, Ed.). Inserm, Paris, 1975, pp. 43-56.
12. G. H. Watson and V. Miller. Arteriohepatic dysplasia familial pulmonary arterial stenosis with liver disease. *Arch. Dis. Child. 48,* 459-466 (1973).
13. E. Passarge and A. J. McAdams. Cerebro-hepato-renal syndrome. *J. Pediatr. 71,* 691-702 (1967).
14. D. M. Danks, P. Tippett, C. Adams, and P. Campbell. Cerebro-hepato-renal syndrome of Zellweger. *J. Pediatr. 86,* 382-387 (1975).
15. S. Goldfischer, C. L. Moore, and A. B. Johnson. Peroxisomal and mitochondrial defects in the cerebro-hepato-renal syndrome. *Science 182,* 62-64 (1973).

4 Diseases of Genetic Origin Associated with Liver Disease in Infancy and Childhood

ANDREW SASS-KORTSAK / University of Toronto, and The Hospital for Sick Children, Toronto, Canada

I. Introduction

There are many diseases of genetic origin (inborn errors of metabolism) that may present in infancy or in childhood with liver disease.

Twelve conditions are listed in Table 1, all of them dependent on genetic factors. The six on the left are single gene defects, and they have the pattern of an autosomal recessive mode of inheritance. The six on the right are less clearly defined as yet.

We could devote a volume to a discussion of these entities, but perhaps by picking out two—$alpha_1$-antitrypsin deficiency and Wilson's disease—we can give you a reasonable illustration of this complex problem. Recent reviews on these two subjects have appeared in the literature [1-4, 5-8].

Table 1 Genetic Defects Associated with Pediatric Liver Disease

Single gene defects	Not yet defined
Galactosemia	Fibrocystic disease
Fructosemia	Familial cholestasis
Tyrosinemia	Congenital hepatic fibrosis
α_1-Antitrypsin deficiency	Porphyria hepatica
Glycogen storage disease (IV)	Polycystic liver disease
Wilson's disease	Hereditary hemorrhagic telangiectasia

II. Alpha$_1$-Antitrypsin Deficiency

Alpha$_1$-antitrypsin (α_1AT) is a serum protein which inhibits the activity of several proteolytic enzymes, including trypsin, chymotrypsin, elastase, thrombin, and leukocyte and bacterial proteases. This is the only known function of this protein, which is an α_1-globulin; it normally makes up 90-95% of this serum protein fraction.

Laurell and Eriksson were the first to report that some individuals have a greatly diminished amount of α_1AT in the serum. They also found that many of these individuals developed chronic obstructive lung disease, emphysema, and that the onset was rather early, about 40 years of age [9]. Then Sharp and colleagues reported that α_1AT deficiency is associated with the development of neonatal hapatitis in infancy [10]. These first reports were extended and confirmed by many workers [11-16]. About one-third of all cases of neonatal hepatitis involved profound α_1AT deficiency. Moreover, the presentation of α_1AT-deficient patients may not always be in the form of neonatal hepatitis; some patients with α_1AT deficiency may present with portal hypertension and/or cirrhosis of the liver without jaundice.

Finally, liver and lung disease may both be present in the same α_1AT-deficient individual either early in life or later. Some of the α_1AT-deficient children with early development of liver disease have obstructive lung disease [15], and some adults presenting with obstructive lung disease have liver disease [17, 18]. Other organs may also be involved in some individuals (for example, the kidneys) [19].

A. Diagnosis of α_1AT Deficiency

The molecular weight of the α_1AT protein is 55,000 daltons It is a glycoprotein containing 8-13% carbohydrate, including six sialic acid residues. Its electrophoretic mobility is that of an α_1-globulin, and it makes up 90-95% of this fraction of proteins in human serum.

A marked deficiency of α_1AT can frequently be picked up by electrophoresis. A useful method for this purpose is electrophoresis of serum proteins on cellulose acetate supporting medium at pH 8.6, with a barbital buffer [20]. Albumin and four globulin fractions (α_1, α_2, β, and γ) can be separated in this manner, and this method is used widely now in many hospital laboratories. In severe α_1AT deficiency the α_1-globulin peak is usually virtually absent (Fig. 1). The difficulty–albeit rare–is that because of infection or other condition, the portion of this fraction (normally 5-10%), which is not α_1AT, may be increased; thus the marked deficiency may be missed by this method. In addition, Pi type ZZ patients may in fact have up to 50% of the normal amount of this protein in their serum, particularly in the presence of liver disease. Further work in this area established much better methods, but at the same time revealed more complications.

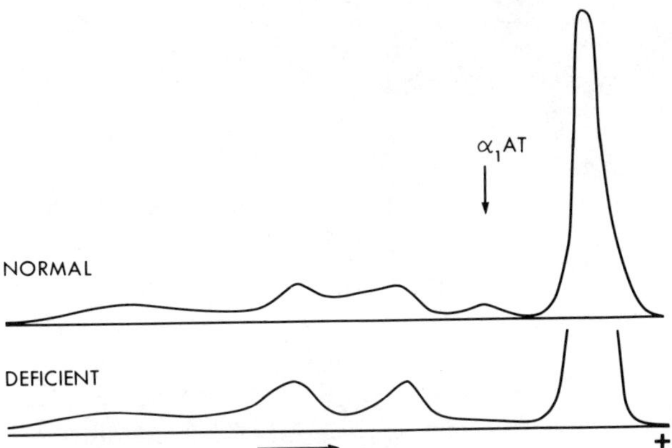

Figure 1 Electrophoretic pattern (pH 8.6) of serum proteins from normal individual (upper) and from α_1AT-deficient individual (lower).

For finer resolution of α_1AT, starch gel can be used as the supporting medium, and the electrophoresis can be carried out at pH 4.9 [21]. At this low pH most proteins move very slowly, and the usual fractions, including serum albumin, are very poorly separated (Fig. 2). However, α_1AT, with a few other proteins present in small amounts, moves ahead of albumin. To detect α_1AT, specific antibody was used against this protein. A vertical strip was cut from each individual "run" and placed between two sheets of agarose in which a suitable concentration of antibody against α_1AT was present. Then electrophoresis was run at a right angle to the previous run [22]. The result was most interesting (Fig. 3A). Precipitation by antibody against α_1AT occurred in two major and at least three minor bands. This was the result with normal sera, with no deficiency of α_1AT.

When there was a marked deficiency of α_1AT, it was difficult to see any protein on the original starch gel run at pH 4.9 (Fig. 2). However when electrophoresis was continued at a right angle to the previous run, and the gel contained antibody against α_1AT, a very different pattern emerged. There were three main bands, all of which ran more slowly than before, and two very small bands, one ahead and one behind (Fig. 3B).

When we ran the serum of the parents of the severely deficient individual, there was a mixture of the two patterns (Fig. 3C). The two main peaks, as in the normal individual, were present, but they were somewhat smaller. Then there was a doubling of the minor peaks behind the two main peaks. Thus there is a homozygous normal pattern (Fig. 3A), a homozygous abnormal one, (Fig. 3B), and a heterozygous pattern (Fig. 3C).

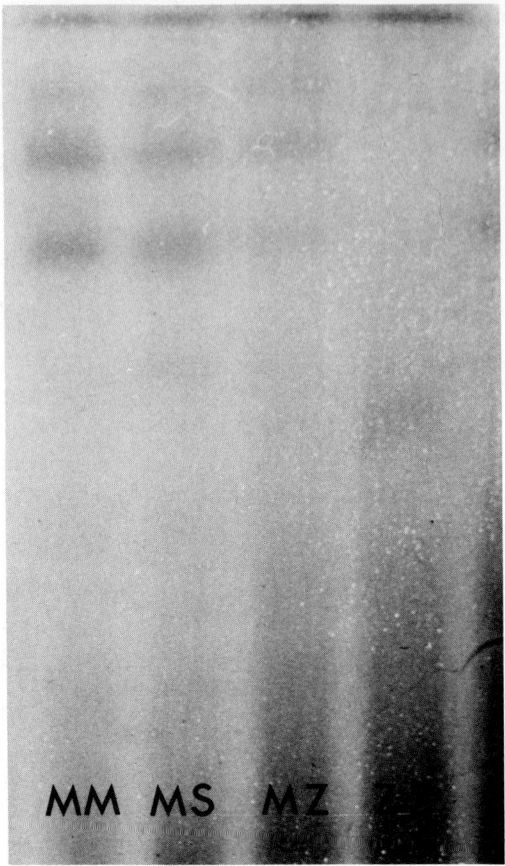

Figure 2 Starch gel electrophoresis (pH 4.9). Separation of serum α_1AT into several bands. Four serum samples were run, which turned out to be Pi types MM, MS, MZ, and ZZ.

Screening large groups of the population then revealed that the markedly deficient variety of α_1AT is just one of the abnormalities of this protein [23]. By now we know of more than 25 variations from the normal pattern (Fig. 4). The normal α_1AT pattern is named "Pi (protease inhibitor) type MM"; the markedly deficient variety "Pi type ZZ," and the heterozygotes "Pi type MZ." In addition to this there are variants moving faster than the M variety (such as Pi type F) and some moving slower (such as Pi type S) [23].

The Pi types of 723 individuals, living in and around Toronto, were determined by Dr. Diane Cox in our laboratories by the methods presented here.

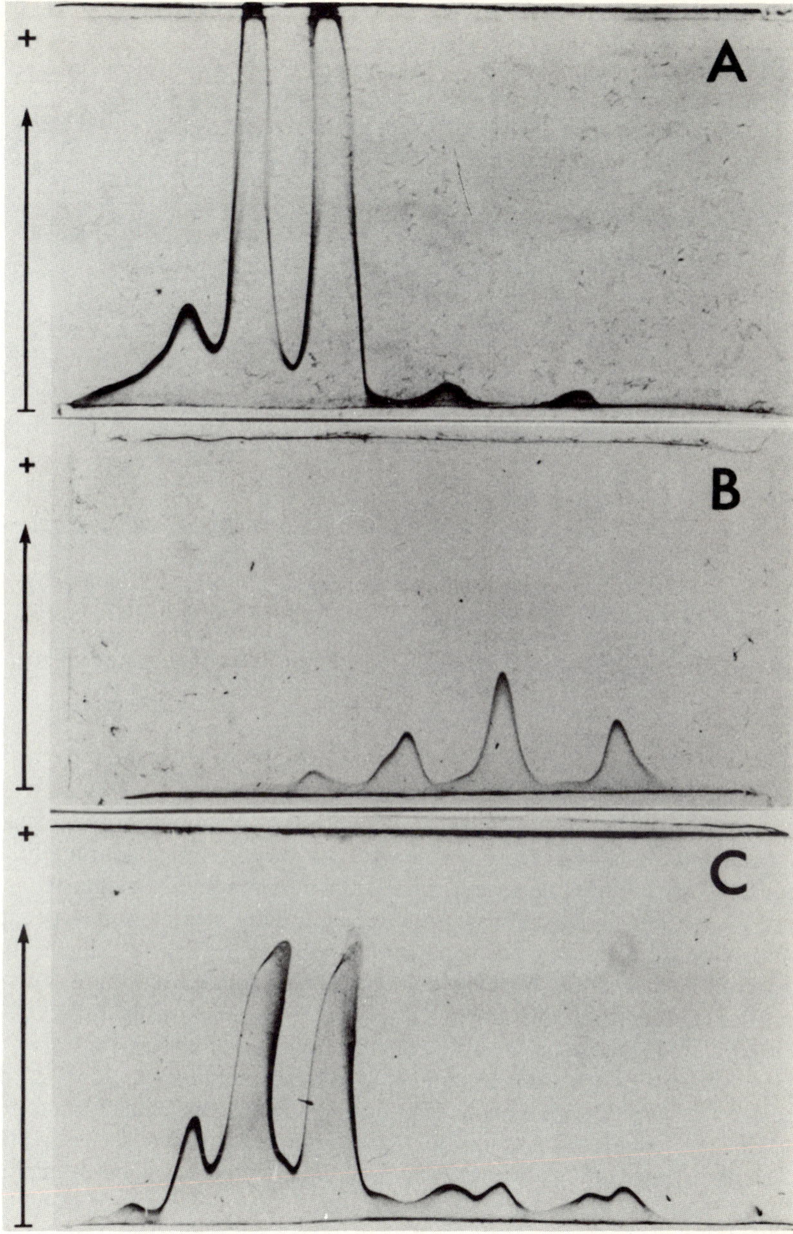

Figure 3 After initial run on starch gel (Fig. 2), and after 90° turn, electrophoresis was rerun into agarose gel impregnated with antibody against α_1 AT. (A) Normal serum–PiMM. (B) α_1 AT-deficient serum–PiZZ. (C) Serum of heterozygote–PiMZ.

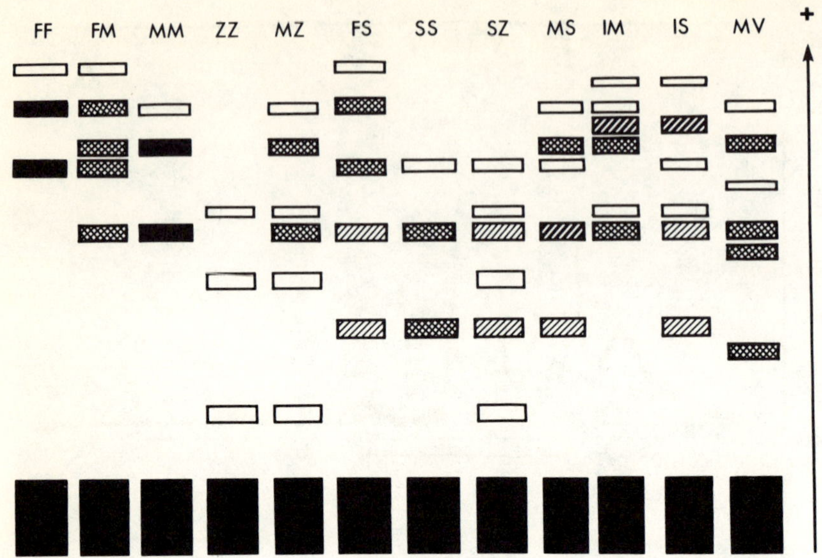

Figure 4 Drawing of electrophoretic runs of serum α_1AT on starch gel in front of serum albumin (pH 4.9). Genotype of each person is indicated at top: FF, FM, MM, etc. Staining intensities are indicated by different shadings of black, increasing from white through hatched, crosshatched, heavily hatched, to black.

Of these, 89.0% were of Pi type MM, 7.8% PiMS, 2.3% PiMZ, and the remaining 0.9% of individuals were of other rare Pi types.

The total amount of α_1 AT in human serum can be determined by an immunochemical method, using a specific antibody against α_1 AT and measuring the amount by radial immunodiffusion, by electroimmunoassay, or by nephelometry. By using a synthetic substrate one can also measure the trypsin-inhibitory capacity of human serum. However, this latter method—although relatively simple—is nonspecific in that 5-10% of the total trypsin-inhibitory activity in human serum is due to factors other than α_1AT (such as α_2-macroglobulin).

Fagerhol [24] has done quantitative studies on the inherited variants of α_1AT by measuring the total amount of α_1AT in serum and determining the Pi type, as well by the methods briefly outlined earlier and described in his paper in more detail. He has reported that a marked deficiency of α_1AT is found only in the homozygous PiZZ type individuals (15% of the normal amount). The heterozygotes (Pi type MZ) have some reduction of α_1AT content (50-60%). The groups of individuals with various other types of α_1AT have a tendency to have moderately reduced amounts of α_1AT, but with all variants the amount of α_1AT is usually between 50 and 100% of the amounts present in Pi type MM individuals.

Table 2 Alpha$_1$-Antitrypsin Deficiency–Mode and Age of Presentation

Mode	No. of patients		Age of patients
Neonatal hepatitis syndrome	14		
with onset of jaundice		8	<1 wk
		4	1-3 wk
		2	1-3 mo
Hepatosplenomegaly	3		4 mo, 6 mo, 6 yr
Hematemesis	1		18 mo
Total	18		

B. Alpha$_1$-Antitrypsin Deficiency and Liver Disease in Children

We have found 18 patients in our own case records who had marked α_1 AT deficiency and liver disease. Most patients were identified by surveying a rather large number of children with liver disease. All of them previously had serum protein electrophoresis performed, using cellulose acetate supporting medium; the results, including the tracings of the electrophoretic patterns, had been kept in their hospital histories. Those patients with markedly reduced amounts of α_1-globulin were then recalled with their families for further study of their α_1 AT type by the methods presented earlier.

The 18 patients selected were found to be of Pi type ZZ. Their sibs and parents were also studied. Of the 18 patients, 14 had presented with the neonatal hepatitis syndrome (Table 2). In eight of these, jaundice had appeared during the first week of life, in four between 1 and 3 weeks of age, and in two between 1 and 3 months of age. The duration of the jaundice was from 2 to 8 months; then the jaundice cleared. There were three additional patients who have not had any jaundice, but who presented at 4 months, 6 months, and at 6 years of age, with a firm and enlarged liver, splenomegaly, and other signs of liver disease. The last of the 18 patients presented at 18 months of age with massive hematemesis, which was then proved to be due to portal hypertension and cirrhosis of the liver. Presentation was therefore at any time between <1 week and 6 years of age. The majority (14 patients) presented with jaundice and the neonatal hepatitis syndrome. But four patients presented without jaundice, with hepatosplenomegaly and portal hypertension.

The current status of these patients is shown in Table 3). Four of the 18 patients died between 5 and 12 years of age. Three others have obvious and advancing chronic liver disease at 1, 4, and 7 years of age. However, 11 of the 18 patients are quite well. Only one of these is less than 1 year of age, four are between 1 and 5 years, two between 5 and 12 years, and four others are

Table 3 Alpha$_1$-Antitrypsin Deficiency—Current Status of Patients

Status	No. of patients		Age of patients
Dead	4		5, 9, 10, 12 yr
Chronic liver disease	4		8, 11 mo; 4, 7 yr
		4	1-5 yr
Well	10	2	5-12 yr
		4	12-18 yr
Total	18		

between 13 and 18 years of age. We assume that a number of these, probably between five and eight patients, will recover and live a reasonably long life. Whether any or all of them will develop emphysema at around 40 years of age remains to be seen.

It seems to us that, after the first reports on this rather serious disease, with the discovery of more patients and perhaps also those who are less severely involved, the prognosis is not as hopeless as it appeared earlier. It is hoped that treatment will be found, and this will make the outlook even better for patients with α_1 AT deficiency.

III. Wilson's Disease: Hepatolenticular Degeneration

The very first description of hepatolenticular degeneration appeared almost 120 years ago, in 1861, by Frerichs [25]. He described a 10-year-old boy with liver disease, who then developed violent tremors and convulsions, and who eventually died. Necropsy revealed cirrhosis of the liver and marked alterations in the brain.

In 1912, Kinnear Wilson, an eminent English neurologist, published his observations on a group of these patients [26]. He recognized the coexistence of liver disease and central nervous system disease. He called attention to the fact that some patients died of liver disease before the central nervous system involvement became obvious.

Kayser-Fleischer rings were not noted by him. These were described 10 years earlier by Kayser [27] and a year later, independently, by Fleischer [28]. The latter proposed in several papers written before Wilson's publication that these rings of the corneae, the liver disease, and the neurological disease were probably due to a single factor, a single metabolic abnormality [29, 30].

In 1913, Rumpel suggested that copper was accumulating in these patients [31]. Siemerling and Oloff [32], and later Glazebrook in 1945 [33], elaborated further on the role of copper in this disease. Finally Scheinberg and Gitlin [34] and, independently, Bearn and Kunkel [35] reported that very low blood levels of the copper-bearing protein, ceruloplasmin, could be found in this condition.

Wilson was the first to notice familial occurrence of this disease [26], and Bearn in 1960 presented definite evidence of autosomal recessive inheritance of hepatolenticular degeneration [36].

Sternlieb et al. [37] and our own group [38] worked out methods using radioactive copper, whereby patients with Wilson's disease and heterozygous carriers of the abnormal gene could be recognized and studied.

A treatment was first suggested and tried by Cumings, who proposed the use of BAL to remove copper [39]. Later John Walshe recognized penicillamine as the drug with which these patients can be most successfully treated [40, 41].

A. Genetic Abnormality

Wilson's disease is caused by the abnormality of an autosomal recessive gene. Patients are homozygous abnormal. Parents of the patients are heterozygous carriers. The disease occurs in sibships. For each sib there is a 1:4 chance of having the disease, a 1:2 chance of being carriers, like the parents, and a 1:4 chance of being homozygous normal. This situation in one of our own families with 18 children is shown in Figure 5.

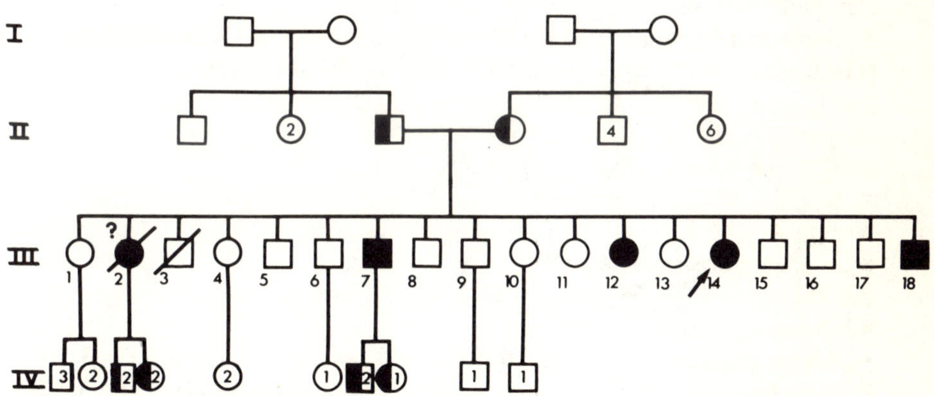

Figure 5 Pedigree of family with Wilson's disease. Propositus, III.14, developed liver disease at 17 years of age. Survey of his sibship (generation III) revealed four additional homozygous abnormals: III.2, presumed, who died earlier of liver disease; III.7 and III.18, presymptomatic with evidence of latent liver disease; and III.12, presymptomatic with no evidence of disease. Parents in generation II and children of patients, in generation IV, are considered obligate heterozygotes. Genotypes of the others are not known.

B. Presentation

The clinical presentation is quite variable, but there is a tendency for the same pattern of appearance of symptoms in sibs. Presentation is usually between 10 and 30 years of age. The earlier the patient presents, the more likely it will be with liver disease; the later the presentation, the more likely it will be with neurological involvement. Presentation with manifest liver and neurological disease together is rare. A more rare form of presentation is with an acute bout of hemolytic anemia and hemolytic jaundice. Other patients, rarely, can present with vitamin D-resistant rickets and bone changes. Another, also rare, form of presentation is with psychiatric problems, usually in the third or fourth decade of life.

C. Diagnosis

The earlier one can make the diagnosis, the better for the patient. The diagnosis can often be made by looking for Kayser-Fleischer rings in the corneae. However, these rings may be absent in the first two decades of life even if the patient has Wilson's disease. The diagnosis cannot be excluded on the basis of not finding these rings despite careful slit lamp examination.

The *serum ceruloplasmin levels* must be determined next (Fig. 6). The normal mean blood level of ceruloplasmin is 31 mg/dl, with a range from 20.6 to 42.0 mg/dl (95% confidence limits).

In approximately 80% of the patients with Wilson's disease the serum ceruloplasmin level is less than 10 mg/dl. In a further 15% of the patients the ceruloplasmin levels are between 10 and 20 mg/dl, but in the remaining 4-5% of patients the ceruloplasmin levels are within the normal range.

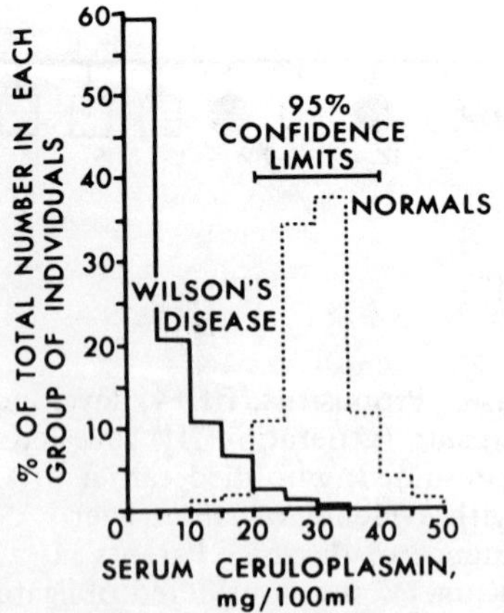

Figure 6. Frequency distribution of serum ceruloplasmin concentrations in 230 patients with Wilson's disease at time of diagnosis (solid line) and in 309 normal controls (interrupted line). Patients are from I. Sternlieb and I. H. Scheinberg (unpublished data) and from A. Sass-Kortsak and D. W. Cox (unpublished data); controls are from D. W. Cox [42].

D. Serum Copper Levels

In normal individuals the serum copper level is 108 μg/dl, with the normal range between 80 and 135 μg/dl. In normals 90-95% of the total serum copper is tightly bound to ceruloplasmin; the remaining 5-10% is more loosely bound to albumin. In Wilson's disease the amount of albumin-bound copper is usually increased to 20-40 μg/dl, but the ceruloplasmin-bound copper is usually much reduced, so that the total amount of copper in the serum is usually reduced.

E. Urinary Copper Excretion

The *24-hr urinary copper excretion* is markedly increased in the patient with Wilson's disease. Normals excrete <40 μg copper per 24 hr. When D-penicillamine is given (0.5 g, b.i.d., q 12 hr) normals excrete 400-800 μg copper per 24 hr. In patients with Wilson's disease, under the same conditions far more copper is excreted, usually 1500-3000 μg per 24 hr.

In 95-97% of instances one can make the diagnosis of Wilson's disease safely and securely on these grounds. The patients present at between 10 and 30 years of age; they have liver or neurological disease or both. Kayser-Fleischer rings of the corneae are present. Serum ceruloplasmin levels are very low; the serum copper levels are somewhat reduced, but the urinary copper excretion is increased. In addition to this there may be other confirmatory findings, especially relating to kidney function. A moderate degree of proteinuria can be present. Uric acid excretion can be increased in the urine, and the blood level of uric acid is reduced. Aminoaciduria can also be present, among other conditions.

However, in 2-5% of the patients, after all this work one may still be uncertain of the diagnosis. Should this situation arise one may have to substantiate the diagnosis of Wilson's disease by investigating the patient with the use of radioactive ^{64}Cu or ^{67}Cu. This investigation should then be carried out without delay to arrive at a definite diagnosis.

F. Treatment

Effective treatment is available for Wilson's disease. Since John Walshe introduced penicillamine for this purpose 20 years ago, there can be little difficulty with the management of patients. However, for treatment to be effective the diagnosis must be made early, before irreversible damage has occurred either in the liver or in the brain.

The drug D-penicillamine (D-dimethylcysteine) is given now for this purpose—0.5 g (per os, b.i.d., q 12 hr) to patients over 15 years of age. For children the dose may be lower—0.5-0.75 g per 24 hr, divided into two doses. During the first year of treatment it may be necessary to increase the dose to 1.5-2.0 g per 24 hr to increase copper removal via the urine, but after 1-1½ years one can usually return to the original dose. With D-penicillamine we always give also 12.5 mg pyridoxine daily.

In addition to drug therapy, copper intake via the diet must be reduced. Normally we take in 3-6 mg copper per 24 hr; this can be easily reduced to 1.0-1.5 mg per 24 hr by not eating liver, nuts, mushrooms, cocoa, chocolate, or shellfish, which have the highest copper content.

Treatment with D-penicillamine may lead to reactions. Some patients develop itching and a rash; they may develop a fever, respiratory symptoms, or other problems. On discontinuation of therapy such problems clear up within a few days. After this one can restart treatment with D-penicillamine but at a much lower dose: 5-10 mg per 24 hr; and one can then double this dose until one achieves 1.0 g per 24 hr. These symptoms usually do not return. However, should this happen, one stops again and—after clearing of the symptoms—one can put the patient on a moderate dose of prednisone or prednisolone and then restart D-penicillamine, gradually increasing the dose. In most instances this should solve the problem, and after this the prednisone can gradually be reduced and discontinued.

Other, more serious, reactions to D-penicillamine treatment (in our opinion) are extremely rare in Wilson's disease. However, very rarely patients may develop increasing proteinuria and eventually the nephrotic syndrome. In other instances a lupus erythematosus-type syndrome or Goodpasture's syndrome may develop. There are other less frequently encountered skin changes as well. These reactions may occur as late as 2-5 years after treatment was started.

Because of the possibility of such reactions, even if these are rare, one has to carefully follow patients with Wilson's disease during the rest of their lives. Periodic clinical assessments, together with checks for protein in urine, hemoglobin, white blood count, and platelet counts, are useful at monthly and then 3-monthly intervals. In rare instances D-penicillamine treatment must be abandoned; these patients can be treated with a new agent, triethylenetetramine-2HCl [43].

References

1. E. Cutz and D. W. Cox. α_1-Antitrypsin deficiency: The spectrum of pathology and pathophysiology. *Perspect. Pediatr. Pathol. 5* (1979). In press.
2. R. A. Norum, A. G. Bearn, W. A. Briscoe, and A. Briscoe. Alpha-1-antitrypsin and disease. *Mt. Sinai J. Med. 44,* 821-827 (1977).
3. R. C. Talamo. Basic and clinical aspects of the alpha-1-antitrypsin. *Pediatrics 56,* 91-99 (1975).
4. F. Kueppers and L. F. Black. α_1-Antitrypsin and its deficiency. *Am. Rev. Respir. Dis. 110,* 176-194 (1974).

5. A. Sass-Kortsak and A. G. Bearn. Hereditary disorders of copper metabolism. Wilson's disease (hepatolenticular degeneration) and Menkes' disease (kindy-hair or steely-hair syndrome). In *The Metabolic Basis of Inherited Disease* (J. B. Stanbury, J. B. Wyngaarden, and D. S. Fredrickson, Eds.), 4th Ed. McGraw-Hill, New York, 1978, pp. 1098-1126.
6. G. W. Evans. Copper homeostasis in the mammalian system. *Physiol. Rev. 53,* 535-570 (1973).
7. J. M. Walshe. The physiology of copper in man and its relation to Wilson's disease. *Brain 90,* 149-176 (1967).
8. I. H. Scheinberg and I. Sternlieb. Wilson's disease. *Annu. Rev. Med. 16,* 119-134 (1967).
9. C.-B. Laurell and S. Eriksson. The electrophoretic α_1-globulin pattern of serum α_1-antitrypsin deficiency. *Scand. J. Clin. Lab. Invest. 15,* 132-140 (1963).
10. H. L. Sharp, R. A. Bridges, W. Krivit, and E. F. Freier. Cirrhosis associated with alpha$_1$-antitrypsin deficiency: A previously unrecognized inherited disorder. *J. Lab. Clin. Med. 73,* 934-939 (1969).
11. A. M. Johnson and C. A. Alper. Deficiency of α_1-antitrypsin in childhood liver disease. *Pediatrics 46,* 921-925 (1970).
12. G. J. Gherardi. Alpha$_1$-antitrypsin deficiency and its effect on the liver. *Hum. Pathol. 2,* 173-175 (1971).
13. H. L. Sharp. Alpha$_1$-antitrypsin deficiency. *Hosp. Pract. 5,* 83- (1971).
14. C. A. Porter, A. P. Mowat, P. J. L. Cook, D. W. G. Hayner, K. B. Shilkin, and R. Williams. α_1-Antitrypsin deficiency and neonatal hepatitis. *Br. Med. J. 3,* 435-439 (1972).
15. J. F. T. Glasgow, M. J. Lynch, A. Hercz, H. Levison, and A. Sass-Kortsak. Alpha$_1$-antitrypsin deficiency in association with both cirrhosis and chronic obstructive lung disease in two sibs. *Am. J. Med. 54,* 181-194 (1973).
16. R. C. Talamo and M. Feingold. Infantile cirrhosis with hereditary alpha$_1$-antitrypsin deficiency. *Am. J. Dis. Child. 125,* 845-847 (1973).
17. M. O. Berg and S. Eriksson. Liver disease in adults with alpha$_1$-antitrypsin deficiency. *N. Engl. J. Med. 287,* 1264-1267 (1972).
18. R. R. Babb, G. A. Lillington, and R. L. Kempson. Cirrhosis in an adult with emphysema and alpha$_1$-antitrypsin deficiency. *Am. J. Dig. Dis. 18,* 803-807.
19. S. P. Moroz, E. Cutz, J. W. Balfe, and A. Sass-Kortsak. Membranoproliferative glomerulonephritis and childhood cirrhosis associated with alpha$_1$-antitrypsin deficiency. *Pediatrics 57,* 232-238 (1976).
20. R. J. Henry, D. C. Cannon, and J. W. Winkelman, Eds. *Clinical Chemistry, Principles and Techniques.* Harper & Row (Med. Dept.), Hagerstown, Md., 1974, pp. 98-102.
21. M. K. Fagerhol. The Pi system. *Ser. Haematol. 1,* 153-161 (1968).

22. M. K. Fagerhol and C.-B. Laurell. The polymorphism of "prealbumins" and α_1-antitrypsin in human sera. *Clin. Chim. Acta 16,* 199-203 (1967).
23. M. K. Fagerhol. Serum Pi types in Norwegians. *Acta Pathol. Microbiol. Scand. 70,* 421-428 (1967).
24. M. K. Fagerhol. Quantitative studies on the inherited variants of serum α_1-antitrypsin. *Scand. J. Clin. Lab. Invest. 23,* 97-103 (1969).
25. F. T. von Frerichs. *Pathologisch-anatomischer Atlas zur Klinik der Leberkrankheiten,* 2nd ed., Vol. 2, Wieweg und Sohn, Weisbaden, Braunschweig (Germany), 1861, p. 62.
26. S. A. K. Wilson. Progressive lenticular degeneration: A familial nervous disease associated with cirrhosis of the liver. *Brain 34,* 295-509 (1912).
27. B. Kayser. Über einen Fall von angeborener grünlicher Verfärbung der Kornea. *Klin. Monatsbl. Augenheilkd. 40,* 22-25 (1902).
28. B. Fleischer. Zwei weitere Fälle von grünlicher Verfärbung der Kornea. *Klin. Monatsbl. Augenheilkd. 41,* 489-491 (1903).
29. B. Fleischer. Die perifäre braun-grünliche Hornhautverfärbung, als Symptom einer eigenartigen Allgemeinerkrankung. *Münch. Med. Wochenschr. 56,* 1120-1123 (1909).
30. B. Fleischer. Über einer der "Pseudosklerose" nahestehende bisher unbekannte Krankheit (gekennzeichnet durch Tremor, psychische Störungen, braunliche Pigmentierung bestimmter Gewebe, insbesondere auch der Hornhautperipherie, Lebercirrhose). *Dtsch. Z. Nervenheilkd. 44,* 179-201 (1912).
31. A. Rumpel. Über das Wesen und die Bedeutung der Leberveränderungen und der Pigmentierungen bei den damit verbundenen Fällen von Pseudosklerose, zugleich ein Beitrag zur Lehre von der Pseudosklerose (Westphal-Strümpell). *Dtsch. Z. Nervenheilkd. 49,* 54-73 (1913).
32. E. Siemerling and H. Oloff. Pseudosklerose (Westphal-Strümpell) mit Corneal-ring (Kayser-Fleischer) und doppelseitiger Scheinkatarakt, die nur bei seitlicher Beleuchtung sichtbar ist und die der nach Verletzung durch Kupfersplitter entstehenden Kataract ähnlich ist. *Klin. Wochenschr. 1,* 1087-1089 (1922).
33. A. J. Glazebrook. Wilson's disease. *Edinburgh Med. J. 52,* 83-87 (1945).
34. I. H. Scheinberg and D. Gitlin. Deficiency of ceruloplasmin in patients with hepatolenticular degeneration (Wilson's disease). *Science 116*, 484-485 (1952).
35. A. G. Bearn and H. G. Kunkel. Biochemical abnormalities in Wilson's disease. *J. Clin. Invest. 31,* 616 (1952).
36. A. G. Bearn. A genetical analysis of thirty families with Wilson's disease (hepatolenticular degeneration). *Am. J. Hum. Genet. 24,* 33-43 (1960).
37. I. Sternlieb, A. G. Morell, C. D. Bauer, B. Combes, S. de Bobes-Sternberg, and I. H. Scheinberg. Detection of the heterozygous carrier of the Wilson's disease gene. *J. Clin. Invest. 40,* 707-715 (1961).
38. A. Sass-Kortsak, B. S. Glatt, M. Cherniak, and I. Cederlund. Observations on copper metabolism in homozygotes and heterozygotes of Wilson's disease. In *Wilson's Disease: Some Current Concepts* (J. M. Walshe and N. J. Cumings, Eds.). Blackwell, Oxford, 1961, pp. 151-167.

39. J. N. Cumings. The copper and iron content of brain and liver in the normal and in hepato-lenticular degeneration. *Brain 71,* 410-415 (1948).
40. J. M. Walshe. Penicillamine, a new oral therapy for Wilson's disease. *Am. J. Med. 21,* 487-495 (1956).
41. J. M. Walshe. Wilson's disease: New oral therapy. *Lancet 1,* 25-26 (1956).
42. D. W. Cox. Factors influencing serum ceruloplasmin levels in normal individuals. *J. Lab. Clin. Med. 68,* 893-904 (1966).
43. J. M. Walshe. Copper chelation in patients with Wilson's disease. A comparison of penicillamine and triethylene tetramine dihydrochloride. *Q. J. Med. N.S. 42,* 441-452 (1973).

5 Reye's Syndrome: A Disease of Incompetent Mitochondria

PETER N. PERINCHIEF / Cornell University Medical College, New York, New York, and North Shore University Hospital, Manhasset, New York

I. Introduction

Fifteen years have elapsed since R. D. K. Reye first described the syndrome that now bears his name, although the disease may have been recognized by others at an earlier date. The article by Reye et al. [1] focused the attention of the scientific community on this enigmatic disease, and a large literature has subsequently accumulated. The primary event that initiates the onset and subsequent progression of the clinicopathologic features of the syndrome is not yet understood.

The aim of this chapter is to acquaint physicians with the modern concepts of the basic pathophysiology of cerebral edema, the function of the blood-brain barrier, and mitochondrial metabolism and bioenergetics within the context of Reye's syndrome. A unifying hypothesis of the pathophysiology is presented, and a discussion of the current therapy is included—together with arguments for routine use of intracranial pressure monitoring.

II. Clinical Manifestations

Reye's syndrome (RS) is not a rare disease, and the incidence may be increasing. In 1971 only acute infectious encephalitis outranked RS as the cause of death in children suffering from virally induced infectious diseases of the central nervous system (CNS) [2].

The disease frequently exhibits a biphasic nature. The initial complaint may begin with a nonspecific, innocuous prodrome that can last 5-7 days. A viral etiology is suggested, since there may be low-grade fever, upper respiratory tract

Table 1 Correlated Laboratory, Clinical, and Pathophysiologic Changes in the

Upper diencephalic (Stage I)	"Mid"-diencephalic (Stage II)	Lower diencephalic-upper midbrain (Stage III)
Behavioral changes, vomiting, lethargy, plantar extensor response. Drowsiness. Seizure activity is rare. EEG type 1; theta waves dominate; delta waves rare unless < 5 yr old. Slowing of rhythmicity.	Disorientation, combativeness, semicoma, increased deep tendon reflexes. Hyperventilation. Cheyne-Stokes respirations. Appropriate responses to noxious stimuli. EEG type 2; delta waves unless < 10 yr old. Dysrhythmic slowing.	Coma, hyperventilation. Decorticate posturing. Pupillary reflex and oculovestibular reflex still present. EEG type 2. Monitor respiratory patterns, ocular and motor signs to assess progression, unless patient is curarized and on ventilator. Intracranial pressure monitoring advisable.
Abnormal liver function. Hypoglycemia, hyperammonemia, abnormal coagulation profile. Nonhypoxic hyperlacticacidemia/hyperpyruvicacidemia. CSF glutamine elevation. Mitochondrial changes in liver biopsy. Acellular CSF. Elevated gluconeogenic amino acids. Elevated short- and medium-chain fatty acids.	Markedly abnormal liver function. Sympathetic nervous system overactivity: sweating, tachycardia, pupillary dilatation with sluggish reaction. Institute intracranial pressure monitoring at this time.	
EEG Type 1	EEG Type 2	EEG Type 2
Onset of cerebral edema (cytotoxic type). Intracranial capacitance spaces nearly collapsed. Pressure increase begins within cranium. Ammonia may disrupt cerebral metabolism.	Intracranial pressure increases (nonlinear)	Capillary perfusion pressure decreases. Cerebral ischemia.
	Decompensation phase of capacitance space. Initiation of steep ascent of pressure curve (Fig. 1).	

Staging based on Lovejoy.

Progression of Reye's Syndrome

Midbrain-upper pons (Stage IV)	Medullary (Stage V)
Coma deepens. Decerebrate posturing. Large fixed pupils. Loss of corneal and oculocephalic reflex (doll's head phenomenon). Oculovestibular reflex (caloric stimulation) produces dysconjugate eye movements. Absent ciliospinal reflex. EEG type 3; disorganized monorhythmic or polyrhythmic delta waves; low voltage with burst suppression. Brief isoelectric intervals	Seizures–loss of deep tendon reflexes. Respiratory arrest. Flaccidity. EEG type 4. Isoelectric EEG (denotes energy failure in the brain). Normal hepatic function.

EEG Type 3	EEG Type 4
Intracranial pressure exceeds perfusion pressure. "A"-type pressure waves–acceleration of ischemic/ Loss of cerebral autoregulation.	Vasogenic cerebral edema develops? (Necrosis and permanent damage.) Brain death

involvement (cough and coryza), gastrointestinal symptoms (abdominal cramping, diarrhea), and occasionally an exanthem. Subtle behavioral changes are observed [3], often retrospectively, with decreased verbal spontaneity, difficulty with routine daily activities such as dressing, and momentary confusion. Following the prodrome the patient appears to recover [4], but subsequently becomes irritable and lethargic and begins to vomit [5]. The latter is a cardinal sign and a warning of progressing pathology. In infants, apnea and seizures are prominent findings [6].

The presence of an influenza A or B or varicella outbreak within the community [7, 8] should raise the index of suspicion. The victims tend to be older Caucasian children in northern rural areas [8, 9], with younger non-Caucasians predominating in the cities [6]. This may reflect demography rather than susceptibility [2]. The sex ratio is close to unity in the two environments [2, 6, 10]. After the prodrome the clinical progression is variable. Occasional emesis may be the only sign. Dehydration with mixed acid-base abnormalities [11] without neurological progression may also obtain. Other victims show variable neurological deterioration (Table 1). A rapid progression is usually associated with a poor prognosis [12]. The disease formerly had a mortality rate of 80-100%, but aggressive therapy has now reduced this to 25-30% in some centers [8, 9]. The diagnosis of milder cases and an earlier institution of therapy may have also contributed to this statistical decline.

Several reports [13-15] have described and quantified the clinical evolution of Reye's syndrome. The clinical staging of Lovejoy et al. [15] is based on Plum and Posner's [16] classification of progressing cerebral dysfunction. Lovejoy divided the neurological status of patients into five stages (I-V) and correlated these with four electroencephalographic (EEG) subcategories (1-4) [17]. The Lovejoy staging is useful, as it provides a standard by which to gauge clinical responses to therapy. The chief problem with this system is the tacit assumption that there is a tight temporal coupling between intracranial events, clinical signs, and chemical parameters. However, experimental [18] and clinical studies [19-21] now indicate that a temporal dissociation can occur between clinical and chemical variables and intracranial pressures—particularly when the latter are in a state of rapid change.

The Lovejoy staging represents the presentation of a progressing but potentially reversible rostral-caudal dysfunction of the brain. Each stage delineates a serial, functional transection of the brain, and the process may culminate in transtentorial diencephalic herniation or cerebellar herniation through the foramen magnum [19, 22, 23]. This devastating progression is driven by an accumulating cerebral edema [19] of cytotoxic origin [24] within an inelastic skull (Section VII.B and Table 1). Since the entire brain is involved [1, 25], lateralizing signs of focal injury or space-occupying lesions are unusual [19, 26], although residual sequelae may be both lateralized and generalized

(Section IX) [12, 20, 26-29]. Table 1 incorporates a modified tabulation of the clinical, electroencephalographic, pathophysiologic, and laboratory correlates of cerebral edema in RS.

III. Differential Diagnosis

There are a number of other conditions besides viral encephalitis that can mimic RS. These include viral hepatitis with encephalopathy, toxin ingestion, inborn errors of metabolism, hypovolemic or endotoxic shock, anoxia, hyperthermia, and purulent meningitis.

The child suspected of having RS should be screened for the presence of barbiturates, amphetamines, hallucinogens, phenothiazines, salicylates [7], and acetaminophen. A careful history may assist in determining whether there has been exposure to toxins that can mimic RS biochemically, histologically, and clinically. These include methyl bromide [30], aflatoxin [7, 31], ingested vegetable matter containing hypoglycin A or related compounds [1, 32], pyrrolizidine alkaloids [33], chlordane [34], disulfiram [35], carbon tetrachloride [1], organophosphates, oleandomycin, and heavy metals

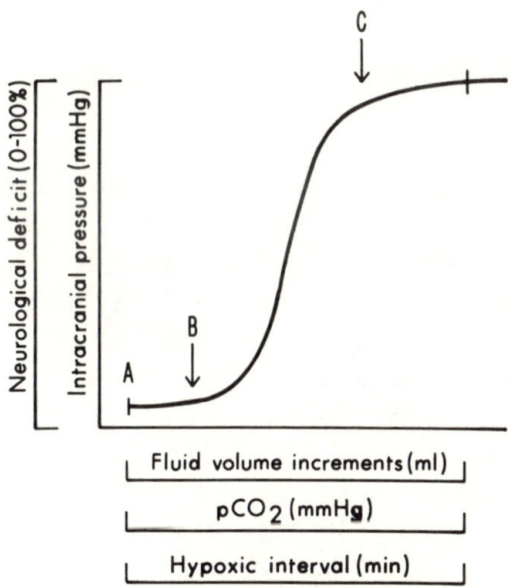

Figure 1 Sigmoid relation exists between intracranial edema pressure (ordinate) and further increments of intracranial fluid (abscissa), derived either exogenously (indwelling subarachnoid or ventricular catheters) or endogenously due to uptake from capillary lumen. Similar relation obtains with arterial pCO_2 in presence of an already elevated intracranial pressure. Permanent neurologic deficits also accumulate rapidly after a critical hypoxic interval. In presence of edema, intracranial pressure does not initially rise (A-B), owing to rapid shifts of fluid out of capacitance compartments within the skull. Subsequently, with small additions of edema fluid (B-C) there is an accelerating rise in pressure until the brain begins to shift downward through the tentorial notch and foramen magnum (C). Plateau ("A") waves appear between points B and C. For further details see text.

[34]. A history of travel to tropical or desert areas respectively is important when hypoglycin or pyrrolizidine ingestion is suspected. The latter is also found in herbal teas. In rare cases the patient may be suffering a second attack of RS [23, 25], and the possibility of rare inborn errors of metabolism (branched-chain amino acids or urea-cycle enzyme defects) must be rule out [35, 36].

The diagnostic lumbar puncture (LP) poses a problem [37]. A child in state I or II may have already entered a phase of rapidly increasing intracranial pressure (ICP) (Table 1 and Fig. 1) and may already be exhibiting a dissociation between the ICP and the clinical signs of progressing cranial hypertension. The patient is therefore at risk of brain herniation when spinal fluid is withdrawn. Examination of the fundi for papilledema can be falsely reassuring, especially when the ICP is rising rapidly. It has been suggested [37] than an LP should be done since the information gained outweighs the definite risk of herniation. Only one LP—to rule out meningitis—should be performed on admission if there are no obvious signs of pressure elevation, such as papilledema, retinal venous engorgement, or deep coma.

IV. Laboratory Data

Establishment of the diagnosis requires laboratory studies that are directed at determining the hepatic and metabolic status of the patient.

Serum electrolytes, urea nitrogen, glucose, ammonia, clotting parameters, and liver enzymes should be measured immediately. In addition, a complete blood count, blood cultures, and acute viral titers (to be followed by convalescent serum at a later date) are required.

The presence of an elevated ammonia level, hypoglycemia, variably elevated values for liver transaminases, and a minimally elevated bilirubin level is commonly found [1], but individually normal values may also been seen. A deficiency of all clotting factors, with the exception of factor VIII has been reported [29]. A liver biopsy will confirm the diagnosis (Section V), but the coagulation profile should be within acceptable limits [29] before a biopsy is performed. There is evidence to suggest that a confirmatory liver biopsy is unnecessary, as it makes no significant difference to the outcome of the disease process once the diagnosis has already been made on the basis of clinical evaluation and laboratory data [6, 38]. In isolated cases the indication for obtaining a biopsy will understandably increase.

V. Histology

The histological changes that characterize the disease have been described in detail elsewhere [7, 22].

The clinical evolution of RS can be rapid, and the histologic changes in the liver must also be viewed as dynamic, time-dependent, and potentially rapidly reversible, particularly after therapy has been started [39].

In tissues that have undergone in vivo biopsy (liver, renal cortex tubular epithelium, and cerebral cortex) [25], three consistent features tend to characterize the syndrome. These are (1) microvesicular fat deposition within cells (with the unique exception of the cerebral parenchyma), (2) absence of inflammation, and (3) marked mitochondrial ultrastructure changes.

Lipid droplets have also been observed in pulmonary histiocytes, skeletal muscle myofibrils pancreatic acinar cells, histiocytic cells of the spleen, and lymph nodes. The myocardium (especially the atria), Purkinje's fibers, cerebellum, and the brain capillary endothelium also display similar fat infiltrates. Hepatic microvesicular fat accumulation alone is insufficient to make a histologic diagnosis since a number of conditions enumerated in Section III may produce the same histopathology. In addition, the tissues listed above are often postmortem specimens, and the fatty changes may not necessarily reflect a unique pathology.

The conspicuous absence of fat infiltration in the cerebral parenchyma is likely the reflection of a fundamentally different metabolic compensation within neurons and glial tissue as compared to other tissues. Conversely, capillary endothelial cells do show fat droplets [1, 9], and if this reflects a metabolic decompensation of the endothelium it may have profound implications in the development of cerebral edema–since the cerebral capillary endothelium provides the structural and functional components of the blood-brain barrier (Section VII.A).

The absence of inflammation is a puzzling phenomenon, particularly when circumstantial evidence suggests an infective process is responsible for the onset of the disease (Section VI, VI.B). Whether inflammatory changes occur and then resolve before the clinical signs appear is not known. It is possible that lack of inflammation may represent an impaired host defense.

Early in the course of the disease the hepatic mitochondria progressively swell and achieve an ameboid form [40]. Loss of structural integrity (inner mitochondrial matrix disruption and loss of density), loss of the matrix dense bodies, and loss or fragmentation of the cristae are commonly observed [7, 40, 41]. These changes often correlate with the severity and outcome of the illness [42]. The mitochondria may appear normal if the biopsy is not performed at the right time.

Mitochondrial changes are generally believed to be rapidly reversible–especially after therapy is begun–but there may be a terminal stage when irreversible damage develops. This is manifested by matrix space expansion, rupture of the outer mitochondrial membrane, complete absence of cytosolic glycogen, nuclear swelling, and dissociation of the ribosomes from the rough endoplasmic reticulum. In such cases, mitochondrial pathology has not reversed even when the patient has been kept alive for 3-4 days. Conversely, fatal cases have also been reported where the mitochondria have reverted to a normal shape, peroxisomes have decreased (see below), and the Golgi apparatus and rough endoplasmic reticulum appear to be functioning normally [39]. Mitochondrial autophagia has not been observed either during the acute illness or 3 months later [40].

Changes within the brain mitochondria at autopsy and upon *in vivo* biopsy, although not invariably present, are similar to those found in the liver. Neuronal myelin sheaths develop blebs, and swelling of astrocytic cell bodies and foot processes is commonly found. Complex inclusion bodies within neurons and vascular pericytes have been reported—whether they are a pathognomonic sign is doubtful. The choroid plexus mitochondria [43] also display swelling and disruption. Within the central nervous system, myelin bleb formation, absence of inflammation, astrocyte swelling, and mitochondrial disruption in the presence of an intact microvasculature may be pathognomonic for RS and other cytotoxic insults. Endothelial fat accumulation may represent either evidence for, or a potential cause of, endothelial mitochondrial dysfunction.

In the hepatocyte, peroxisomes are increased in number and size [39, 40]. The role of peroxisome proliferation in Reye's syndrome is unclear. The metabolic role of peroxisomes in higher animals is also enigmatic, but it is suspected to be, in part, protective—by degrading hydrogen peroxide and thus shielding the cell from the harmful oxidizing effects of hydrogen peroxide and ultimately superoxide radicals [7]. Whether peroxisome proliferation is real or only apparent is not clear. The normal hepatocyte peroxisome–mitochondrion ratio is 1:4 [44]. A loss of mitochondria by attrition (Section VI.B) would produce a relative increase of peroxisomes. They may be nonfunctional in RS [42] and therefore incapable of degrading cytosol-generated hydrogen peroxide, which could then functionally damage the mitochondria through oxidation of membrane lipids. Peroxisomes may play a central role in lipid metabolism [44], and the possibility that peroxisomes degrade fat is an intriguing concept within the context of RS—particularly in view of the fact that some hypolipemic drugs induce peroxisome proliferation [44]. Disrupted mitochondrial fat oxidation, with accumulation of intracellular fat may act as a trigger to peroxisomal proliferation. Salicylates [42] have also been implicated in peroxisome proliferation. Since children in the early stages of Reye's syndrome may have been treated with salicylates, this drug may frequently be present as an additional stimulus to proliferation.

VI. Pathophysiology

The fundamental question that has yet to be answered is how the disease process is initiated. Histologic and enzymatic [45-48] analysis of the liver suggests that hepatic mitochondria are the site of primary cellular dysfunction. The hepatocytic fatty infiltration and early hyperammonemia and hypoglycemia of RS support this view, as do the elevated levels of lactate, pyruvate, and glucogenic amino acids in the serum. Defective gluconeogenesis and ureagenesis likely play a pivotal role in the disease's progression. The hepatic mitochondria play a central role in the rate control of glucose and urea formation, and an inhibition of these pathways may influence mitochondrial function elsewhere in the body.

The theory that an environmental toxin (e.g., aflatoxin) initiates the disease is questionable [49], although in experimental animals viral agents and organic toxins may act synergistically to produce a Reye's-like syndrome [50].

Most evidence, albeit circumstantial, indicates that a viral infection is responsible. Influenza A and B and varicella viruses display the most consistent temporal and epidemiologic association with onset of the syndrome, but a direct cause-effect relation has not been demonstrated. Other viral agents such as echoviruses, adenoviruses, and parainfluenza viruses have also been implicated [2]. The reports of viral particles in biopsy material adds support to an infectious etiology, but these may be artifacts or merely coincidence. Koch's postulates have yet to be fulfilled.

Whether victims have a predisposition to develop the disease after a viral infection is moot, although recurrence of the syndrome with subsequent viral infections would support this contention. Studies of host defenses have not been forthcoming; HLA typing of victims would be of considerable interest, as some viruses apparently bind to cell surface HLA antigens prior to cellular invasion [51].

A. Mitochondrial Bioenergetics

The chemosmotic hypothesis [52] provides the conceptual framework on which to build a logical explanation of the development and progression of the pathophysiology of RS.

Mitochondria behave simultaneously as electrical generators, transducers, and capacitors. The electron transport chain (ETC) acts as a proton pump and drives the transport of matrix-compartment hydrogen ions outward across the inner mitochondrial membrane (IMM)—leaving hydroxyl ions within the matrix—thus generating an electrochemical potential of protons. The IMM, in which the ETC is embedded, acts as a capacitor and a transducing machine. The electrochemical energy is converted (transduced) directly into covalent bond synthesis (ATP formation) and, indirectly, drives the transport of key anionic and cationic substrates [53-56] of intermediary metabolism, via stereospecific carrier proteins that are themselves embedded in the IMM. Mitochondria also behave as osmometers in that they have a propensity to take up water and therefore swell. Continual removal of water from the mitochondrial matrix is indirectly coupled, via sodium transport, to the proton gradient. *Uncontrolled* swelling is therefore prevented.

In order for the IMM to function efficiently, it must exist as a topologically closed system; otherwise the proton gradient will collapse. Stated somewhat differently: if the IMM is nonspecifically "leaky" to protons–for any reason –the proton potential will be short-circuited; the transducing and translocation functions will "run down." It follows that the histologic appearance of incompetent mitochondria would be that of swelling and disorganization.

B. Origin of Hepatic Mitochondrial Dysfunction (Hypothesis)

The cause of hepatocyte mitochondrial swelling (Section V) and the reduction of mitochondria-associated enzyme systems [45-48] is not known. The disruption of hepatic function may reflect a decrease in absolute numbers of hepatocyte mitochondria, but this possibility does not seem to have been raised. Abnormal mitochondria-peroxisome ratios may reflect such an event (Section V). Alternatively, the formation of a critical mass of mitochondria that were structurally abnormal on a molecular level, and therefore functionally incompetent, would have the same consequences as a decline in absolute numbers.

Within a susceptible host, RS may represent the consequences of a direct or indirect attack by certain viruses on hepatic mitochondria. As mitochondria arise from preexisting mitochondria, the following postulated influences may account for mitochondrial dysfunction.

1. Following viral infection cytoplasmic protein synthesis is inhibited (shutoff phenomenon) [57]. A number of structural proteins of the IMM that are programmed by the nuclear genome and are synthesized in the cytoplasm may also be subject to the shutoff phenomenon.

2. Interferon can inhibit intramitochondrial protein synthesis directed by the mitochondrial genome. These proteins are incorporated in the IMM and also influence the incorporation of the cytosol-derived IMM proteins [58]. The mitochondrial replication process may therefore be affected as an "innocent bystander." The nucleic acid RNA is a particularly effective inducer of interferon. The RNA-containing myxoviruses, of which influenza A and B are members, may exhibit such properties.

3. Viruses may directly alter mitochondrial membrane function. They have been shown to rapidly alter membrane systems [59] that display a number of the characteristics of mitochondria [60].

4. Mitochondria may be involved in the process of viral replication [61] and thus be subject to disruption of their normal synthetic processes.

5. The half-life of hepatic mitochondria (5-7 days) is suspiciously close to the temporal lag between the prodrome and the onset of hepatic failure with concomitant neurologic deterioration. If normal hepatic mitochondrial biogenesis or assembly is inhibited in RS as suggested above, then the collapse of hepatic urea and glucose synthesis should be a function of the half-life

phenomenon. Recovery of hepatic mitochondrial function would also reflect half-life kinetics.

6. The above postulates do not preclude a viral influence on nonhepatic mitochondrial biogenesis.

7. The acquisition of a population of mitochondria that are structurally defective on a molecular level, with respect to the assembly of the IMM, has several predictable metabolic consequences.

a. The mitochondrial IMM could not generate and maintain an adequate electrochemical potential.

b. The synthesis of ATP should therefore become inefficient [62]. Urea and glucose synthesis will decline.

c. Transport of ornithine into the matrix space [56] will decline, and urea synthesis will therefore display a substantial rate decrease [5].

d. Inefficient translocation of gluconeogenic precursors from the mitochondria to the cytosol (and vice versa) will occur [53-55].

e. The alkaline matrix pH [52] will drift toward neutrality. This event may promote the dissociation of at least one of the key urea-cycle enzymes—ornithine transcarbamylase. This enzyme is of particular interest because it exists as a trimer and appears to operate optimally at the alkaline pH generated within the matrix. The trimer tends to dissociate with pH shifts, and its interaction with carbamyl phosphate synthetase may also be alkaline pH-dependent. This phenomenon would be reflected mainly as a decline in the amount of functional enzyme rather than by the presence of structural variants with altered substrate affinities.

f. Mitochondria will display various degrees of swelling. This event may then enhance postulates (a-e) as the IMM is further distorted topologically. A positive-feedback system would be generated.

g. Only hepatic mitochondrial enzymes should be affected. Enzymes associated with the matrix space and the IMM have been shown to be less active in RS, whereas cytosolic enzymes are normal, and this finding appears to be *restricted* to the liver [45]. The available data on ornithine transcarbamylase, carbamyl phosphate synthetase, cytochrome oxidase, the terminal electron transport chain, succinic dehydrogenase, pyruvate dehydrogenase and carboxylase, citrate synthetase, and glutamic dehydrogenase—all mitochondrial enzymes—indicate that there is a deficiency of these enzymes rather than the presence of structural variants [34, 45-48, 63]. These deficiencies apparently disappear after recovery [47]. The mitochondrial enzyme that synthesizes acetyl glutamate [64] has not been measured. Acetyl glutamate is necessary for organic trapping of ammonia by mitochondrial carbamyl phosphate synthetase.

The consequence of the hepatic mitochondrial abnormalities outlined above would be hypoglycemia, hyperammonemia, inhibition of fat oxidation with fatty acidemia, and a compensatory increase of anaerobic glycolysis. These abnormalities have been documented in RS. Hepatic-derived ammonia and short- and medium-chain fatty acids are theoretically able to collapse the mitochondrial proton gradients in other organ systems, and salicylate has similar capabilities. These three classes of compounds behave as proton ionophores (acidic uncouplers) in that they can ferry protons across the IMM—in effect they short-circuit the IMM.

A fourth agent has been isolated from the serum of RS patients. Its origin and identity are not known, but it apparently blocks the terminal ETC and can cause mitochondrial swelling in vitro [63, 65].

The available evidence indicates that the liver is indeed the primary site of metabolic disruption, and that the production of hepatic-derived mitochondrial toxins then leads to the major complications of the disease.

Whether the mitochondria of other organs besides the liver are simultaneously and similarly affected is not clear. The kidney and brain undergo similar morphological changes (Section V), and they also depend upon intact mitochondrial function. The apparent primary liver involvement may reflect different rates of turnover of the respective mitochondrial population in each organ system. Conceivably a short mitochondrial half-life within an organ (liver) might make it more susceptible to a viral inhibition of mitochondrial biogenesis.

VII. Brain Edema

A. The Blood-Brain Barrier

The main body of the blood-brain barrier (BBB) consists of the capillary endothelium and its basement membrane. There are compelling reasons to consider that one of the chief functions of the BBB is the active removal of water from the brain parenchyma and interstitium. The available information listed below suggests that the BBB acts like a transporting epithelium.

1. The endothelium is ultrastructurally and enzymatically similar to epithelia (gut and kidney) specialized for transport of organic and inorganic ions and water. These epithelia and the cerebral endothelium are sealed by tight junctions and have high levels of γ-glutamyl transpeptidase. This enzyme has not been demonstrated in the capillary endothelium of other organs. Abundant mitochondria are also found in the above epithelia, but the cerebral endothelium is unique as it contains three to five times the number of mitochondria found in noncerebral endothelial cells.

2. Cerebral endothelium demonstrates an "A"-type, sodium gradient-coupled, concentrative transport of small, neutral amino acids. This system appears to be outwardly polarized (vectorial) across the endothelium from the parencymal side into the capillary lumen (Fig. 2) [66].

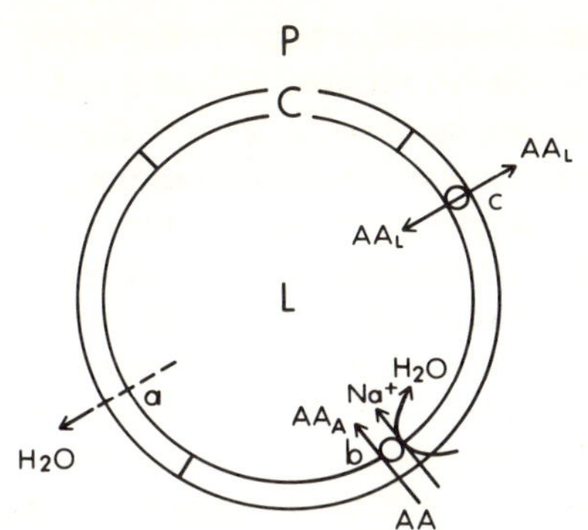

Figure 2 Illustration of essential components of the capillary endothelium as a transporting "epithelium." Skull encloses brain parenchyma (P). Endothelium (C) forms structurally tight monolayer enclosing capillary lumen (L). Continual, passive movement of water across endothelium (a) is balanced by sodium-coupled covectorial transport in opposite direction (b). Sodium gradient is maintained by vectorial, lumen-directed sodium pump, $(Na^+\text{-}K^+)$-ATPase, probably mounted on juxtaluminal membrane (b). Cotranslocation of sodium and amino acids occurs on juxtaparenchymal membrane, but for simplicity it is shown here as part of the ATPase complex. Functional coupling between ATPase and amino acid transport is therefore mediated by sodium-ion gradient. The L-system translocase (AA_L) is shown at (c), and bidirectional arrows indicate nonconcentrative, equilibrative transport. See text for details. (Section VII.A,B).

3. In most biological systems the generation of a sodium gradient across an epithelium automatically couples a co-vectorial movement of water. This coupling probably occurs across the cerebral endothelium–water will flow from the brain into the capillary lumen.

4. Rapid back-flux of water and ions into the parenchyma is probably prevented by the continuous, tight junctional complex [67] which welds consecutive endothelial cells together to form an integrated "epithelial" monolayer.

5. Vectorial, sodium-dependent transport systems require the presence of an electrochemical gradient of sodium ions, and in the BBB this is probably generated by a juxtaluminal membrane sodium-potassium ATPase ($Na^+\text{-}K^+$ ATPase) (Fig. 2).

6. The energy source (ATP) of the $Na^+\text{-}K^+$ ATPase is likely provided by the uniquely abundant endothelial mitochondria (Section VI.A).

7. It follows that toxic inhibition of mitochondrial ATP synthesis (Section VI.B) will uncouple water and amino acid transport out of the cerebral parenchyma and thus generate a cytotoxic edema.

8. The inhibition of the active removal of small, neutral amino acids that are putative neurotransmitters [68] may also have a profound effect on cerebral neural activity in RS.

9. In addition to concentrative transport, the BBB contains stereospecific, saturable translocase systems that mediate a nonconcentrative, bidirectional transport of glucose as well as acidic, neutral, and basic amino acids (L-system translocases, Fig. 2). The glucose transport system has an apparent K_m of 6-9 mM [69], which is "poised" near physiologic serum levels. Under normal conditions, transport of sugar is not a rate-limiting step [69]. However, when neuronal anaerobic glucose metabolism develops in (a) postictal states, (b) hyperammonemia, or (c) cerebral ischemia (secondary to cerebral edema), the endothelial transport system is probably unable to translocate glucose at a rate fast enough to supply the parenchyma; transport therefore becomes rate limiting. Hypoglycemia will understandably add to the problem. The maintenance of serum glucose and the prevention of cerebral ischemia-anoxia are therefore essential in RS (Section VIII).

B. Cerebral Edema in Reye's Syndrome

The brain can become edematous in the presence of agents that are toxic to cellular metabolic reactions but do not distort the structural integrity of the capillary endothelium (cytotoxic edema) [24]. The parenchyma of the brain therefore appears to function as an osmometer in that it is always tending to take up free water from the vascular system.

The maintenance of normal intracranial pressures probably demands the presence of a transendothelial equilibrium between the passive, inward flux of water and its active transport in the opposite direction (Section VII.A). The endothelium may therefore act to keep the brain "dry," thus providing the principal defense of the CNS parenchyma against water overload. The neuronal and glial tissue may be ill-equipped to maintain their entire osmotic homeostasis if unaided by a "first-line defense." Unfortunately there has been insufficient research into this aspect of cerebral edema.

In RS there are at least four different classes of compounds that can interfere with cerebral parenchymal and endothelial mitochondrial function (Section VI.B). In the brain and its capillaries the ultimate effect of all agents may be similar—the inhibition of ATP synthesis and an obligatory shift of cell metabolism to inefficient cytosolic anaerobic glycolysis. Thus in RS, the cytotoxic edema could arise solely from the inability of the BBB to maintain an equilibrium between the opposing vectors of transendothelial water flux and active transport (Fig. 2) because of inefficient synthesis of ATP. This does not preclude a similarly derived loss of osmotic control within parenchymal cells. Ammonia has long been suspect as an agent toxic to cerebral function [70], and recent experiments [71] show a close temporal relationship between serum ammonia levels and intracranial edema.

All the available evidence indicates that the initial cerebral edema in RS is of the cytotoxic type [1, 7, 13, 22]. There is frequently no evidence of vascular injury or inflammation, and even in advanced stages the BBB has remained structurally intact [13].

In some victims of RS who had deep coma and high intracranial pressure (ICP), the surprising lack of residual brain damage in the form of focal neurological defects indicates a lack of permanent damage to the structural integrity of the brain parenchyma and capillary endothelium. When permanent neurological sequelae are found in survivors [19, 20, 26-28], the children have usually advanced beyond clinical stage III coma in the course of their illness [15, 28]. In these cases permanent complications may reflect a vasogenic edema superimposed on cytotoxic edema.

C. Intracranial Pressure and Brain Perfusion

Increases in intracranial parenchymal volume either from cytotoxic or vasogenic mechanisms are not initially accompanied by sustained elevations of intracranial pressure. This is due to rapid shifts of fluid out of the cerebrospinal fluid (CSF) and cranial vascular compartments (particularly the venous sinuses). These compartments function as a capacitance system and thus compensate for cellular swelling.

Once these mechanisms are exhausted, the ICP elevates in an exponential (sigmoid-shaped) fashion in response to small increments of intracranial edema fluid, blood, or exogenous fluid delivered to the subarachnoid space (Fig. 1).

In the presence of rising ICP the cranial contents will begin to shift along paths of least resistance–specifically through the tentorium and then the foramen magnum. In this way the edema drives the clinical manifestations of rostral-caudal dysfunction [15, 16] of Reye's syndrome (Table 1).

Once the ICP begins to rise, the cerebral blood flow encounters increasing resistance. As only a fraction of the aortic pressure may be transmitted to the capillary bed, a mild increase in ICP can markedly diminish the capillary blood flow. Ischemic anoxia can then develop with loss of vasomotor tone (autoregulation) in precapillary sphincters. Reflexive hypertension (Cushing's reflex) or loss of autoregulation permits the influx of space-occupying blood into the cranial vault. In the presence of exhausted capacitance spaces a precipitous rise in ICP will occur. These are termed "A" or plateau waves, and they can halt the flow of blood within the brain.

It is not clear how long the brain can withstand complete circulatory arrest without suffering permanent damage. In humans, it is suggested to be 4-5 min, although in other animals it may be 14-15 min. A sigmoidal relationship exists between the production of neurologic defects and the duration of global ischemia. A nearly vertical rise in permanent damage is observed in primates after 14-15 min of global ischemia, reaching almost total neurologic deficit by 18-19 min (Fig. 1) [72]. A waves may last this length of time. If the capillary sphincters are still responsive to hypocarbia (Fig. 1), acute hyperventilation and osmotic diuresis may terminate a plateau wave. Such A waves occur in RS, and they should be viewed as a major medical emergency.

VIII. Treatment

All children with RS should be transferred to a tertiary care hospital and admitted to the intensive care unit. The patient should be clinically staged [15] by an experienced group of physicians interested in the disease. It is advisable that a team leader be appointed, and that this physician should "orchestrate" the entire treatment program until the child is out of danger.

A universally acceptable therapy has not yet been determined. It is clear, however, that intracranial hypertension is responsible for the morbidity and mortality. An adequate cerebral perfusion must be maintained in order to prevent permanent brain damage or death, and ultimately all therapy is directed at achieving this goal through cerebral decompression. Early, aggressive intervention appears to reduce mortality and lessen the permanent neurologic complications of the disease.

Direct monitoring of pressure changes within the skull by intracranial pressure monitoring (ICPM) shows considerable promise in that this technique provides an instanteous assessment of intracranial status and eliminates clinical temporal lags. Studies using ICPM in RS have already confirmed the suspicion that marked pressure changes in either direction can occur without any obvious change in the patient's status. Acute elevations of pressure can be precipitated by seemingly innocuous nursing procedures [20]. More importantly, ICPM promises to resolve a number of therapeutic dilemmas [19, 27, 73]–once carefully controlled studies are instituted.

Stage I patients who are stable should be closely monitored for neurologic or chemical deterioration. The latter parameters may herald an approaching crisis before clinical changes become apparent. The treatment of stage I is essentially a matter of fluid restriction, maintenance of serum glucose, and regular administration of vitamin K, neomycin (via nasogastric tube or enema), and steroids. Frequent assessment of blood sugar, liver enzymes, clotting factors, and serum ammonia is advisable.

An intracranial pressure monitor should be placed as soon as possible in all patients who have advanced to stage II and beyond [74]. Curarization, intubation, and assisted ventilation are also advocated when ICPM is utilized. Mechanical ventilation allows rapid changes in arterial pCO_2 to be made in an attempt to reduce acute pressure elevations. Curarization and barbiturate or diazepam administration inhibit muscular and cerebral seizure activity respectively. Such seizures may aggravate intracranial hypertension to a degree sufficient to reduce the brain perfusion pressure to zero [20] and can also shift brain metabolism to anaerobic glycolysis. The consequences of this are outlined in Section VII.

Concomitant monitoring by an electrocephalogram provides an assessment of cerebral electrical activity. Branchial or radial artery cannulation provides easy access to arterial blood in order to assess arterial pressure, acid-base balance, oxygenation, and other laboratory parameters. Pulmonary artery wedge pressure is also utilized in some studies [74].

Intracranial pressures may be measured by epidural or subarachnoid monitors [75, 76] or by ventricular catheters [20, 73, 75]. The latter involve the risk of infection or the development of porencephalic tracts and cysts. The epidural monitor is preferable, as it is easy to insert and maintain and does not violate the brain tissue.

Intracranial pressure should be maintained below 10-15 mmHg [73]. Any elevation above 15 mmHg or acute A wave formation requires the immediate induction of hypocarbia or mannitol diuresis.

Mannitol and hypocarbia alone may be sufficient to terminate a gradual rise in cerebral hypertension or to abort A wave formation if the former fails. Continual elevation of the patient's head may act to reduce intracranial hydrostatic pressure by promoting venous drainage.

Prior to the use of ICPM, osmotic diuretics were administered regularly every 4-6 hr or in response to clinical deterioration. The epidural monitor now permits the administration of these agents when specifically required and, in addition, allows the monitoring of potential rebound phenomena after diuretic administration.

Should these agents fail, the intravenous administration of glycerol may be of benefit [20]. Glycerol gavage does not appear to be effective [19] and may cause gastric irritation. The effectiveness of glycerol may depend upon an intact blood-brain barrier and upon the properties of glycerol as a metabolizable substrate in the cerebral capillary endothelium. It should, however, be used with caution. Individual and combined use of barbiturates and hypothermia may also be of benefit in maintaining cerebral decompression or reducing anoxic damage [27, 75]. As a last resort, some centers resort to craniectomy.

In cases reported [77] one cause of equivocal and adverse effects of exchange methods may have been a discrepancy between the exchange fluid osmolality (fresh blood or Dianeal in exchange or peritoneal dialysis respectively) and that of the patient's serum. Cerebral capacitances are likely to have been exhausted in a number of patients who had reached the point of requiring exchange, and the pressure response of the brain to small increments of intracranial fluid would have reached the steep ascending portion of the pressure-volume curve (Fig. 1).

The introduction of an exchange blood that is hypotonic relative to the patient's serum (especially if the patient has already been deliberately dehydrated) will be tantamount to the administration of a bolus of free water.

Conversely, Dianeal is markedly hyperosmolar and has the potential to cause hypernatremia and hyperosmolarity, with potentially disastrous consequences to the brain. Controlled studies utilizing ICPM will now be absolutely necessary in order to determine the real benefits of exchange transfusion.

During exchange transfusion it may be expedient to match the osmolalities of the patient's serum and the exchange blood. Alternatively the pretransfusion and posttransfusion serum osmolalities should be compared, and osmotic diuresis instituted immediately if there has been a reduction of osmolality. The use of ICPM may help to dispel any confusion surrounding the problem of a serum osmolality shift in the wrong direction and its effect on cerebral edema.

There is little evidence to warrant the administration of steroids in an effort to control the cerebral edema of RS. The precedent was set by Reye and his co-workers [1], and it has now become a part of the routine supportive care in the management of the disease. Steroids have been shown to be of benefit in cerebral edema of vasogenic origin (trauma, tumor, inflammation, and prolonged exposure of the brain to air), but they seem to have no effect on cytotoxic-type cerebral edema once it is established [26]. Documentation of their beneficial effects is lacking [75]. Steroids may complicate therapy by causing stress ulceration and gastrointestinal bleeding.

The administration of urea-cycle intermediates (citrulline) in an attempt to circumvent the mitochondrial dysfunction is probably futile. Ammonia trapping is mainly an intramitochondrial event [64] and requires the potentially rate-limiting active transport of ornithine into the organelle. Citrulline is not likely to influence ureagenesis in the presence of mitochondrial dysfunction. Carefully controlled experiments will be required to assess the efficacy of citrulline and steroids.

General supportive measures for all stages of the disease include restriction of fluids, administration of vitamin K, and maintenance of the serum glucose level in order to supply the brain (and other tissues) with sufficient nutrient (Section VII.A). The concomitant infusion of insulin promotes peripheral glucose utilization and inhibits lipolysis [78]. It should be noted that Vitamin K may be useless in the presence of hepatic failure.

Some centers routinely decompress the upper gastrointestinal tract. Cleansing enemas and neomycin have been used in an attempt to reduce ammonia production by gut flora. Enemas may provoke an elevation of ICP, owing to absorption of water by the colonic mucosa.

IX. Complications

There are a number of complications that may occur during therapy. They may arise from the disease process itself or as a result of treatment. Radial nerve palsy may follow arterial cannulation [26]. Paralysis of the vocal cords and subglottic stenosis [12], as well as pneumonia, may develop as a result of prolonged intubation. Hypophosphatemia and hypokalemia may occur when glucose metabolism is enhanced by insulin infusion. Cranial hypertension may cause pituitary infarction or inappropriate antidiuretic hormone secretion which could worsen the cerebral edema. Acute tubular necrosis, renal failure, gastrointestinal bleeding, clotting factor deficits, disseminated intravascular coagulation [29], mixed metabolic and respiratory alkalosis, chronic respiratory failure, and simple metabolic acidosis or respiratory alkalosis have also been reported.

Following recovery from the cerebral edema of RS, the observed complications involve damage sustained by the brain as a result of hypoxic-ischemic insult. There may be focal defects or more global involvement. A number of documented clinical sequelae of RS can be explained on the basis that the occipital and calcarine cortices and the basal ganglia are more susceptible to anoxic damage than either the frontal or temporal cortices [72]. Temporary defects include third-nerve palsy with diplopia, memory deficits, hemiparesis, hemiballismus, and akinetic mutism. Persisting complications have included marked deficits of intelligence, cranial-nerve palsies, cortical blindness, seizure disorders, spastic quadriplegia, global psychomotor retardation, marked personality changes, emotional lability, and extrapyramidal damage.

Earlier reports did not measure subtle changes that reflect mild neocortical damage. It is now evident that significant neuropsychologic sequelae-hitherto ignored–are present in children who have sustained marked elevations of intracranial pressure [28]. These deficits may go unnoticed unless a specific battery of tests is used. These include the preschool language test, social maturity scale testing, tests of receptive function, and the Denver Developmental Screening Test (DDST).

The tests show that recovered victims of RS may have deficits of intelligence, loss of short-term memory, abnormal visual-motor integration, decreased vocabulary, and impairments in speech articulation and grammatical usage. Age is a factor in the development of "soft" neurologic deficits; younger children are more severely affected. The degree of recovery does not correlate with parental education, socioeconomic status, or residential setting. Older children may derive some benefit from physical and language therapy. The effect of ICPM in the prevention of soft neurologic deficits will be of particular interest.

X. Summary

Reye's syndrome appears to be caused by a reversible dysfunction of mitochondria in at least three essential organ systems–the liver, brain, and kidneys. A viral infection or toxic agent may initiate the process. Since the liver malfunction produces such dramatic biochemical and physiologic changes, studies on this tissue have predominated. Much circumstantial evidence suggests that the liver is the primary site of "attack" by an unknown agent (possibly more than one); however it is equally conceivable that all vital organs are influenced simultaneously. The production of secondary mitochondrial dysfunction by "hepatic toxins" in other tissues is an attractive hypothesis, particularly in the light of what is known about the effects of such agents on brain metabolism in general and on mitochondria in particular. Cerebral edema—largely responsible for the mortality of the victims—probably evolves as a result of energy depletion in the blood-brain barrier and neuronal tissue. The unique structure and function of the blood-brain barrier make it particularly susceptible to agents that adversely influence mitochondrial function. Residual complications of RS reflect the ravages of cerebral edema. Treatment of the syndrome must be directed at an early, rapid, and sustained reduction of intracranial hypertension.

Acknowledgment

The research for and preparation of this chapter was supported in part by a grant from the Robert Stigwood Organization Medical Research Fund.

References

1. R. D. K. Reye, G. Morgan, and J. Baral. Encephalopathy and fatty degeneration of the viscera. *Lancet 2,* 749-752 (1963).
2. L. Corey, R. J. Rubin. Reye's syndrome 1974: An epidemiological assessment. In *Reye's Syndrome* (J. D. Pollack, Ed.). Grune & Stratton, New York, 1975, pp. 179-187.
3. D. C. DeVivo, J. P. Keating, and M. W. Haymond. Acute encephalopathy with fatty infiltration of the viscera. *Pediatr. Clin. North Am. 23,* 527-540 (1976).
4. S. E. Landsay. Varicella hepatitis and Reye's syndrome: An interrelationship? *Pediatrics 60,* 746-748 (1977).
5. P. R. Huttenlocher, A. D. Schwartz, and G. Klastskin. Reye's syndrome. Ammonia intoxication as a possible factor in the encephalopathy. *Pediatrics 43,* 443-453 (1969).
6. P. R. Huttenlocher and D. A. Trauner. Reye's syndrome in infancy. *Pediatrics 62,* 84-90 (1978).
7. W. K. Schubert, R. C. Bobo, J. C. Partin, and J. S. Partin. Reye's syndrome. In *Disease-A-Month* (H. F. Dowling, Ed.). Year Book Med. Pub., Chicago, 1975, pp. 1-30.
8. L. Corey, R. J. Rubin, M. A. W. Hattwick, G. Noble, and E. Cassidy. A nationwide outbreak of Reye's syndrome. *Am. J. Med. 61,* 615-625 (1976).

9. J. S. Haller. Clinical experience with Reye's syndrome. In *Reye's Syndrome* (J. D. Pollack, Ed.). Grune & Stratton, New York, 1975, pp. 3-14.
10. L. Corey, R. J. Rubin, and T. R. Thompson. Influenza B-associated Reye's syndrome: Incidence in Michigan and potential for prevention. *J. Infect. Dis. 135,* 398-407 (1977).
11. D. C. Shannon, R. DeLong, B. Bercu, T. Glick, J. T. Herrin, F. M. B. Moylan, and I. D. Todres. Studies on the pathophysiology of encephalopathy in Reye's syndrome: Hyperammonemia in Reye's syndrome. *Pediatrics 56,* 999-1004 (1975).
12. F. H. Lovejoy, M. J. Bresnan, C. T. Lombroso, and A. L. Smith. Anti-cerebral oedema therapy in Reye's syndrome. *Arch. Dis. Child. 50,* 933-937 (1975).
13. D. C. DeVivo, J. P. Keating, and M. W. Haymond. Intensive supportive approach to the management of Reye's syndrome. In *Reye's Syndrome* (J. D. Pollack, Ed.). Grune & Stratton, New York, 1975, pp. 315-327.
14. E. S. Sherard, Jr., and R. F. Cooper. Multiphasic diagnosis of Reye's syndrome. In *Reye's Syndrome* (J. D. Pollack, Ed.). Grune & Stratton, New York, 1975, pp. 27-37.
15. F. H. Lovejoy, A. L. Smith, M. J. Bresnan, J. N. Wood, D. I. Victor, and P. C. Adams. Clinical staging in Reye's syndrome. *Am. J. Dis. Child. 128,* 36-41 (1974).
16. F. Plum and J. B. Posner. The pathological physiology of signs and symptoms of coma. In *Diagnosis of Stupor and Coma* (F. Plum and J. B. Posner, Eds.). Davis, Philadelphia, 1972, pp. 1-118.
17. J. M. Hockaday, F. Potts, and E. Epstein. Electroencephalographic changes in acute cerebral anoxia from cardiac or respiratory arrest. *Electroencephalogr. Clin. Neurophysiol. 18,* 575-586 (1965).
18. B. Ljunggren, L. Granholm, H. Schutz, and B. K. Siesko. Energy state of the brain during and after compression ischemia. In *Intracranial Pressure* (M. Brock and H. Dietz, Eds.). Springer-Verlag, New York, 1972, pp. 90-95.
19. B. A. Shaywitz, J. M. Leventhal, M. S. Kramer and J. L. Venes. Prolonged continuous monitoring of intracranial pressure in severe Reye's syndrome. *Pediatrics 59,* 595-605 (1977).
20. J. J. Mickell, D. R. Cook, D. H. Reigel, M. J. Painter, and P. Safar. Intracranial pressure monitoring in Reye-Johnson syndrome. *Crit. Care Med. 4,* 1-7 (1976).
21. G. W. Kindt, J. Waldman, S. Kohl, J. Baublis, and R. P. Tucker. Intracranial pressure in Reye's syndrome. *JAMA 231,* 822-825 (1975).
22. D. C. DeVivo and J. P. Keating. Reye's syndrome. *Adv. Pediatr. 22,* 175-229 (1976).
23. M. van Callie, C. L. Morin, C. C. Roy, G. Geoffroy, and B. McLaughlin. Reye's syndrome—Relapse and neurological sequelae. *Pediatrics 59,* 244-249 (1977).
24. R. A. Fishman. Brain edema. *N. Engl. J. Med. 293,* 706-711 (1975).

25. J. S. Partin, W. K. Schubert, R. L. McLaurin, and J. C. Partin. Brain ultrastructure in Reye's syndrome. In *Reye's Syndrome* (J. D. Pollack, Ed.). Grune & Stratton, New York, 1975, pp. 159-168.
26. L. Corey, R. J. Rubin, and M. A. W. Hattwick. Reye's syndrome. Clinical progression and evaluation of therapy. *Pediatrics 60,* 708-713 (1977).
27. L. F. Marshall, H. M. Shapiro, A. Rauscher, and N. M. Kaufman. Pentobarbital therapy for intracranial hypertension in metabolic coma. Reye's syndrome. *Crit. Care Med. 6,* 1-5 (1978).
28. P. W. Davidson, R. H. Willoughby, L. A. O'Tuama, C. N. Swisher, and D. Benjamins. Neurological and intellectual sequelae of Reye's syndrome. *Am. J. Ment. Defic. 82,* 535-541 (1978).
29. C. Pegelow, R. Goldberg, S. Turkel, and D. Powers. Severe coagulation abnormalities in Reye's syndrome, *J. Pediatr. 91,* 413-416 (1977).
30. L. K. Shield, T. L. Coleman, and W. R. Markesbery. Methylbromide intoxication. Neurologic features including simulation of Reye's syndrome. *Neurology 27,* 959-962 (1977).
31. C. H. Bourgeois. Encephalopathy and fatty viscera: A possible response to acute aflatoxin poisoning. In *Reye's Syndrome* (J. D. Pollack, Ed.). Grune & Stratton, New York, 1975, pp. 131-134.
32. K. Tanaka, E. A. Kean, and B. Johnson. Jamaican vomiting sickness. Biochemical investigation of two cases. *N. Engl. J. Med. 295,* 461-467 (1976).
33. D. W. Fox, C. M. Hart, P. S. Bergeson, P. B. Jarrett, A. E. Stillman, and J. R. Huxtable. Pyrrolizidine (senecio) intoxication mimicking Reye's syndrome. *J. Pediatr. 93,* 980-982 (1978).
34. K. E. Bove. The character and specificity of the hepatic lesion in Reye's syndrome. In *Reye's Syndrome* (J. D. Pollack, Ed.). Grune & Stratton, New York, 1975, pp. 93-116.
35. M. E. Pichichero and E. R. B. McCabe. Recurrent Reye's syndrome. *Am. J. Dis. Child. 132,* 1097-1099 (1978).
36. C. Bachmann. Urea cycle. In *Heritable Disorders of Amino Acid Metabolism* (W. Nyhan, Ed.). John Wiley, New York, 1974, pp. 361-386.
37. R. K. Byers. To tap or not to tap. *Pediatrics 57,* 561 (1973).
38. L. Corey, R. J. Rubin, D. Bregman, and M. B. Gregg. Diagnostic criteria for Influenza B-associated Reye's syndrome. Clinical vs. pathologic criteria. *Pediatrics 60,* 702-707 (1977).
39. J. C. Partin. Liver ultrastructure in Reye's syndrome. In *Reye's Syndrome* (J. D. Pollack, Ed.). Grune & Stratton, New York, 1975, pp. 117-129.
40. J. C. Partin, W. K. Schubert, and J. S. Partin. Mitochondrial ultrastructure in Reye's syndrome (encephalopathy and fatty degeneration of the viscera). *N. Engl. J. Med. 285,* 1339-1343 (1971).
41. P. L. Lantos, P. P. Anthony, and C. R. A. Clarke. Unusual cerebral inclusions in Reye's syndrome. *Br. Med. J. 2,* 1176 (1976).

42. E. J. Bradel and C. B. Reiner. The fine structure of hepatocytes in Reye's syndrome. In *Reye's Syndrome* (J. D. Pollack, Ed.). Grune & Stratton, New York, 1975, pp. 147-158.
43. R. E. Brown and G. E. Madge. The pathology of Reye's syndrome: An overview. In *Reye's Syndrome* (J. D. Pollack, Ed.). Grune & Stratton, New York, 1975, pp. 77-92.
44. C. Masters and R. Holmes. Peroxisomes: New aspects of cell physiology and biochemistry. *Physiol. Rev. 57,* 816-882 (1977).
45. B. H. Robinson, J. Taylor, E. Cutz, and D. G. Gall. Reye's syndrome: Preservation of mitochondrial enzymes in brain and muscle compared with liver. *Pediatr. Res. 12,* 1045-1047 (1978).
46. F. Sinatra, T. Yoshida, M. Appelbaum, W. Mason, N. J. Hoogenraad, and P. Sunshine. Abnormalities of carbamyl phosphate synthetase and ornithine transcarbamylase in liver of patients with Reye's syndrome. *Pediatr. Res. 9,* 829-833 (1975).
47. T. Brown, G. Hug, L. Lansky, K. Bove, A. Scheve, M. Ryan, H. Brown, W. K. Schubert, J. C. Partin, and J. Lloyd-Still. Transiently reduced activity of carbamyl phosphate synthetase and ornithine transcarbamylase in liver of children with Reye's syndrome. *N. Engl. J. Med. 294,* 861-867 (1976).
48. P. J. Snodgrass and G. R. DeLong. Urea cycle enzyme deficiencies and an increased nitrogen load producing hyperammonemia in Reye's syndrome. *N. Engl. J. Med. 294,* 855-860 (1976).
49. J. D. Pollack, Ed. *Reye's Syndrome.* Discussion (Glasgow). Grune & Stratton, New York, 1975, pp. 169-176.
50. J. F. S. Crocker, K. R. Rozee, R. L. Ozere, S. C. Digout, and D. Hutzinger. Insecticide and viral interaction as a cause of fatty visceral changes and encephalopathy in the mouse. *Lancet 2,* 22-24 (1974).
51. A. Helenius, B. Morein, E. Fries, K. Simons, P. Robinson, V. Schirrmacher, C. Terhorst, and J. L. Strominger. Human (HLA-A and HLA-B) and murine (H-2K and H-2D) histocompatability antigens are cell surface receptors for Semliki Forest virus. *Proc. Natl. Acad. Sci. USA 75,* 3846-3850 (1978).
52. P. Mitchell. Vectorial chemistry and the molecular mechanics of chemiosmotic coupling: Power transmission by proticity. The Ninth CIBA Medal Lecture. *Biochem. Soc. Trans. 4,* 399-430 (1974).
53. E. Shrago, A. Shug, and C. Elson. Regulation of cell matabolism by mitochondrial transport systems. In *Gluconeogenesis: Its Regulation in Mammalian Species* (R. W. Hanson and M. A. Mehlman, Eds.). John Wiley, New York, 1976, pp. 221-238.
54. J. R. Williamson. Role of anion transport in the regulation of metabolism. In *Gluconeogenesis: Its Regulation in Mammalian Species* (R. W. Hanson and M. A. Mehlman, Eds.). John Wiley, New York, 1976, pp. 165-220.
55. J. B. Chappell. Systems used for the transport of substrates into mitochondria. *Br. Med. Bull. 24,* 150-157 (1968).
56. J. G. Gamble and A. L. Lehninger. Transport of ornithine and citrulline across the mitochondrial membrane. *J. Biol. Chem. 248,* 610-618 (1973).

57. L. Carrasco. The inhibition of cell functions after viral infection. *FEBS Lett. 76,* 11-15 (1977).
58. A. Kortsaris, J. T. Papadimitriou, and J. G. Georgatsos. Interferon inhibition of protein synthesis by isolated mitochondria. *Biochem. Biophys. Res. Commun. 68,* 1317-1322 (1976).
59. J. R. Britton and R. Haselkorn. Permeability lesions in male *Escherichia Coli* infected with bacteriophage T_7. *Proc. Natl. Acad. Sci. USA 72,* 2222-2226 (1975).
60. J. M. Palmer and D. O. Hall. The mitochondrial membrane system. *Recent Prog. Biophys. Mol. Biol.,* 125-176 (1972).
61. V. M. Zhdanof. Transfection methods. In *Methods in Virology* (K. Maramorosch and H. Koprowski, Eds.). Academic Press, New York, 1977, pp. 283-321.
62. P. Hinkle and McCarty. How cells make ATP. *Sci. Am. 238,* 104-123 (March 1976).
63. G. K. Asimakis and J. R. Aprille. Reye's syndrome: The effect of patient serum on mitochondrial respiration in vitro. *Biochem. Biophys. Res. Commun. 79,* 1122-1129 (1977).
64. V. E. Shih. Urea cycle disorders and other congenital hyperammonemic syndromes. In *The Metabolic Basis of Inherited Disease* (J. B. Stanbury, J. B. Wyngaarden, and D. S. Fredrickson, Eds.). McGraw-Hill, New York, 1978, pp. 362-386.
65. J. R. Aprille. Reye's syndrome. Patient serum alters mitochondrial function and morphology in vitro. *Science 197,* 908-910 (1977).
66. A. L. Betz and G. W. Goldstein. Polarity of the blood-brain barrier: Neutral amino acid transport into isolated brain capillaries. *Science 202,* 225-226 (1978).
67. H. J. Manz. The pathology of cerebral edema. *Hum. Pathol. 5,* 291-313 (1974).
68. G. A. R. Johnston. Neuropharmacology of amino acid inhibitory transmitters. *Annu. Rev. Pharmacol. Toxicol. 18,* 269-289 (1978).
69. W. M. Partridge and W. H. Oldendorf. Transport of metabolic substrates through the blood-brain-barrier. *J. Neurochem. 28,* 5-12 (1977).
70. S. P. Bessman and A. N. Bessman. The cerebral and peripheral uptake of ammonia in liver disease with an hypothesis for the mechanism of hepatic coma. *J. Clin. Invest. 34,* 622-628 (1955).
71. M. A. Hanid, R. L. Mackenzie, R. E. Jenner, R. A. Chase, P. J. Mellow, P. N. Trewby, I. Janota, M. Davis, D. B. A. Silk, and R. Williams. Intracranial pressure in pigs with surgically induced acute liver failure. *Gastroenterology 76,* 123-131 (1979).
72. E. M. Nemoto, A. L. Bleyaert, S. W. Stezoski, J. Moossy, G. R. Rao, and P. Safar. Global brain ischemia, a reproducible monkey model. *Stroke 8,* 558-564 (1977).
73. W. Berman, F. Pizzi, L. Schut, R. Raphaely, and P. Holtzapple. The effects of exchange transfusion on intracranial pressure in patients with Reye syndrome. *J. Pediatr. 87,* 887-891 (1975).

74. A. Boutros, J. Hoyt, A. Menezes, and W. Bell. Management of Reye's syndrome. A rational approach to a complex problem. *Crit. Care Med. 5,* 234-238 (1978).
75. P. Safar, A. Bleyaert, E. M. Nemoto, J. Moossy, and J. V. Snyder. Resuscitation after global brain ischemia-anoxia. *Crit. Care Med. 6,* 215-227 (1978).
76. H. E. James, L. Bruno, L. Schut, and W. Bell. Intracranial subarachnoid pressure monitoring in children. *Surg. Neurol. 3,* 313-315 (1975).
77. F. J. Samaha and E. Blau. The role of peritoneal dialysis in Reye's syndrome. In *Reye's Syndrome* (J. D. Pollack, Ed.). Grune & Stratton, New York, 1975, pp. 295-299.
78. C. C. Roy, A. Silverman, and F. J. Cozzetto. *Pediatric Clinical Gastroenterology.* C. V. Mosby, St. Louis, Mo., 1975, pp. 490-501.

74. A. Rongas, J. Hoyt, [illegible] and W. Bell, Management of Reye's syndrome: A rational approach to a complex problem. Crit. Care Med. 3: 2[illegible]-246 (1978).

75. [illegible] Bleyaert, [illegible] Nemoto, [illegible] Moossy, and [illegible] Snyder, Resuscitation after global brain ischemia-anoxia. Crit. Care Med. 6: 215-[illegible] (1978).

76. [illegible] Shapiro, [illegible] Bruce, and [illegible] Bell, [illegible] intracranial pressure monitoring in children. Surg. Neurol. [illegible] 313-315 (1978).

77. [illegible] and [illegible] The role of peritoneal dialysis in Reye's syndrome. In Reye's Syndrome II (J. D. Pollack, Ed.). Grune & Stratton, New York, 1979, pp. 285-[illegible].

78. [illegible] Reye's Syndrome [illegible] New York, [illegible] 1979, pp. [illegible]

6 Biliary Atresia: Current Perspectives in Surgical Treatment

R. PETER ALTMAN / George Washington University School of Medicine, and Children's Hospital National Medical Center, Washington, D.C.

I. Introduction

The application of Kasai's portoenterostomy procedure for infants with extrahepatic biliary atresia has modified the outlook for this formerly hopeless condition. When the surgery is performed before the age of 3 months, bile drainage can be anticipated [1]. For those patients in whom bile drainage is not achieved, or in whom cirrhosis with hepatic failure is progressive despite bile drainage, liver transplantation has provided an additional hope for salvage [2]. Since 1972, 45 infants have had the portoenterostomy procedure at Children's Hospital, National Medical Center, Washington, D.C. The operative results are summarized in this chapter. The current status of hepatic transplantation in infants with biliary atresia, based on experience at the University of Colorado, is also presented.

II. Diagnostic Procedures

In the infant presenting with conjugated hyperbilirubinemia, emphasis is placed upon a thorough but expeditious diagnostic evaluation. The more common intrauterine infections are excluded by serologic Torch titers. The Rose Bengal scan is particularly useful to *exclude* a diagnosis of biliary atresia if the isotope is excreted into the gastrointestinal tract [3]. However, hepatic retention is consistent with extrahepatic biliary atresia or severe intrahepatic cholestasis. The alpha_1-antitrypsin level is determined routinely to rule out this metabolic deficiency disorder, which can result in intrahepatic cholestasis and can mimic extrahepatic biliary atresia clinically [4, 5]. In our experience, therapeutic trials with choleretic agents have not been helpful in discriminating between infants with cholestatic syndromes and those with obstruction, and therefore such trials cannot be recommended. Serial percutaneous needle biopsy of the liver has been valuable for identification and follow-up of infants with cholestasis. Surgical exploration is advised for any infant in whom the etiology of conjugated hyperbilirubinemia remains unexplained.

III. Surgical Technique

The technical details of portal exploration and biliary reconstruction have been described elsewhere [6, 7], and only the general approach will be considered here. Operative cholangiography is performed if the gallbladder is obviously patent. If the gallbladder exists only as a fibrous remnant, X-ray studies are a useless expenditure of operative time.

The bile ducts are not absent in infants with biliary atresia; rather they exist as fibrous cords. These fibrous remnants have been identified in every patient. When the diagnosis of biliary atresia has been confirmed, a thorough portal exploration is undertaken. The distribution of ductal atresia is variable (Fig. 1). In 26 of the 45 infants studied, the entire extrahepatic ductal system was involved. In 12 infants the gallbladder, cystic duct, and common bile duct were patent to the duodenum, but the proximal hepatic radicles were present only as fibrous remnants. The remaining patients had isolated cystic structures in the porta hepatis, but the hepatic ducts were fibrous in each patient.

After transection of the fibrous ductal remnants, preparatory to extablishing a conduit to the intestine, frozen-section examination of the ductal structures at the porta hepatis is carried out. The histologic characteristics of these ductal remnants have prognostic significance. When the presence of

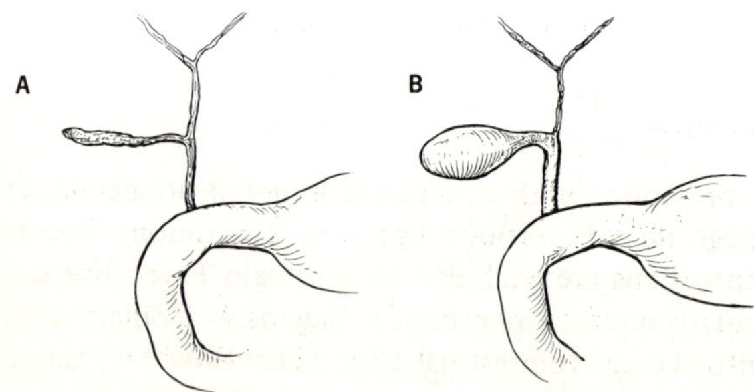

Figure 1 Most frequent operative findings in infants with extrahepatic biliary atresia. A. Entire extrahepatic duct system involved (26 of 45 cases). B. Patency of gallbladder, cystic duct, and common bile duct with atresia of hepatic ducts (12 of 45 cases).

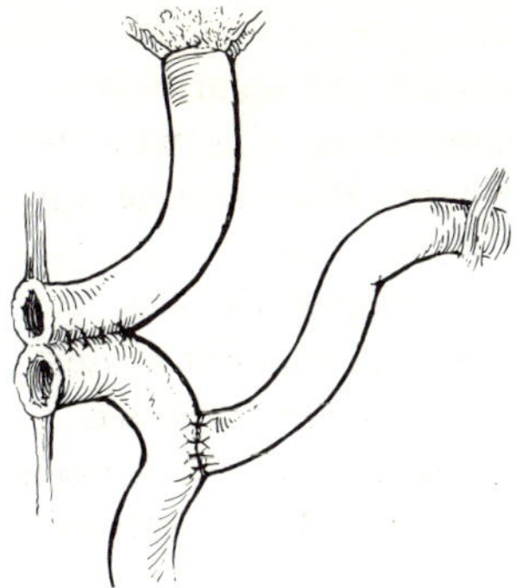

Figure 2 Portojejunostomy (Roux-en-Y) with double-barrel cutaneous diversion (Mikulicz).

biliary epithelium has been confirmed histologically, the portojejunostomy is created. For establishment of the biliary intestinal conduit, we currently favor the Roux-en-Y portojejunostomy with double-barrel Mikulicz enterostomy diversion (Fig. 2).

For those patients with exterioized conduits, the drainage of bile is seen first as the passage of a few plugs of green mucus. By the end of the first week bile drainage is usually in the range of 20-30 cc. By the end of 1 month, bile output is in the range of 120 to 250 cc in patients who are relieved of jaundice. Parenteral antibiotics are used routinely in the postoperative period. Oral antibiotics are instituted and continued indefinitely when bile drainage is obtained.

The levels of serum bilirubin, cholesterol, phospholipids, and bile salts remain elevated for several months. The trend toward normal is apparent by the third month, and normal levels are reached by the end of the first year in those infants who do well [8].

IV. Histopathologic Correlation

Examination of the fibrous duct transected at the porta hepatis demonstrates microscopically patent ductular structures lined by biliary epithelium in the majority of patients. These ducts have been the subject of study at our institution and have been classified histologically into three types: type I—epithelium-lined channels measuring 150 μm or greater; type II—ductular structures usually measuring between 60 and 120 μm, lined by biliary epithelium; type III—ductal structures showing concentric fibrosis without evidence of biliary epithelium. The histologic characteristics of these ductal structures can be correlated with the clinical outcome [9]. Thus eight of the nine patients having type I ducts and 21 of the 26 patients having type II ducts had extended biliary drainage postoperatively, whereas only one of the nine patients with type III ducts had bile drainage.

Other histologic features of the liver and bile ducts did not seem to bear directly upon the clinical outcome. Giant cell transformation of hepatocytes was seen in 24 patients and was not present in 19 others. Bile drainage was accomplished in approximately equal proportions of both groups (17 of 24, 11 of 19). Similarly, the degree of hepatic fibrosis observed in the liver biopsy specimens obtained at the time of portoenterostomy was not related to postoperative bile drainage. Of the 12 patients whose biopsies showed only mild fibrosis, 6 had drainage. Fifteen of the 18 patients whose biopsies were graded as showing moderate fibrosis and 7 patients of 13 with severe fibrosis had postoperative bile drainage.

V. Results

Although extended bile drainage was achieved in 31 of the 45 infants, a progression of fibrosis confirmed by follow-up biopsy was observed in many [10]. This histologic finding was present even in patients whose serum bilirubin, liver function, and growth and development were apparently normal or near-normal. Of the 31 patients having bile drainage, 17 are currently alive and jaundice-free 1-6 years postoperatively. The remaining 12 patients are alive with jaundice [6] or have died with liver failure despite bile drainage [6].

VI. Reoperations for Biliary Atresia

Reoperations were carried out in 18 patients. In eight of these infants, the first operation, performed elsewhere, consisted of exploration and diagnostic

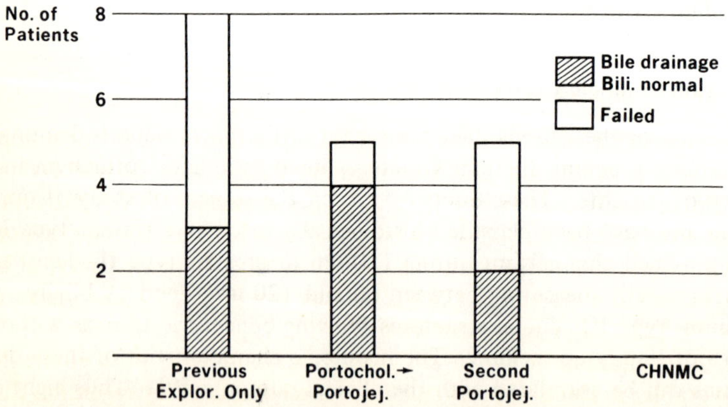

Figure 3 Reoperations for biliary atresia (18 cases). Bile drainage achieved in 3 of 8 patients having previous exploration; 4 of 5 portocholecystostomy cases converted to portojejunostomy; 2 of 5 patients having second portojejunostomy. Total 9 of 18 cases (50%).

liver biopsy only. Five patients had an initial portocholecystostomy which drained bile temporarily, but was subsequently converted to a portojejunostomy. In five additional patients, the first portojejunostomy failed, and reoperation was undertaken. Nine of these reoperations were successful in providing bile drainage, with return of the serum bilirubin to normal (Fig. 3). These results justify the additional operative effort [11].

VII. Discussion

Kasai and others have demonstrated that the course of biliary atresia is modified by the portoenterostomy procedure [12, 13]. However, provision of bile drainage cannot be equated with "cure." Despite the many structural modifications of the biliary intestinal conduit, progressive cirrhosis and postoperative cholangitis continue to exact their toll [14, 15].

The etiology of biliary atresia remains obscure. Landing's hypothesis that the disease is a dynamic, obliterative process may be supported by the operative observations from this group of infants [16]. The varying extent of involvement of the extrahepatic duct system may support the concet of an acquired inflammatory process rather than a single congenital insult. The ductular patency within the fibrous remnants at the porta hepatis is probably lost at about 3 months. This would account for the discrepancy in operative results between patients operated upon before and after 12 weeks of age.

The outcome for patients with biliary atresia is affected by: (1) their age at the time of surgery; (2) the histologic characteristics of the bile ducts at the porta hepatis; (3) the incidence and severity of postoperative cholangitis; and (4) the progression of fibrosis after biliary drainage is established. We conclude from our experience with 45 patients that the prognosis has been favorably altered in 19 (42%) and therefore can recommend further application and study of the portoenterostomy procedure.

VIII. Transplantation

Starzl's pioneering efforts in liver transplantation have brought new hope for those infants in whom the portoenterostomy fails to provide bile drainage or for those having liver failure despite biliary drainage. Forty patients with endstage liver disease secondary to biliary atresia have undergone orthotopic liver transplantation at the University of Colorado. Extended survival has been achieved in eleven cases (28%). In this group, seven remain alive as long as 5½ years after transplantation .*

For those children in whom the clinical outcome after portoenterostomy is unfavorable, it seems appropriate to counsel the families regarding the availability of organ transplantation. The portoenterostomy procedure in some instances may be regarded as a temporizing measure, allowing additional

*T. E. Starzl and J. R. Lilly, personal communication, 1978.

time for growth while the patient awaits hepatic transplantation. The pool of donors for infant and child recipients is restricted, and it is anticipated that the availability of hepatic homografts will continue to be a serious limiting factor. Nonetheless, liver transplantation must be regarded as a legitimate therapeutic endeavor for patients in whom the alternative is irreversible liver failure.

References

1. M. Kasai, S. Kimura, Y. Asakura, H. Suzuki, Y. Taira, and E. Ohashi. Surgical treatment of biliary atresia. *J. Pediatr. Surg. 3,* 665-675 (1968).
2. T. E. Starzl, K. A. Porter, C. W. Putnam, G. Schroter, C. Halgrimson, R. Weil, M. Hoelscher, and H. Reid. Orthotopic liver transplantation in ninety-three patients. *Surg. Gynecol. Obstet. 142,* 487-505 (1976).
3. F. B. Becker and D. F. Hoeffler. The radioactive Rose Bengal test. Its value in the diagnosis of extrahepatic biliary atresia. *Clin. Pediatr. 3,* 715-717 (1967).
4. R. C. Talamo. Basic and clinical aspects of the alpha-1-antitrypsin. *Pediatrics 56,* 91-99 (1975).
5. R. P. Altman and R. Chandra. Biliary hypoplasia consequent to alpha-1-antitrypsin deficiency. *Surg. Forum 27,* 378-379 (1976).
6. R. P. Altman and J. R. Lilly. Technical details in the surgical correction of extrahepatic biliary atresia. *Surg. Gynecol. Obstet. 140,* 952-956 (1975).
7. M. Kasai. Treatment of biliary atresia with special reference to hepatic portoenterostomy and its modifications. *Prog. Pediatr. Surg. 6,* 5-52 (1974).
8. J. R. Lilly and N. B. Javitt. Biliary lipid excretion after hepatic portoenterostomy. *Ann. Surg. 184,* 369-375 (1976)
9. R. S. Chandra and R. P. Altman. Ductal remnants in extrahepatic biliary atresia: A histopathologic study with clinical correlation. *J. Pediatr. 93,* 196-200 (1978).
10. R. P. Altman, R. Chandra, and J. R. Lilly. Ongoing cirrhosis after successful porticoenterostomy in infants with biliary atresia. *J. Pediatr. Surg. 10,* 685-691 (1975).
11. R. P. Altman. Reoperations for correction of extrahepatic biliary atresia. *J. Pediatr. Surg. 14,* 305, 1979.
12. M. Kasai, I. Watanabe, and R. Ohi. Follow-up studies of long term survivors after hepatic portoenterostomy for "non-correctable" biliary atresia. *J. Pediatr. Surg. 10,* 173-182 (1975).
13. J. R. Lilly and R. P. Altman. Hepatic portoenterostomy (the Kasai operation) for biliary atresia. *Surgery 78,* 76-86 (1975).
14. M. Kasai, Y. Asakaura, and H. Suzuki. Modifications of hepatic portoenterostomy to prevent postoperative ascending cholangitis. *Proc. Pacific Pediatr. Surgeons 5,* 83-88 (1972).

15. A. Kobayashi, T. Utsunomiya, Y. Ohbe, and K. Shimizu. Ascending cholangitis after successful surgical repair of biliary atresia. *Arch. Dis. Child. 48,* 697-703 (1973).
16. B. H. Landing. Considerations of the pathogenesis of neonatal hepatitis, biliary atresia, and choledochal cyst—The concept of infantile obstructive cholangiopathy. *Prog. Pediatr. Surg. 6,* 113-139 (1974).

PART II

Gastrointestinal Disorders

7
Intestinal Defenses in Health and Disease

W. ALLAN WALKER / Harvard Medical School, and Massachusetts General Hospital, Boston, Massachusetts

I. Introduction

An important adaptation of the gastrointestinal tract to the extraauterine environment is its development of a mucosal barrier against the penetration of harmful substances (bacteria, toxins, and antigens) present within the intestinal lumen. At birth, the newborn infant must be prepared to deal with bacterial colonization of the gut, with formation of toxic by-products of bacteria and viruses (enterotoxins and endotoxins), and with the ingestion of antigens (milk proteins). These potentially noxious substances, if allowed to penetrate the mucosal epithelial barrier under pathologic conditions, can cause inflammatory and allergic reactions which may result in gastrointestinal and systemic disease states [1].

To combat the potential danger of invasion across the mucosal barrier, the infant must develop an elaborate system of defense mechanisms within the lumen and on the luminal mucosal surface—which act to control and maintain the epithelium as an impermeable barrier to uptake of macromolecular antigens. These defenses include a unique local immunologic system adapted to function in the complicated milieu of the intestine, as well as other nonimmunologic factors such as a gastric barrier, intestinal surface secretions, peristaltic movement, and natural antibacterial substances (lysozyme, bile salts), which also help to provide maximum protection for the intestinal surface [2].

Unfortunately, during the immediate postpartum period, particularly for premature and small-for-date infants, this elaborate local defense system is incompletely developed. As a result of the delay in the maturation of the mucosal barrier, newborn infants are particularly vulnerable to pathologic penetration by harmful intraluminal substances. The consequences of altered defense are a susceptibility to infection and a potential for hypersensitivity reactions and the formation of immune complexes. With these reactions comes the potential for developing life-threatening diseases such as necrotizing enterocolitis, sepsis, and hepatitis. Fortunately, "nature" has provided a means for passively protecting the "vulnerable" newborn against the dangers of a deficient intestinal defense system; i.e., human milk. It is now increasingly apparent that human milk contains not only antibodies and viable leukocytes, but many other substances which can interfere with bacterial colonization and prevent antigen penetration.

II. Antigen Transport in the Small Intestine

Several clinical studies suggest that macromolecules can cross the mucosal barrier under normal physiologic conditions in humans [3]. Since the pinocytotic process of antigen absorption most likely represents a residual and premature absorptive mechanism in the alimentary canal [4], the capacity to absorb large molecules may be more extensive in the immature small intestine than in the mature and more highly developed intestine. In fact, this observation is supported by evidence suggesting that premature and newborn infants can absorb greater quantities of ingested food antigens than older infants or adults [5]. Rothberg [6], for example, has measured bovine serum albumin (BSA) in the serum of premature infants fed quantities of this protein normally present in the daily milk requirement. In contrast, circulating BSA could not be detected in serum samples from older children fed equivalent quantities of protein. Several groups [7, 8] have also reported a larger percentage of infants with serum samples containing antibodies to food antigens–suggesting that food proteins are absorbed intact into the circulation of infants in sufficient quantities to evoke a systemic immune response.

The implication of these studies is that the neonatal intestine may absorb antigenic quantities of ingested protein more readily than the more mature adult intestine. To support this hypothesis, Lev and Orlic [9], in recent morphological studies with fetal monkeys, and Moxey and Trier [10] with human fetuses, have shown an excessive uptake of large molecules by intestinal epithelial cells. They also described morphologic features of epithelial cells suggesting structural immaturity. This same immaturity of gastrointestinal function and structure may persist beyond fetal life into the newborn period, at a time when the small intestine is exposed to increased quantities of both bacterial and food antigens. In addition to increased antigen uptake, it is also possible that a greater quantity of protein ingested by intestinal epithelial cells escapes intracellular proteolysis as a result of immature lysosomal function, and therefore more protein becomes available for subsequent transport out of the cell and into the circulation.

Although infants may absorb greater quantities of antigens, evidence also exists to suggest a limited but nonetheless measurable absorption of macromolecular antigens from the small intestine of older children and adults. Korenblat et al. [8] showed that an appreciable percentage (15-30%) of normal adults developed milk precipitins after a physiologic load of milk proteins. In earlier studies, Wilson and Walzer [11], using immunologic methods to measure circulating food proteins, reported upon the uptake and transport of undigested protein (egg albumin); they also demonstrated precipitins to food proteins in the serum of adults fed physiologic quantities of the same proteins.

III. Factors Contributing to Pathologic Absorption of Antigens and Development of Host Defenses

Although macromolecular antigens can traverse human intestinal mucosa in small, nutritionally insignificant quantities, the vast majority of humans show no ill effects as a result of this apparently natural phenomenon. However, when increased quantities of antigenic or toxic substances gain access to the body because of an alteration in the intraluminal digestive process, or because of a defect in the mucosal barrier, macromolecular absorption may be increased to pathologic proportions–which may in turn contribute to the pathogenesis of either local intestinal or systemic clinical disease. It would now appear that certain factors may, in fact, predispose to abnormal or pathologic transport of macromolecules (Table 1).

The factors listed are meant to be representative and not comprehensive. Many of the factors to be discussed are altered during the neonatal period, when gastrointestinal defense mechanisms are incomplete, and when the developing enterocyte may retain an enhanced capacity to engulf large molecules. The increased intestinal permeability to antigens noted during this period may therefore be potentially dangerous to the neonate.

Table 1 Factors Contributing to Pathologic Absorption of Intestinal Antigens

Selective immunoglobulin-A deficiency
Alteration in mucosal barrier
Increased adherence of antigens
Inflammation
Ulceration
Lysosomal dysfunction
Abnormal intraluminal digestion
Achlorhydria
Pancreatic insufficiency

A. Immunologic Defenses

The mature gastrointestinal tract is replete with lymphoid tissue capable of mounting an immunologic response to protect against the penetration of antigens across the epithelial barrier. Lymphocytes and plasma cells are present in abundance, either as aggregates in Peyer's patches in the ileum and appendix or as a diffuse population of cells in the lamina propria of the small and the large intestine. During the past decade, several classic studies have established the local immunologic system as a unique, protective process present at all epithelial surfaces in direct contact with the external environment (bronchial tree, genitourinary tract, and intestine [12]. Research studies have demonstrated that the local immunologic response is governed by an antigen stimulus at the epithelial surface. Furthermore, the plasma cell population responsible for antibodies in external secretions is, in large part, located in close proximity to the epithelial surface. In addition, the antibodies produced by local plasma cells are delivered to the epithelial surface by a unique transport system. These antibodies have properties adapted for optimum function in the complicated milieu of intestinal secretions containing proteolytic enzymes and other digestive substances. These observations suggest that the immunologic defenses of the gastrointestinal tract are uniquely suited for protecting the host against the penetration of microorganisms and antigenic material at that site [13].

1. Secretory Immunoglobulin A (SIgA). Although all classes of immunoglobulins are represented in intestinal secretions, the predominant secretory immunoglobulin is IgA, which exists in a dimeric form. In the absence of IgA (e.g., selective IgA deficiency), there is a compensatory increase in the luminal secretion of another polymer immunoglobulin, namely, IgM. These observations suggest that polymeric immunoglobulins are the preferred form of secretory antibody. The process of delivering polymeric antibodies into intestinal secretions involves transport through the intestinal epithelium by a specific intracellular glycoprotein-carrier system (secretory component, SC) localized to secretory columnar cells in the crypt region of the intestinal villus. Strong evidence suggests that dimeric IgA and polymeric IgM are completely assembled within local plasma cells, and that the joining chain (J chain) participates in the formation of polymeric immunoglobulins. After release from the plasma cells in the crypt region of intestinal villi and diffusion across the basement membrane, these antibodies become linked to SC, either during contact with this protein on the basal-lateral surface of the epithelial cells or during passage through the epithelial cells. Following combination with SC, the completed secretory immunoglobulin is released from the epithelial cell by reverse pinocytosis. Linkage of SC to the IgA dimer protects it against breakdown by lysosomal enzymes on the intestinal surface. The cooperation between plasma cells producing the IgA dimer and epithelial cells producing SC represents an unusual cellular interaction to provide most mammals with antibody molecules that can coexist with the proteolytic enzymes of intestinal secretions [14]. Figure 1 depicts this process.

Although a number of mechanisms of action have been suggested for secretory antibodies, including opsonization and complement fixation, there is now substantial evidence that a major function of intestinal antibodies is the

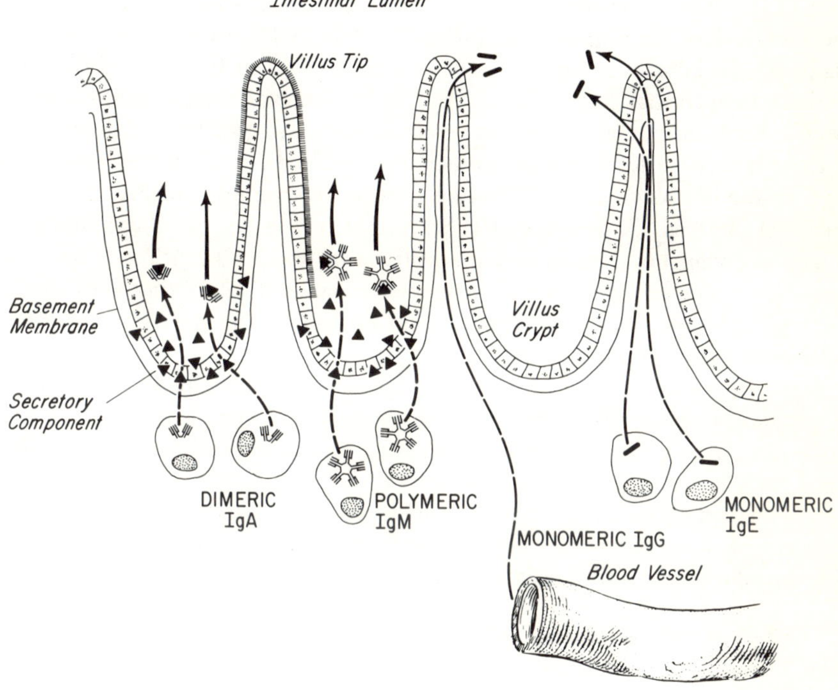

Figure 1 Transport mechanisms for intestinal antibodies. Polymeric immunoglobulins (IgA and IgM) are assembled and secreted in polymeric form by local plasma cells adjacent to crypt secretory cells. After diffusion across basement membrane, these molecules interact with a receptor, on the surface of or within intestinal cells, and are transported as complete secretory antibodies by specific carrier process through cell onto intestinal surface. Monomeric immunoglobulins are synthesized locally (IgE), or transported to lamina propria via the circulation (IgD and IgG), and diffuse across villus epithelial cells by nonspecific mechanism common to other plasma proteins entering intestinal lumen. (Reprinted by permission from *N. Engl. J. Med. 297,* 767, 1977.)

process of immune exclusion at the mucosal surface [13]. Several specific properties of secretory antibodies are enhanced in their effectiveness within the gastrointestinal tract. After transport from the lamina propria onto the intestinal surface, secretory antibodies are retained within the mucous coat on the surface of epithelial cells by interaction with cystine residues contained in mucins present within the glycocalyx [15]. This stationary location of antibodies in juxtaposition to the intestinal epithelial cell allows for more effective interaction with intestinal antigens coming in contact with the mucosal barrier. This property of secretory antibodies has lead to the term "antiseptic paint" to describe the mucous barrier of the gastrointestinal tract [13]. Recent investigations have provided direct evidence for the immune exclusion function of intestinal antibodies. Williams and Gibbons [16] examined the adherence properties of oral pathogens, such as *Streptococcus viridans,* to epithelial cells before and after exposure of these organisms to specific SIgA antibodies. They observed a significant decrease in adhesion of these bacteria after exposure to secretory antibodies. They concluded that SIgA antibodies block specific binding sites on the bacterial adherence to epithelial surfaces. A decrease in adherence results in decreased colonization, as well as enhancing clearance of the bacteria by surface secretions. The presence or absence of intestinal antibodies capable of interfering with specific bacterial adherence may also be important in determining the nature of the indigenous bacterial flora of the gut.

Intestinal antibodies can also protect against the effects of toxic bacterial by-products (e.g., enterotoxins). Secretory antitoxins complexing with cholera toxin can prevent toxin binding to receptors on intestinal microvillus membranes —and thereby can interfere with the activation of adenylate cyclase, a necessary step in the active secretion associated with toxigenic diarrhea [17]. In like manner, intestinal antibodies interfere with the uptake of nonviable antigens introduced directly into the gastrointestinal tract [18].

2. Cell-Mediated Immunity. Although considerably less attention has been focused on the nature of cell-mediated immunity (CMI), this aspect of intestinal immunity may also be independent of a comparable systemic CMI response. Research in this area has been largely experimental, and therefore extrapolation into clinical areas remains highly speculative. Nevertheless, the data suggest that epithelial surfaces develop an independent CMI response, and the nature of the immune response depends on the mode of immunization (oral versus parenteral). Although investigations in this area have largely involved the lung, recent studies reported by Muller-Schoop and Good [19] suggest that lymphocytes committed to a CMI are present in Peyer's patches of the ileum and are capable of responding to antigens present within the intestinal lumen.

3. Role of Secretory Immunity in Local Defenses. Monomeric immunoglobulins (IgD, IgE, IgG) also present in intestinal secretions, appear to function in a secondary capacity as secretory antibodies, since their concentrations in secretions reach protective levels only with intestinal inflammation [13]. In contrast to polymeric intestinal antibodies, monomeric immunoglobulins are transported into secretions by a nonspecific process shared by other proteins entering the intestinal lumen from the systemic circulation (Fig. 1). The IgD and IgG antibodies, synthesized by peripheral lymphoid tissues, as well as local lymphoid cells, enter the lumen by transudation or by direct diffusion across the epithelial surface. However, IgE antibodies are produced locally by IgE-producing plasma cells present along epithelial surfaces. Regardless of the site of synthesis, all monomeric immunoglobulins are transported across epithelial surfaces at the villus tip. These antibodies do not interact with SC and therefore are not protected from intracellular and intraluminal degradation as are polymeric immunoglobulins. As a result of nonspecific transport and degradation, minimal monomeric immunoglobulins can be detected in secretions. When the gastrointestinal tract becomes inflamed, increased quantities of monomeric immunoglobulins, particularly IgG, are noted in secretions. This increase in secondary secretory antibodies probably results from chemotactic factors released by inflammatory cells, which enhance the exudation of immunoglobulins from the intravascular space. The process has been referred to as the "secondary line of defense" of intestinal epithelial surfaces [13].

B. Nonimmunologic Defenses

A number of nonimmunologic factors, present either within the intestinal lumen or on the intestinal mucous surface, exist and are of importance as an adjunct to more classic host defense mechanisms of the gut [2]. These nonspecific defenses help to control the proliferation of microorganisms present in the gastrointestinal tract, aid in decreasing the adherence of organisms to the gut surface, and are important in limiting the available antigen mass that may otherwise overwhelm local immunologic defense mechanisms and penetrate the mucosal barrier or enter the systemic circulation. Taken individually, these factors contribute very little to the overall protection of epithelial surfaces. However, when all nonspecific defenses are operational, their combined contribution provides important additional protection.

1. Intestinal Secretions. Numerous factors that exist in saliva and intestinal secretions are of importance in preventing proliferation of specific organisms within the gut. Gibbons and van Houte [20] have stressed the role of mucins (glycoproteins in mucus) and salivary polymers in controlling the adherence of streptococcal, staphylococcal, and lactobacillus organisms to the epithelial surface of the intestinal mucosa. If these organisms can be inhibited from adhering to an epithelial surface, their proliferation can also be controlled, and they may be cleared from the mouth by the natural washing effect of saliva. When operational, this initial encounter with gram-positive organisms from the external environment provides an excellent means of minimizing the passage of these microorganisms into the gastric reservoir.

Mucins, the glycoproteins and glycolipids present in the mucous coat lining epithelial surfaces, have a molecular structure similar to that of components of the epithelial cellular surface which act as receptors for microorganisms. Mucins apparently interact with organisms migrating through the mucous coat and provide a competitive inhibition for the attachment of these flora to the epithelial surface. Without a specific receptor on the cellular surface, organisms can be readily removed from the intestinal cavity by mechanical means (peristalsis). These same mucins exist in secretions throughout the gastrointestinal tract and presumably function in a similar fashion to help control both bacterial and viral proliferation. In addition to providing microbial protection, mucins may also interact with allergens, enterotoxins, and other biologically active substances, to prevent their penetration across the epithelium [21]. Recent work from this laboratory has shown that an enhancement of goblet cell mucus release occurs in association with immunologic reactions on the intestinal surface (Fig. 2) [22].

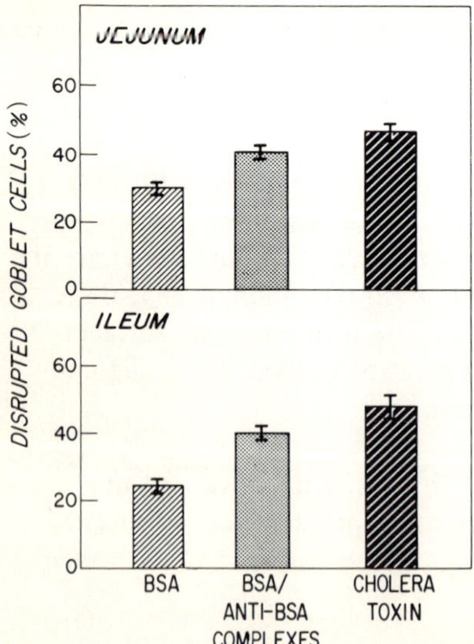

Figure 2 Average percentage of disrupted goblet cells (± standard error) in 20 villi from each jejunal and ileal section of intestine from three groups of rats exposed to BSA, complexes of BSA with rat antibodies to BSA, or cholera toxin. Significant increase in number of disrupted goblet cells was noted in rat jejunum and ileum exposed to immune complexes, compared with those exposed to BSA alone ($P < 0.001$). Difference in percentage of disrupted goblet cells in intestine exposed to complexes or cholera toxin was not significant ($P > 0.1$). (From W. A. Walker, M. Wu, and K. J. Bloch. *Science 197*, 370, 1977; copyright 1977 by the American Association for the Advancement of Science.)

2. *Gastric Barrier.* The concept of the gastric barrier to bacterial, viral, and antigen penetration of the small-intestinal cavity is an important consideration in the nonimmunologic defense of the gut. Several studies have shown that achlorhydria may be associated with an increased proliferation of gram-positive microorganisms within the small-intestinal cavity and with an increased incidence of gastrointestinal infections [23]. In addition to intestinal flora, excessive quantities of ingested food antigens may gain access to the small intestine in the absence of a gastric barrier. Kraft et al. [24] have reported an increased incidence of circulating antibovine serum albumin (anti-BSA) antibodies in adults with achlorhydria, suggesting that the BSA may not be degraded in the stomach and therefore may be present in greater concentrations for absorption by the small intestine. These studies suggest that the digestive effect of gastric acid and pepsin may provide an important limit to antigenic material to the intestinal tract.

3. *Indigenous Intestinal Flora.* In addition to nutrition per se, normal bacterial and viral populations in the gastrointestinal tract are valuable deterrents to the overgrowth of pathogens that may be of potential importance in infectious disease states. After birth, the newborn infant's intestine becomes rapidly colonized with a mixture of organisms which make up the normal or indigenous microbial population of the gut. The nature of the intestinal flora is determined by a number of factors, including diet [25] (nursing versus bottle feeding) and competitive interactions with other organisms [26]. Certain naturally occurring factors in the succus entericus may also limit the growth of intestinal microorganisms.

4. *Peristaltic Movement.* Many invesitgators feel that the mechanical movement of the intestine as part of peristalsis provides the most important factor in controlling proliferation of bacteria within the small intestine [27]. The importance of normal peristaltic activity within the intestine is apparent when one considers the consequences of clinical states in which peristalsis has been disrupted. The serious disruption of gastrointestinal function and the extensive proliferation of bacteria within the small intestine as a result of stagnation of intestinal contents are consistent components of the blind-loop syndrome [28]. The differences in bacterial growth within the small and the large intestine may be directly related to the mechanical movement of these two segments of intestine. In the small intestine, peristalsis is vigorous and frequent, and bacterial growth is limited. In contrast, the large intestine is less mobile, and peristaltic movement is episodic, resulting in prolonged periods of stagnation of luminal contents. The outcome is extensive proliferation of bacterial flora. These

observations underscore the importance of mechanical cleansing as a defense mechanism of the gut.

5. Hepatic Filtration. Approximately 30% of the total liver mass is composed of reticuloendothelial cells [29]. This organ, which receives the major component of serum filtrate from the gastrointestinal tract, has an enormous capacity to phagocytize noxious substances which may gain access to the portal circulation. Therefore, it is reasonable to consider the liver as an "internal line of defense" against invasion of the biologically active substances from the external environment of the gut. Evidence exists that biologically active macromolecules [30] and endotoxins can traverse the small intestine and enter the portal circulation. Yet under usual physiologic circumstances no ill effects (disease states) are apparent. This observation suggests that the liver or, more specifically, Kupffer cells in the liver may act as a filter to deter substances absorbed from the gut from entering the systemic circulation. When the reticuloendothelial system of the liver is blocked in experimental animals or is malfunctioning in certain destructive liver disease states, this filter system is defective, and endotoxins/antigens may cause symptoms of clinical disease (fever, autoimmunity) [31].

6. Miscellaneous Factors. Numerous substances with potential inhibitory properties against bacteria have been reported within the succus entericus and on mucus-coating, epithelial surfaces. These substances may also contribute to the control of bacterial growth within the intestinal cavity. Lysozyme, isolated from the gastrointestinal tract, has been suggested to contribute to lysis of microorganisms within the gut when combined with complement and specific (SIgA antibodies [32]. Many microorganisms grow poorly in medium containing bile salts [33]. This observation suggests that the paucity of bacterial growth within the small intestine may be due in part to high concentrations of bile at that site. In addition to these substances, "natural antibodies" which have been isolated from intestinal contents have generalized inhibitory properties against a number of intestinal pathogens but not against indigenous flora.

C. Development of Intestinal Host Defense

From the brief review of intestinal protective mechanisms in the foregoing paragraphs, it is apparent that numerous immunologic and nonimmunologic processes must function together in order to provide complete protection from the external environment. At birth, these processes are not completely developed and therefore do not work effectively to protect the neonate. A lack of intrauterine stimulation results in an underdeveloped local secretory antibody system at birth. Shortly after birth, however, the ingestion of food antigens and the colonization of the gut with indigenous flora provide sufficient antigenic stimulation to evoke a rapid SIgA response. Selner et al. [34] have documented the development of local immunity in newborns. They have shown that very little response occurs for 2 weeks post partum, but by 28 days almost 100% of infants studied have demonstrable salivary SIgA levels. In contrast to the rapid response of SIgA to antigenic stimulation, serum IgA does not reach adult levels until after several years of life, suggesting that secretory antibodies are more important in neonatal host defense than is serum IgA. It is of importance to note that the local immune response in premature infants to oral antigen stimulation may not be as effective as that of full-term infants [35]. The appearance of antibodies in intestinal secretions most likely lags behind that of full-term infants, making the premature group more vulnerable to adverse environmental factors. Although no studies have been reported on local cell-mediated immunity in premature and newborn infants, Silverstein [36] suggests that an intact and functioning cellular immune system may be operating in utero to prevent a possible graft-versus-host response of maternal leukocytes after gaining access to the fetal circulation. It is, therefore, probable that local CMI develops in response to local antigenic stimuli during the newborn period.

Very little is known about the developmental aspects of other host defenses in the human gastrointestinal tract. However, experimental animal [1, 13] and human fetal studies have suggested that the small-intestinal tract in utero and during initial extrauterine premature existence remains underdeveloped. The intestinal epithelial cell lacks a well-defined brush border and retains a primitive transport mechanism for endocytosis of macromolecular substances [1, 13]. Under these conditions antigens present in the intestinal lumen and on the intestinal surface are engulfed more readily and transported to the intestinal interstitial space (lamina propria) or into the systemic circulation. Rothberg [37] has actually measured circulating foreign antigens in serum samples from premature infants. After a short period of extrauterine life (2 weeks), the capacity to engulf antigens and microorganisms decreases, presumably because of a maturation of epithelial cellular function. It is likely that the absence of an established intestinal flora, the decrease in an effective gastric barrier, and the lack of mucins or other antibacterial substances in the mucous coat of the small intestine contribute to the transient period of increased antigen penetration. Whatever the reason, the premature remains vulnerable for a transient period of extrauterine existence. During this period, the infant may develop a life-threatening disease or become sensitized to disease states which may manifest themselves immediately or in later life. Furthermore, it has recently been reported [38] that pathologic *Escherichia coli* organisms can be attracted more readily to the immature small intestine than to the intestine of the mature animal. This suggests an objective basis for increased infection potential during the premature perinatal period. The concept of *physiologic* and *pathologic* uptake of intestinal macromolecules in association with immunologic and nonimmunologic host defenses is explained by Figure 3.

IV. Passive Protective Function of Human Milk in the Developing Intestine

As stated in the foregoing discussion, newborn infants lack many specific and nonspecific intestinal features that are necessary to adequately protect them in the extrauterine environment. Because of a functionally immature gastrointestinal tract, the perinatal period represents a time when increased susceptibility to the development of clinical disease states may occur. Fortunately, nature has provided an excellent substitute to passively protect the vulnerable neonate during this critical period. This substitute, human milk, contains many factors which can compensate for processes lacking in the infant and at the same time can stimulate the maturation of the gut toward independent function.

It is increasingly apparent that human milk contains not only important nutrients and protective factors for the newborn, but also factors which can facilitate intestinal maturation. In recent studies, several investigators [39, 40] have reported that the ingestion of colostrum can facilitate the maturaation of mucosal epithelial cells, enhance absorption of digested foods, and perhaps accelerate the development of an intact mucosal barrier. Widdowson et al. [39] and others [40] have shown that the gastrointestinal epithelium proliferates and matures more rapidly in experimental animals given maternal milk than in those given isocaloric substitute formulas. It has been shown [40] that brush border enzymes (lactase, sucrase, alkaline phosphatase) are enhanced after the ingestion of colostrum. The investigators have suggested that milk may contain a "mucosal growth factor" which facilitates the early maturation of the gut.

The implication of these observations with respect to intestinal host defenses are obvious. As mentioned earlier, the premature infant, because of an immature intestinal epithelial surface, is more vulnerable to the adherence of bacteria and the absorption of intestinal antigens. If the maturation of epithelial cells is accelerated, the period of vulnerability becomes shortened and the susceptiblity to disease lessened.

A. Milk Antibodies

1. Nonhuman Mammalian Species. Intestinal uptake and transport of proteins has been most extensively studied in animals that acquire passive immunity either in part or entirely from the passage of maternal antibodies across the small-intestinal tract [1]. Animals such as ruminants, which receive all their maternal immunoglobulins in the postpartum period, have a short period of increased permeability to all macromolecules coming in contact with the intestinal mucosa. Maternal colostrum ingested during this period of increased permeability contains an increased concentration of IgG antibodies, the predominant immunoglobulins present in serum. During this same period, γ-globulin levels in neonatal serum increase from virtually undetectable amounts to adult levels, and marked proteinuria can be demonstrated, to support this observation of enhanced macromolecular transport. After the period of enhanced uptake, which lasts only a few days, the intestinal tract quickly "closes" to prevent the further bulk passage of proteins. "Closure" is related to a morphological and functional maturation of small-intestinal epithelial cells.

In contrast to the bulk transport of macromolecules in ruminants, animals such as rodents, which derive passive immunity in part from the intrauterine transport of maternal antibodies and in part from the postpartum intestinal uptake of immunoglobulins, have a prolonged period of selective transport of γ-globulins. The concept of selectivity in transport is supported by the observation that the uptake and transport of γ-globulin proteins are much greater than the absorption of other proteins, such as albumin. The period of enhanced transport in rodents ceases abruptly at 20 days. Morphological studies during the period of enhanced absorption and afterwards demonstrate that the ultrastructural appearance of intestinal epithelial cells changes from the more primitive-appearing cell of the newborn (containing multiple membrane invaginations and vesicles in the apical cytoplasm) to the characteristic appearance of an adult intestinal epithelial cell (with its typical microtubular cytoplasmic network).

2. Human-Milk Antibodies. In humans, passive immunity is derived almost entirely from the intrauterine transport of maternal antibodies [1]. Accordingly, there is very little absorption of γ-globulins across the intestinal tract. This is partly due to the nature of the immunoglobulins in the ingested colostrum. Unlike the colostrum of ruminants and rodents, which contains IgG antibodies, the colostrum of humans primarily contains SIgA antibodies [14]. This class of immunoglobulins cannot be readily transported across intestinal barriers because of the presence of secretory component on the γ-globulin molecule [14]. Although specific antibodies can be detected in the serum of newborn infants fed human colostrum, in contrast with those on formula feedings, the antibody levels detected suggest a nonselective intestinal permeability to macromolecules rather than a selective transport of γ-globulins as demonstrated in the newborn rodent.

B. Additional Protective Factors

In addition to the immunologic factors demonstrated in human milk, several substances have been demonstrated to provide additional protection against systemic and gastrointestinal infection in newborn infants [41]. Lactoferrin, an iron-binding protein present in large concentrations, has been shown to possess inhibiting effects on the growth of *E. coli* and staphylococci by robbing these organisms of iron needed for their metabolism. However, the bacteriostatic effect is abolished by iron saturation. Lysozyme is found in significant amounts in the stools of breast-fed infants and is known to possess powerful bacteriolytic properties. Its concentration in human breast milk is 300 times that in cow's milk. Growth factors contributing to *Lactobacillus bifidus* proliferation include nonspecific conditions, such as the low buffering capacity of human milk and the high lactose content, which promote an acid milieu within the colon and thereby prevent overgrowth of shigella, *E. coli* and candida organisms. In addition to these nonspecific factors, glycoproteins in milk are thought to promote the proliferation of these organisms. Other factors include an antistaphylococcal factor which helps to control the low-grade contamination present in all samples of human milk and to prevent pathologic contamination of the small intestine. Complement components have also been demonstrated in human milk.

Many as yet undiscovered factors are undoubtedly present in human milk, particularly in colostrum, which maintain additional control over bacterial and viral proliferation in the gut. For example, mucinlike glycoproteins which interfere with bacterial attachment to the immature intestinal surface may be an effective control for the microbial environment. It is not inconceivable that adjuvants which promote local intestinal immunity may be discovered by future investigators. It would appear that nature has provided for the newborn a passive means of protecting itself from the environment. Virtually every deficiency or delay in the maturation of host defenses is countered by a factor discovered in human milk—which compensates for the deficiency.

V. Disrupted Host Defenses and Human Disease States

Having briefly reviewed the development of basic host defense mechanisms within the gastrointestinal tract, we may now consider some clinical conditions in pediatrics which may result from the temporary derangement in host defense occurring in the perinatal period. This section is meant to be representative and not comprehensive of all conditions resulting in altered host defense.

The conditions will be considered in two categories, one associated with an immediate manifestation of disease and a second associated with a delayed manifestation. Table 2 lists those conditions probably associated with disrupted intestinal defenses.

A. Immediate Disease States

1. Necrotizing Enterocolitis. In the newborn period, particularly during prematurity, it seems likely that numerous clinical disease states, particularly infectious diseases, might result from a pathologic penetration of the mucosal barrier of the gut by bacteria and antigens. A comprehensive discussion of diseases such as neonatal sepsis and allergy is not indicated. However, one clinical disease state, common among premature infants, should be considered, to illustrate the association of altered host defense and pathogenesis of clinical disease. This condition, necrotizing enterocolitis (NEC), in all likelihood is directly related to defective mechanisms for detaining bacteria on the surface of the small intestine. Clinical signs of NEC begin after infants have started on formula feedings, particularly elemental formulas [42]. Presumably, bacterial colonization of the intestinal tract occurs after feedings have begun. The condition usually progresses rapidly with signs of vomiting, abdominal distension, obstruction, and finally, if severe enough, perforation. The x-ray findings are diagnostic, showing air pockets within the distal small-intestinal wall (pneumatosis intestinalis) [42]. Despite an extensive epidemiologic investigation, no specific bacterial species has been implicated in the condition. In fact, Virnig and Reynolds [43] suggest that "organisms involved in NEC are normal bowel flora that enter the peritoneum and bloodstream through an altered gut mucosa." Investigators [42] using experimental animal models have suggested that bacterial penetration relates to an absence of local immunologic defenses. Barlow et al. [44] have direct evidence that macrophages present in maternal milk may provide passive protection against bacterial penetration.

Table 2 Clinical Conditions in Newborns Possibly Associated with Disrupted Intestinal Host Defenses

Immediate disease states
Necrotizing enterocolitis
Gastrointestinal allergy
Sudden infant death syndrome
Dermatitis enteropathica
Delayed disease states
Inflammatory bowel disease
Chronic active hepatitis
Nephritis
Autoimmune diseases

Other factors, such as intestinal ischemia and the use of elemental diets, both of which can cause direct damage to the intestinal mucosa, have been implicated in the pathogenesis of this disease. Although numerous unrelated precipitating events may predispose to the classic syndrome of NEC, each factor seems to relate directly to altered protection of the intestinal mucosal surface against penetration by intestinal microflora. Thus, it would seem the NEC represents a classic example of clinical disease associated with altered intestinal defenses in premature infants.

2. *Gastrointestinal Allergy*. As stated above, during the neonatal period the gut has an increased permeability to macromolecules [1]. Furthermore, a much higher percentage of infants than of older children or adults have serum and secretory antibodies against dietary proteins, suggesting that antigenic quantities of protein are absorbed during the neonatal period. It is as yet unclear whether this observation can best be explained simply by the fact that larger quantities of these food antigens are ingested during infancy, or whether some additional intraluminal intestinal mucosal factor contributes to the increased transport of macromolecules. A very small percentage of infants will manifest clinical symptoms suggestive of gastrointestinal allergy. Therefore, predisposing factors—in addition to increased intestinal permeability—play a significant part in the clinical expression of allergic states. Yet several clinical syndromes have been described which appear to relate directly to the ingestion of specific foods (particularly cow's milk) [45].

Although the mechanism of gastrointestinal allergies is not completely understood, it would appear that the intestinal transport of macromolecules is a necessary initial step in the process. During the period of increased neonatal permeability, susceptible individuals may become sensitized to ingested proteins. With reexposure at a time when much less macromolecular absorption is occurring, minute but sufficient quantities of allergen may be adsorbed and result in allergic symptoms. Furthermore, an additional alteration in the natural barrier to intestinal uptake of antigens may also contribute to the allergic state. For example, an altered mucosal epithelium after gastroenteritis may predispose susceptible newborns to sensitizing quantities of allergens, or an underdeveloped secretory immune system may also allow for the uptake of critical amounts of sensitizing proteins.

3. *Other Diseases*. Additional newborn diseases which are related to altered defense or dysfunction of the immature gastrointestinal tract include the sudden infant death syndrome [46], which has been reported in association with decreased secretory component in a select population of infants—with resultant prolonged SIgA deficiency and acrodermatitis enteropathica [47], now related to zinc deficiency and malabsorption of this ion during infancy.

B. Delayed Disease States

1. Inflammatory Bowel Disease. The pathogenesis of this pleomorphic condition, inflammatory bowel disease, which includes chronic ulcerative colitis and Crohn's enterocolitis, remains evasive. One of the current hypotheses is that bacterial antigens taken up from the intestine lead to a local hypersensitivity reaction. This, in turn, causes local intestinal inflammation, mucosal ulceration, and granulomatous reaction [1]. Shorter et al. [48] suggest that a deranged permeability of the gut mucosa allows for the passage of macromolecules and nonenteropathic gram-negative bacteria into the gut wall containing gut-associated lymphoid tissues previously sensitized to these antigens. In turn, this penetration results in a hypersensitivity reaction in the gut wall, which ultimately causes inflammatory bowel disease.

These authors suggest that the initlal sensitization may begin during the neonatal period when the mucosal barrier is incomplete, continue with the uptake of undigested macromolecules, and progress to the penetration of proliferating *E. coli* organisms (Fig. 3). After this initial sensitization, a reexposure to bacteria and intestinal antigens may occur in later life when a temporary breakdown of the mucosal barrier results from acute gastroenteritis or from specific substances which can damage the mucosal surface directly. This reexposure causes the local primary cellular immune-mediated hypersensitivity reaction resulting in inflammatory bowel disease. In support

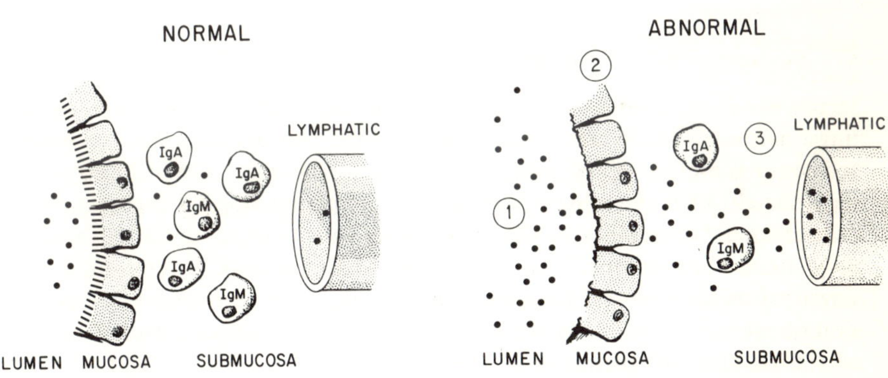

Figure 3 Physiologic and pathologic transport of antigens across intestinal mucosal barrier into systemic circulation. Under normal conditions (left), factors within intestinal lumen, on surface of epithelial cells, and within lamina propria combine to limit access of antigens to systemic circulation. However, when these natural defenses are disrupted (right), excessive quantities of antigenic material may enter circulation and contribute to clinical diseases. Factors contributing to pathologic absorption of antigens include (1) decreased intraluminal digestion, (2) disrupted mucosal barrier, or (3) decrease in IgA-producing plasma cells in lamina propria. (From W. A. Walker, *Pediatr. Clin. North Am. 22,* 731, 1975.

of this hypothesis, antibodies cytotoxic to normal colonic cell suspensions have been reported in the serum of patients with inflammatory bowel disease [1]. Lymphocytes isolated from the serum of patients with inflammatory bowel disease can cause destruction of normal colonic cells [48]. These immunologic responses constitute a cross-reaction of shared antigenic determinants between nonpathologic *E. coli* present in the intestinal contents and mucosal cell membranes. This suggests that bacterial penetration of the gut wall predisposes to the autoimmune response. Why some individuals are more susceptible than others to inflammatory bowel disease has not yet been answered by this hypothesis.

In addition to local intestinal inflammation, the systemic manifestations of inflammatory bowel disease could represent an increased uptake of antigen across a denuded mucosal barrier. These antigens might, in turn, react with antibody and complement to cause inflammation in a vulnerable target organ. The systemic manifestations of the disease lessen after removal of the inflamed gut. This suggests that, with decreased antigen uptake, the systemic manifestations subside [49].

2. *Other Diseases.* In recent clinical reports, the suggestion has been made that milk antigens absorbed during infancy may predispose to immune complex diseases such as chronic active hepatitis and nephritis at a later time [50]. There is also increasing evidence that endotoxin uptake from the small intestine in infancy may predispose to chronic liver disease in later life [51].

VI. Summary and Conclusions

In this review of the development of host defense mechanisms of the gastrointestinal tract, I have attempted to develop the concept of a mucosal barrier to the uptake of intestinal antigens and microorganisms. Alterations in the development of immunologic defenses and nonimmunologic defenses result in an increased vulnerability to clinical disease in the pediatric patient, particularly the newborn infant. The passive role of human milk in promoting intestinal maturation and protecting the newborn gut from pathologic penetration of macromolecules has been discussed. The prediction is made that many as yet undiscovered factors will be reported in future years, to further underscore the importance of human milk in perinatal host defense. Immediate and delayed disease states resulting from an altered defense are considered.

Acknowledgments

Supported in part by grants GM21700 and AM16269 from the National Institutes of Health. The author is the recipient of Research Academic Career Development Award KO4-AM00025 from the National Institutes of Health.

References

1. W. A. Walker and K. J. Isselbacher. Uptake and transport of macromolecules by the intestine: Possible role in clinical disorders. *Gastroenterology 67,* 531-550 (1975).
2. W. A. Walker. Host defense mechanisms in the gastrointestinal tract. *Pediatrics 57,* 901-916 (1976).
3. W. A. Walker. Antigen absorption from the small intestine and gastrointestinal disease. *Pediatr. Clin. North Am. 22,* 731-740 (1975).
4. S. L. Clark. The ingestion of proteins and colloidal materials by columnar epithelial cells of the small intestine in suckling rats and mice. *J. Biophys. Biochem. Cytol. 5,* 41-61 (1959).
5. A. F. Anderson, O. M. Schloss, and C. Meyers. The intestinal absorption of antigenic protein by normal infants. *Proc. Soc. Exp. Biol. Med. 23,* 180-187 (1925).
6. R. M. Rothberg. Immunoglobulin and specific antibody synthesis during the first weeks of life of premature infants. *J. Pediatr. 75,* 391-397 (1969).
7. J. Katz, H. M. Spiro, and T. Herskovic. Milk precipitating substance in the stool in gastrointestinal milk sensitivity. *N. Engl. J. Med. 278,* 1191-1197 (1968).
8. R. E. Korenblat, R. M. Rothberg, P. Minden, and R. S. Farr. Immune response of human adults after oral and parenteral exposure to bovine serum albumin. *J. Allergy 41,* 226-232 (1968).
9. R. Lev and D. Orlic. Uptake of protein swallowed in amniotic fluid by monkey fetal intestine in utero. *Gastroenterology 65,* 60-65 (1965).
10. P. C. Moxey and J. S. Trier. Structural features of the mucosa of human fetal small intestine. *Gastroenterology 68,* 1002-1007 (1975).
11. S. J. Wilson and M. Walzer. Absorption of undigested proteins in human beings. *Am. J. Dis. Child. 50,* 49-57 (1935).
12. T. B. Tomasi, E. M. Tau, A. Solomon, and R. A. Prendergast. Characteristics of an immune system common to certain external secretions. *J. Exp. Med. 121,* 101-111 (1965).
13. W. A. Walker and K. J. Isselbacher. Intestinal antibodies. *N. Engl. J. Med. 297,* 767-773 (1977).
14. M. E. Lamm. Cellular aspects of immunoglobulin A. *Adv. Immunol. 22,* 223-229 (1976).
15. J. Beinenstock. The local immune response. *Am. J. Vet. Res. 36,* 488-501 (1975).
16. R. C. Williams and R. J. Gibbons. Inhibition of bacterial adherence by secretory immunoglobulin A: A mechanism of antigen disposal. *Science 177,* 697-698 (1972).
17. A. L. Wu and W. A. Walker. Immunological control mechanism against cholera toxin: Interference with toxin binding to intestinal receptors. *Infect. Immun. 14,* 1034-1042 (1976).

18. W. A. Walker, J. J. Isselbacher, and K. J. Bloch. Intestinal uptake of macromolecules: Effect of oral immunization. *Science 177,* 608-610 (1972).

19. J. W. Muller-Schoop and R. A. Good. Functional studies of Peyer's patches: Evidence for their participation in intestinal immune responses. *J. Immunol. 114,* 1757-1763 (1975).

20. R. J. Gibbons and J. van Houte. Bacterial adherence in oral microbial ecology. *Annu. Rev. Microbiol. 29,* 19-44 (1975).

21. D. R. Stombeck and D. Harrold. Binding of cholera toxin to mucins and inhibition by gastric mucin. *Infect. Immun. 10,* 1266-1272 (1974).

22. W. A. Walker, M. Wu, and K. J. Bloch. Stimulation by immune complexes of mucus release from goblet cells of the rat small intestine. *Science 197,* 370-375 (1977).

23. F. Goldstein, C. W. Wirtis, and L. Josephs. Bacterial flora of the small intestine. *Gastroenterology 42,* 755-769 (1962).

24. S. C. Kraft, R. M. Rothberg, C. M. Kramer, A. C. Svoboda, L. S. Monroe, and R. S. Farr. Gastric output and circulating antibovine serum albumin in adults. *Clin. Exp. Immunol. 2,* 321-330 (1967).

25. J. R. Porter and L. F. Rettger. Influence of diet on distribution of bacteria in stomach, small intestine and cecum of white rat. *J. Infect. Dis. 66,* 104-111 (1940).

26. S. L. Gorbach. Intestinal microflora. *Gastroenterology 60,* 1110-1129 (1971).

27. G. M. Back and E. Petran. Bacterial activity in different levels of intestine and in isolated segments of small and large bowel in monkeys and in dogs. *J. Infect. Dis. 54,* 204-215 (1934).

28. R. W. Reilly and J. B. Kirsner. Blind loop syndrome. *Gastroenterology 37,* 491-501 (1959).

29. H. Popper and F. Schaffner. *Progress in Liver Diseases.* Grune & Stratton, New York, 1972, pp. 201-220.

30. D. H. Alpers and K. J. Isselbacher. Protein synthesis by the rat intestinal mucosa: The role of ribomilease. *J. Biol. Chem. 242,* 5617-5620 (1967).

31. D. R. Triger and R. Wright. Studies on hepatic uptake of antigen II. The effect of hepatotoxins in the immune response. *Immunology 25,* 951-960 (1973).

32. M. Adinolfi, A. A. Glynn, M. Lindsay, and C. M. Milne. Serological properties of IgA antibodies to *Escherichia coli* present in human colostrum. *Immunology 10,* 517-524 (1966).

33. R. C. Williams, R. Showalter, and F. Kern, Jr. In vivo effect of bile salts and cholestyramine on intestinal anaerobic bacteria. *Gastroenterology 69,* 483-491 (1975).

34. J. C. Selner, D. A. Merrill, and H. N. Claman. Salivary immunoglobulin and albumin: Development during the neonatal period. *J. Pediatr. 87,* 515-519 (1975).

35. C. H. L. Rieger and R. M. Rothberg. Development of the capacity to produce specific antibody to an ingested food antigen in the premature infant. *J. Pediatr. 87,* 515-518 (1975).

36. A. M. Silverstein. Immunological maturation in the fetus: Modulation of the pathogenesis of congenital infection and disease. In *Ontogeny of Acquired Immunity: A CIBA Foundation Symposium.* Elsevier North-Holland, Amsterdam, 1972, pp. 17-20.
37. R. M. Rothberg. Immunoglobulin and specific antibody synthesis during the first weeks of life of premature infants. *J. Pediatr. 75,* 391-397 (1969).
38. M. Hirschberger, D. Mirelman, and M. M. Thaler. Mechanisms of attachment by a pathogenic strain of *E. coli* (0111/B4) to intestinal mucosa in pre- and post weanling rats. *Pediatr. Res. 11,* 500-507 (1977).
39. E. M. Widdowson, V. E. Colombo, and C. A. Artavams. Changes in the organs of pigs in response to feeding for the first 24h after birth. II. The digestive tract. *Biol. Neonate 28,* 272-279 (1976).
40. W. C. Heird and I. H. Hansen. Effect of colostrum on growth of intestinal mucosa. *Pediatr. Res. 11,* 406A (1977).
41. A. S. Goldman and C. W. Smith. Host resistance factors in human milk. *J. Pediatr. 82,* 1082-1090 (1973).
42. A. Lake and W. A. Walker. Neonatal necrotizing enterocolitis: A disease of altered host defense. *Clin. Gastroenterol 6,* 463-472 (1977).
43. N. L. Virnig and J. W. Reynolds. Epidemiologic aspects of neonatal necrotizing enterocolitis. *Am. J. Dis. Child. 128,* 186-192 (1974).
44. B. Barlow, T. V. Santulli, W. C. Heird, J. Pitt, W. A. Blanc, and J. N. Schullinger. An experimental study of acute necrotizing enterocolitis—The importance of breast milk. *J. Pediatr. Surg. 9,* 587-594 (1974).
45. E. J. Eastham and W. A. Walker. Effect of cow's milk on the gastrointestinal tract: A persistent dilemma for the pediatrician. *Pediatrics 60,* 477-486 (1977).
46. P. L. Ogra, S. S. Ogra, and P. R. Loppola. Secretory component and sudden-infant-death syndrome. *Lancet 2,* 387-390 (1975).
47. C. D. Eckhert, M. V. Sloan, J. R. Duncan, and L. S. Hurley. Zinc binding. A difference between human and bovine milk. *Science 195,* 789-794 (1977).
48. R. G. Shorter, R. A. Huizenga, and R. J. Spencer. A working hypothesis for the etiology and pathogenesis of non-specific inflammatory bowel disease. *Am. J. Dig. Dis. 17,* 1024-1033 (Nov. 1972).
49. S. Kraft and J. B. Kirsner. Immunological apparatus of the gut and inflammatory bowel disease. *Gastroenterology 60,* 922-930 (1971).
50. D. F. Davies, B. W. G. Pees, A. P. Johnson, and P. C. Elwood. Food antibodies and myocardial infarction. *Lancet 1,* 1012-1018 (1974).
51. A. I. Jacob, P. K. Goldberg, N. Bloom, G. A. Degenshein, and P. J. Kozinn. Endotoxin and bacteria in portal blood. *Gastroenterology 72,* 1268-1276 (1977).

8
Esophageal Motility Disorders

SIDNEY COHEN / University of Pennsylvania School of Medicine and Hospital of the University of Pennsylvania, Philadelphia, Pennsylvania

I. Introduction

The concepts in this chapter of esophageal motility disorders pertain to the young adult and to the adult, though most of the comments concerning the clinical disorders may also be relevant for the pediatric age group. We shall discuss the clinical disorders of esophageal motility and the treatment of these disorders, with specific recommendations and suggestions for the management of achalasia and gastroesophageal reflux in children.

II. Motility Disorders of the Esophagus

A. Pathophysiology

The esophagus serves two very important functions: first, the transport of material from the mouth to the stomach; and second, the prevention of regurgitation of gastric content from the stomach back into the esophagus. Most disorders of the esophageal function reflect abnormalities in one or both of these primary functions. The function of transport is served by peristalsis, which allows food and secretions to progress down the esophagus. Primary peristalsis occurs in the act of swallowing. Secondary peristalsis occurs during distension of the esophagus after swallowing. There are two dimensions to peristalsis. First, the rhythmicity of the peristalsis and second, the amplitude or force of the peristaltic wave. Thus, there may be diseases involving the amplitude or force of this wave or abnormalities of the rhythm. The other important function of the esophagus is served by the physiological lower esophageal sphincter. The lower esophageal sphincter is a zone of elevated pressure. This zone is about 3 cm in length and is interposed between the positive, intraabdominal pressure cavity and the negative, intrathoracic pressure cavity. This sphincteric high-pressure zone in normal individuals is about 15-30 mmHg in pressure. The sphincter also relaxes or opens in response to swallowing. The relaxation of the sphincter to its nadir very closely approximates the gastric pressure.

B. Classification of Esophageal Motility Disorders

In Table 1, the frequent esophageal motility disorders are shown. The two major clinical disorders that occur in humans are achalasia, which is seen in all age groups, and diffuse esophageal spasm, which is rarely seen in children [1]. In addition, there may be abnormalities of the esophagus with normal peristaltic function, but a decreased force of peristalsis. This is most commonly seen in patients with scleroderma or other collagen diseases. Here there is a normal peristaltic sequence, but the force of the peristaltic wave gradually diminishes and finally disappears as the disease progresses. This disorder may occur in young patients who present with very prominent reflux symptoms and the classic features of Raynaud's disease without having the peripheral manifestations of scleroderma. The classic skin changes may develop at some later date. In looking at these patients in retrospect, it has been found that many such individuals had presented at an early age with esophageal reflux symptoms and sometimes an esophageal stricture, together with Raynaud's phenomenon. This symptom complex should be a clue to collagen disease. In adult life these patients may develop the classic picture of scleroderma.

The abnormalities of the lower esophageal sphincter may be classified as those where the pressure is decreased and those where sphincter relaxation is abnormal (Table 2) [1]. The most common disorder is idiopathic sphincteric incompetence with or without a hiatus hernia. There is another entity which is called chalasia of infancy. It is believed that this is a transient disorder which will be discussed in detail below (C). In about 80% of patients with

Table 1 Abnormalities in Esophageal Peristaltic Function

Dysrhythmia with increased or decreased contractile pressure
Achalasia
Diffuse esophageal spasm
Normal peristaltic sequence with decreased force
Scleroderma

Table 2 Abnormalities in Lower Esophageal Sphincter Function

Decreased sphincter pressure
Idiopathic sphincteric incompetence with or without a hiatus hernia
Chalasia of infancy
Scleroderma
Iatrogenic conditions (surgical or medical)
Hypothyroidism
Abnormal sphincter relaxation with normal or increased pressure
Achalasia
Diffuse esophageal spasm

scleroderma there may be sphincteric incompetence. There are other causes of sphincteric incompetence of an iatrogenic (medical or surgical) origin: e.g., Heller myotomy and the surgically sectioned sphincter at the gastric junction; atropine-like drugs, as well as other drugs such as isoproterenol or the beta-adrenergic drugs. Also, sphincteric incompetence is seen, rarely, in hypothyroidism. Disorders that cause abnormalities due to partial sphincter relaxation include achalasia and diffuse esophageal spasm.

C. Achalasia

Achalasia is a disorder of esophageal motility that occurs in any age group. It may occur late in life, as well as in individuals below 10 years of age. It has been reported down to the age of 2 years. In achalasia, there is a classic X-ray appearance, and patients show dysphagia for both solids and liquids. Patients may have nocturnal regurgitation and even pulmonary aspiration with complications of lung disease. Of all the esophageal diseases, achalasia is the disorder where the majority of pulmonary complications occur. It is extremely rare to encounter pulmonary disorders in patients with gastroesophageal reflux or other types of esophageal disease in either young or old patients.

The esophagus in achalasia shows no primary peristalsis; the gastroesophageal junction has a smooth, tapered narrowing to a birdbeak deformity. However, the endoscope can be easily passed into the stomach. The body of the esophagus loses its normal rhythm of peristalsis and no longer has a single contraction that progresses down the esophagus. Esophageal manometry shows a series of repetitive contractions which may be high or low in amplitude. All the esophageal contractions are nonperistaltic. The esophageal contractions may occur spontaneously and are repetitive. The other abnormality that occurs in achalasia is at the lower esophageal sphincter where two alterations are seen. The sphincter pressure is elevated, and there is partial sphincter relaxation [2]. The mean esophageal pressure in patients with achalasia is about 50 mmHg, rarely below 40 mmHG. Normals have a range of about 15-30 mmHg with a mean of about 20 mmHg. Thus, the pressure is elevated in achalasia, and it decreases only partially, without approximating gastric pressure. It is the residual pressure that causes the obstruction, the dysphagia, and the retention of food in the body of the esophagus.

Lower esophageal sphincter function is markedly different in the patients with achalasia as compared to normal individuals. In normals, regardless of how high the sphincter pressure is elevated, a residual pressure does not occur because the sphincter relaxation is always 100%. In a patient with achalasia, the sphincter relaxation may be only 30% [2]. Since the level of the sphincter pressure and the resting sphincter tone determines the obstruction at the lower esophageal sphincter, reducing the pressure surgically or medically should produce similar results. This simple relationship between pressure and obstruction is maintained in this particular disease entity and is correlated best with symptoms.

It is important to emphasize that, in achalasia, there is no modality for treating the abnormality in the body of the esophagus, and there is no mechanism for restoring normal sphincter relaxation. The only modality for treatment available to us is the reduction in the basal sphincter tone. In adults, the modality of treatment used most successfully is pneumatic dilation. The Brown-McHardy dilator is passed through the mouth. It is positioned straddling the diaphragm, with one part above and one part below the diaphragm. This is inflated with 8-15 lb pressure. This procedure reduces the sphincter pressure. Surgery may also be used as a primary modality of therapy for children as well as adults. It has been reasonably successful in children, and they tolerate the procedure well. The level of esophageal pressure can be brought toward the normal range if the surgical procedure is successful.

A successful therapeutic procedure should result in a normal pressure. If not, one must repeat dilation or surgery. Esophageal dilation has become a primary modality of therapy in individuals with achalasia, regardless of age. The problems of surgery and its complications are avoided. Many individuals who had surgery 10 or more years ago are now returning as adults with severe complications of gastroesophageal reflux or stricture formation. These are very difficult patients to manage.

The one abnormality of the esophagus which is a contraindication to pneumatic dilation has been any form of epiphrenic diverticulum. Such patients are more prone to perforation. This finding should be considered as a primary indication for a Heller myotomy.

D. Gastroesophageal Reflux Disease

Gastroesophageal reflux disease is a syndrome of gastroesophageal reflux with or without clinical complications. There has been considerable progress in the study of this entity during the past decade, particularly in adults [1-4]. Patients with gastroesophageal reflux disease have three basic abnormalities in the function of the lower esophageal sphincter mechanism. They have an abnormality in the resting tone of the sphincter, and they have an abnormality in both the neural and humoral mechanisms at the lower esophageal sphincter.

The normal resting sphincter tone, which is about 15-30 mmHg, is usually diminished in most patients with reflux disease. There may be some overlap in pressure with normals, but for the most part patients have a pressure below 10 mmHg. When the pressure is above 15 mmHg patients do not have any symptoms. However, it should be pointed out that there may be problems with the methodology of recording pressure.

This resting abnormality in sphincter pressure must be viewed in relation to the other possible abnormalities. Normally there is a mechanism which allows the sphincter to increase its pressure to a greater degree than the increase in intraabdominal pressure. During any maneuver where intraabdominal pressure is increased, the sphincter pressure can increase about twofold in normal individuals. When the intraabdominal pressure goes up by 30 or 40 mmHg, the esophageal sphincter pressure can go up by 50-80 mmHg. In the patients with reflux there is an abnormality whereby the sphincter pressure increases only about one-half as much as the change in intraabdominal pressure. Therefore, the change in intraabdominal pressure exceeds the change in sphincter pressure in patients with reflux. During normal daily activities such as bending, the increase in intraabdominal pressure can be as high as 60 mmHg, sometimes even higher; but the esophageal sphincter pressure, even if it has a response of only 15-20 mmHg, is overcome by the increase in abdominal pressure.

There is also an abnormality in the release of the hormone gastrin in these patients. Gastrin is released from the antrum and the duodenum and acts to increase sphincter pressure after eating. It has been shown that patients with reflux release a reduced amount of gastrin.

The three abnormalities in sphincter function would account for reflux during the resting stage while lying down, during physical activities, and following eating.

Some time ago, it was suggested that hiatus hernia is a very important component in gastroesophageal reflux. It was suggested that, if the sphincter were moved from its abdominal positive pressure into the thoracic negative pressure, one would produce sphincter incompetence in all individuals, due to the net difference of pressures (about −10 mmHg). This possibility has been evaluated by studying patients with and without reflux and with and without hiatus hernias. It was found that patients without hiatus hernia had normal sphincter pressure in a range from 15 to 30 mmHg. Patients with hernia in whom no symptoms of reflux were present also had normal ranges of sphincter pressure. However, all patients with reflux had reduced sphincter pressure, usually below 6 mmHg. These studies, as well as others showing no link between reflux and hiatus hernia, should lead physicians to concentrate their efforts on demonstrating reflux rather than hiatus hernia [3].

Gastroesophageal reflux may be due to different mechanisms in different types of diseases [4]. The potential mechanisms that may exist are abnormal sphincter muscle tone, an abnormality in the excitatory neurohumoral factors, or some increase in inhibitory neurohumoral factors. There could be an abnormality where there is less muscle mass; this has been suggested to be one of the factors in the developmental changes in infants. There may also be abnormalities of mechanical properties of the muscle or in the neurohumoral responsiveness of the muscle. There are a host of excitatory factors acting on the sphincter; these may be reduced. For example, gastrin is decreased in patients with reflux disease. Or, one may have an increase in inhibitory factors, of which there are many that have been shown to act on the lower esophageal sphincter.

1. Diagnosis. There are many diagnostic tests that are worthwhile in patients with gastroesophageal reflux. Generalizations can now be made concerning the specificity of the tests—as a summation of the sensitivity and the accuracy of the given diagnostic study (Table 3).

Sphincter pressure determination is quite useful if one has standards and the range of normals for comparison. A pressure below 10 mmHg is a good indication of reflux. Certainly pressure below 6 mmHg shows an excellent correlation. A pressure above 20 mmHg rules out the presence of gastroesophageal reflux. A conventional barium esophagogram may pick up this disorder only in about 20-30% of patients. It is accurate but not very sensitive. It has been known that some of the provocative tests, such as the water-siphon test, are not very good, because they take advantage of a relaxing sphincter while applying pressure to the abdomen. This maneuver should produce reflux in a very high percentage of normal individuals. Indeed, one has a very high false-positive response with this study.

There has been some work now with scintiscanning using radioisotopes. This may be an ideal way to make the diagnosis. However, this has not become widely used in all centers.

Table 3 Clinical Tests of Esophageal Competence and Function

Test	Accuracy[a,b]	Sensitivity[a,c]
Tests of esophageal function		
Barium swallow	+++	++
Esophageal manometry	+++	+++
Gastroesophageal reflux studies		
pH Monitoring	++	+++
Scintiscan	++	+++
Water-siphon test	+	++
Acid clearing tests	+	+
Tests of esophageal mucosal integrity		
Barium swallow	+	+
Esophagoscopy	++	+++
Biopsy	++	+++
Provocative tests for esophageal pain		
Bernstein test	++	+++
Esophageal manometry, using cold water	++	+++
Acid-barium swallow	+	+

[a]+ = fair; ++ = good; +++ = very good.

[b]Accuracy: the ability of a test to distinguish one disease from another, i.e., the number of false-positives.

[c]Sensitivity: the likelihood that a test will give a positive result in patients with a given esophageal disease, i.e., the number of false-negatives.

The acid reflux test is quite accurate. However, one has to be aware of physiologic reflux. In infants, for example, one may have reflux up to 20-25% of the time. It is very difficult to say that reflux is significant. In a normal control population there may be a very high frequency of reflux, though the individuals are totally asymptomatic, without any serious consequences of reflux. Physiologic reflux changes some of our opinions concerning the interpretation of the acid reflux test, especially in the newborn infant, where it seems to be more common than in the adult population and seems to be unrelated to position.

There are also indirect measurements of the function of the esophagus. Endoscopy is quite good if there are gross changes. Biopsy is very sensitive, but mucosal suction biopsies are required. We have found that the ordinary punch biopsies were not interpretable when given to several pathologists. Accurate diagnosis requires multiple biopsies, which, for the most part, may not be used in a young age group. The changes in the esophagus that are found in reflux patients include: a loss in the thickness of the squamous epithelium and an increase in the height of the basilar pegs. These changes may occur in infants as well as in adults. But, again, it is hard to get adequate specimens with anything other than an actual suction biopsy.

In patients with reflux, about 10% of biopsies are false-positive and about 10% false-negative. As reflux changes progress in the esophagus, mucosal hemorrhage, friability, inflammation, and ulceration are seen.

One of the areas that we have now been evaluating is the air-contrast barium swallow. This has been an advance because it allows one to determine the mucosal changes and to pick up changes of esophagitis that were not previously seen on regular barium swallow. The granular changes of the mucosa in a patient with esophagitis may be seen. Fine spiculations or ulcerations of the body of the esophagus may also be observed.

Ulceration of the body of the esophagus may also occur with an actual peptic ulcer of the distal esophagus in a patient with reflux. The ulceration of the lower portion of the esophagus may be present with normal mucosa surrounding it. However, the ulceration is usually seen in association with more severe inflammation.

2. Treatment. In terms of the treatment of gastroesophageal reflux (Table 4), we have had some significant advances that apply to the pediatric age group (stage I). Dietary studies show that certain foods produce reductions in esophageal pressure. Some recent data show that the position of the patient does not have much effect in infants with reflux. Obviously, smoking is not a problem in the pediatric age group. Certain contraindicated drugs may be a problem.

Table 4 Therapy for Gastroesophageal Reflux Disease

Stage I
Bed elevation
Diet (high protein, low fat)
Stop drugs that reduce lower esophageal sphincter pressure
Antacids
Stage II
H_2 antagonists
Drugs that increase sphincter pressure (metoclopramide, Urecholine)
Stage III
Specific antireflux surgery

We now have two types of drugs that I have classified as stage II therapy. These drugs should be considered very seriously in the treatment of stage I failures. These are the H_2 antagonists, such as cimetidine, and the other type of drugs that increase sphincter pressure. In treating patients with reflux, we have found drugs that increase sphincter pressure and diminish the amount of reflux. The H_2 antagonist diminishes the amount of secretory volume, giving the patient much less reflux. These drugs should be considered as an intermediate step prior to considering surgery.

The drugs that increase sphincter pressure raise the pressure from a low range to a high range—and can maintain this pressure at the elevated level for prolonged periods of time, diminishing reflux. These drugs should be considered as a modality of therapy in pediatric as well as adult patients.

The data with cimetidine are of importance. During the nighttime period the secretory volumes were diminished, so that the antacid requirements were reduced. Also, the symptoms decreased, and pain-free periods increased dramatically in the patients receiving cimetidine as compared with placebo-treated patients. However, it is very important to note, in discussing gastrointestinal g.i. disease, that in all the studies in the United States where we tested cimetidine and other drugs, there was a large placebo response in reflux disease (as well as in peptic ulcer disease). One has to be careful when discussing the clinical response in these individuals, since one can expect about a 30-40% pure placebo response in individuals with reflux disease. Patients with severe reflux, given a placebo tablet, dropped their antacid requirements markedly, suggesting the emotional component as well as the physiologic abnormality.

Regarding surgery, there are significant advances in antireflux surgery which can restore sphincteric competence [4]. It was suggested that these procedures restore the normal length-tension characteristics of the sphincter, allowing the muscles to contract, generating greater pressure at lower degrees of stretch. This suggestion has been the working hypothesis as to how these new antireflux surgical procedures work. There is very impressive evidence that these operations diminish reflux and give symptom relief. Surgery also diminishes reflux objectively, whereas the old hiatus hernia repair did not have these effects. At the present time we would do operative procedures in only about 5% of patients presenting with reflux. The indications for surgery are stricture and hemorrhage, with intractable symptoms being the most difficult indication to evaluate. In individuals with intractable symptoms, one must have good evidence of reflux by an incompetent sphincter, positive Bernstein test, free reflux on barium swallow, or free reflux during the pH-monitoring study [4].

The indications for surgery that have not been proven are: symptoms of a hernia, unexplained iron deficiency anemia, and globus hystericus. Chronic pulmonary disease, when it occurs, may also be very difficult to associate with esophageal motility disorders and should not be a basis for surgery as a primary form of treatment.

References

1. R. S. Fisher and S. Cohen. Disorders of the lower esophageal sphincter. *Annu. Rev. Med. 26,* 373-390 (1975).
2. S. Cohen and W. Lipshutz. Lower esophageal sphincter dysfunction in achalasia. *Gastroenterology 61,* 814-820 (1961).
3. S. Cohen and L. D. Harris. Does hiatus hernia affect competence of the gastroesophageal sphincter? *N. Engl. J. Med. 284,* 1053-1056 (1971).
4. W. J. Snape, Jr., and S. Cohen. Gastroesophageal reflux: Advances in medical and surgical treatment. In *Progress in Gastroenterology,* Vol. 3 (G. B. J. Glass, Ed.). Grune & Stratton, New York, 1977, pp. 695-716.

9 The Development of the Exocrine Pancreatic Function and its Effect on Infant Nutrition

EMANUEL LEBENTHAL / State University of New York at Buffalo School of Medicine, and Children's Hospital of Buffalo, Buffalo, New York

I. Introduction

Pancreatic exocrine enzyme activity within the duodenum of infants up to 6 months of age, in both fasting and stimulated state, is deficient as compared with that of adults. This functional pancreatic insufficiency of infancy results in a compromised ability to digest starches and long-chain fatty acids. Definitive evidence for a secretory adaptation of the exocrine pancreas to these substrates is lacking. This type of information would make possible appropriate decisions concerning the ideal composition of the infant's diet.

Histologic studies of the fetal pancreas reveal the presence of differentiated zymogen granules in the pancreatic acinar cells by the fifth month of gestation. The various enzymes and proenzymes of pancreatic origin become apparent during midgestation, and each displays a characteristic pattern of maturation. The factors responsible for the timing of their appearance and the ability of the enzymes to be secreted are only scantily characterized. Certainly, this process of maturation is a continuous one, not limited to the period of gestation, as functional levels or adult levels of functional activity are achieved only at various times after birth.

This chapter will describe the various studies which have led to an understanding of this developmental process. The techniques of study have included the evaluation of pancreatic tissue enzyme content, the assay of exocrine enzyme activity in the intestinal lumen, and the evaluation of pancreatic function by more formal testing with the pancreozymin-secretin stimulation test. The topic of infantile starch digestion and the specific pancreatic amylase activity in infancy will be discussed extensively, with a review of the literature and the presentation of some data developed in our unit. Lipolytic function will be mentioned only briefly because of the paucity of available data. An analysis of the available data on the development of pancreatic enzymes and the corresponding impact on infant nutrition will be discussed. In addition, the adaptation of pancreatic exocrine enzymes to the diet will be discussed.

II. Starch Digestibility and the Development of Pancreatic Amylase

Interest in the digestibility of starches and modified food starches used in infancy arises from two principal concerns. The first relates to the bioavailability of the starch, and the second is the potential of undigestible starch for producing diarrheal symptoms and malabsorption.

There have been no long-term studies to delineate the digestibility of starches and the effect of starch feeding on the growth of young infants. Nonetheless, over the past half-century there has been an increasing tendency to introduce solid foods (beikost) to infants very early in life, and today many infants are started on cereal, and other carbohydrate-containing foods, as early as the first, second, or third week of life [1, 2].

A. Starch Digestibility

The question of starch and modified food starch digestibility is pertinent in view of the lack of duodenal α-amylase activity in infants younger than 3 months of age and the very low amylase activity in infants up to 6 months of age. Experimental approaches to the study of starch digestion and absorption include the following:

1. Clinical evaluation of starch tolerance (signs and symptoms of intolerance include abdominal bloating, nausea and vomiting, abdominal colic, and diarrhea)
2. Measurement of coefficients of apparent absorption
3. Measurement of degradation products (organic acids, glucose, maltose, and alpha-dextrins) in the duodenum, jejunum, ileum, and feces
4. Measurement of long-term growth velocity in infants fed starches from the first month of life

There are reports in the literature indicating that starches are digested in infants as early as 3 days of age. Anderson et al. [3], in a study of five infants at 3 days of age, claimed that the feeding of various cornstarch derivatives, in a dosage of 2 gm/kg body weight, caused a mean rise of 5 mg% in the blood glucose. The ingestion of another type of starch was found to produce a rise of 11 mg% in the blood sugar in the tested infants. These results were compared to those in fifteen infants who received glucose and demonstrated a rise of 66 mg% in the blood sugar and in five infants who were fed maltose and experienced a mean elevation of 46 mg% in the blood sugar. One might explain the observation of Anderson et al. as being within the margin of laboratory error for glucose determinations (approximately 5-10%). In reviewing these data, our interpretation is that the evidence for starch absorption is quite weak, and that little or no starch digestion or absorption has taken place. Devizia et al. [4] examined normal infants 30-50 and 90-100 days of age, receiving a diet containing wheat, corn, and tapioca starches, during three consecutive metabolic study periods, each lasting 3 days. During the balance periods, a cow's milk-based formula was administered at 100 ml/kg body weight. The concentration of carbohydrates in the formula was 6 and 7% respectively for the 1- and 3-month-old infants. Starches–derived from wheat, corn, tapioca, potato, or rice, cooked in water for 10 min–were fed to the infants in concentrations varying from 2 to 3½ g%. Devizia et al. [4] claimed that the wheat, tapioca, corn, potato, and rice starches were almost completely digested by the 1- and 3-month-old infants. This conclusion was supported by the findings of extremely low fecal excretion of lactic acid, glucose and dextrin metabolites of starch, and undigested starch. The absorption coefficient of starch was greater than 98% in all infants studied. No alteration was observed in the fecal excretion of fat or nitrogen. In reviewing these results, it is important to note that of five infants fed 6 g% starch solutions (40 g per day or 170 g/m^2 per day), two developed a severe fermentative diarrhea with high fecal excretion of lactic acid, glucose, dextrins, and undigested starch. A very important question raised by this study is the adequacy of the fecal measurement of lactic acid, glucose, dextrins, and polysaccharide as a definitive indicator of starch digestion and absorption. Obviously, intestinal microflora might well utilize starch without producing an increase in the fecal excretion of lactic acid or other hydrolytic products of the polysaccharide. An interesting observation presented in the paper by DeVizia et al. [4] was that, of the starches used, rice starch had the best coefficient of absorption.

B. Starch Maldigestibility

Many infants are now started on cereal and fruit during the first, second, or third week of life, and abnormally loose stools are not uncommon in these young infants. Severe iatrogenic diarrhea and growth failure due to physiologic absence of pancreatic α-amylase has been described [5]. In this report, dietary starch appeared to be a significant factor in impairing the infant's weight gain. The failure to thrive was not due to an exogenous caloric deficiency in the ingested food, even excluding the calories derived from starch. This suggests that the undigested starch interfered with the absorption of other food ingredients and represents an exaggeration of the physiologic pancreatic amylase deficiency, which occurs to some degree in all infants. Auricchio et al. [6] showed that, in infants up to 6 months of age, the hydrolysis of amylopectin is incomplete, and large amounts of dextrins containing 30 or more glucose units are detected in the jejunum [6]. This is in direct contrast to infants at the end of the first year of life, where amylopectin is rapidly hydrolyzed into glucose, maltose, maltotetrose, and branch dextrins [6]. Starch fed as 18% of caloric intake was not completely digested by some infants [7]. A current unreported study is investigating the relationship of starch feeding to normal growth of young infants. A significantly greater proportion of infants fed in this manner have weights below the tenth percentile [7].

Acute gastroenteritis may result in mucosal injury of the small intestine, which might last from several days to a few months and further affect the ability of the infant to tolerate starch feeding. These considerations are even more important for infants in developing countires, where, because of recurrent gastrointestinal infections and malnutrition, the use of starches and modified food starches might be contraindicated.

C. Modified Starches

Starch is a polymer of anhydroglucose units linked together to form either the linear polymer, amylose, or the branched polymer, amylopectin. An abundance of hydroxyl groups imparts an affinity for water to the starch and results in associations between molecules through hydrogen bonding. This bonding results in the formation of an intermolecular network in which water is entrapped, producing a gel. Starches such as corn, tapioca, and potato contain about 18-27% amylose; the remainder is amylopectin. When starch granules in water are heated with agitation, the granules undergo irreversible swelling. Modified starches were developed primarily to overcome the high viscosity, opacity, and tendency to gel-formation of native starch, which has an undesirable texture that limits consumer acceptability. The basic premise behind the modifications is to alter the starches so they can meet the critical needs of the baby food industry in terms of quality, processing, packaging, and distribution, while retaining the nutritive value of the native starch.

Modified food starches in baby food can be simply described as effective stabilizers. A stabilizer is an essential component of baby foods, required to suspend the finely divided food particles and provide a desirable product from the standpoint of food consistency, texture, appearance, distribution of nutrients, and storage stability. Flexibility in caloric density is also provided, as well as flavor intensity in highly flavored foods. If modified food starches had not had significant advantages to the food industry, they would never have assumed the role that they have in the production of baby foods. Modified food starch concentrations in baby foods are from 5 to 6½%, and their addition is considered to be "good manufacturing practices" [7].

There are four basic types of modifying treatments: bleaching, conversions, cross-linking, and stabilizing [7, 8]. By subjecting waxy maize and tapioca to one or more of these modifying treatments, one may produce various modified food starches. The starch modifications used at the present time in the United States include several obtianed from waxy maize (distarch phosphate, acetylated distarch adipate, and acetylated distarch phosphate) and from tapioca (distarch phosphate and acetylated distarch phosphate). As used, modified food starches supply 10-32% of the total energy available from these foods. Pertinent information concerning modified food starch use includes data on total consumption and estimates of the utilization ranges of specific modified food starches. It is possible to calculate that jars of individual foods could contain as high as 9.4 g modified starch per strained-food jar, and 15.4 g per junior-food jar. Intakes as high as 29 g per day of modified starch could be derived from this source [9].

It is claimed by the food industry that the degree of cross-linking used in modified food starches does not change their in vivo digestibility in animal studies [7]. However, in these studies, it was also shown that marked reductions in the in vitro digestibility occurred when higher degrees of cross-linking were used. At the present time, no clinical data are available assessing modified food starch digestibility in human infants.

D. Pancreatic Amylases

Pancreatic α-amylases attack most glycosidic linkages in an α-D-1,4-glycan; they will not catalyze maltose degradation or α-D-1,4 linkages close to α-D-1,6 branch points. The α-D-1,4 linkages nearest nonreducing end groups of a linear glycan are attacked with difficulty. Similarly, trioses are slowly hydrolyzed, but oligosaccharides larger than a tetrose are catalyzed at the same rate as starch.

This enzyme is also sensitive to steric hindrance. Pancreatic α-amylase yields only a small proportion of maltose from amylose which has 40% of its primary hydroxyl groups substituted with methyl groups. The presence of phosphorous in an amylopectin substrate also is a barrier to α-amylase activity. Degradation end products are small dextrins with phosphate groups and unattached α-D-1,4 linkages.

It is not known whether α-amylase is composed of subunits. However, the evidence that the hog pancreas enzyme has two binding sites [10] implies that such a structure is possible. Also, the occurrence of human pancreatic isoenzymes could be explained if the enzymes were capable of splitting into smaller units during gel electrophoresis.

Mammalian α-amylases are generally stable in the pH range of 5.5-8.0. Optimal pH values are species specific. Similarly, optimal pH will also depend on the presence of chloride ion. This is important in assessing in vitro studies of digestibility.

The α-amylases are calcium-containing enzymes, and removal of this ion will reversibly inactivate the enzyme. Calcium also serves to heat-stabilize the enzyme, as will the presence of inert proteins; heavy metals such as mercury, silver, lead, or copper will inhibit activity. In spite of the fact that mercury is the most potent inhibitor, no evidence for the presence of sulfhydryl groups in the active center has been reported.

Amylases differ among species and among tissues of the same species. The molecular weight derived from sedimentation and diffusion properties is 45,000 for hog pancreas and 69,000 for human salivary amylase. The amino acid composition also differs; e.g., serine content is 50% higher in human salivary amylase than in hog pancreas amylase. Recently, structural differences between human salivary and pancreatic amylases have been distinguished by electrophoretic techniques [11].

Keene and Hewer [12] investigated the presence of digestive enzymes in the human fetus. Amylase activity was detected in the fetal pancreas initially at 22 weeks of gestation. Wolf and Taussig [13] characterized the isoamylases present in human amniotic fluid. They detected pancreatic isoamylases in amniotic fluid at 16 weeks of gestation. Auricchio et al. [14] described intestinal glycosidase activity in the human fetus and newborn; they claimed that term infants possessed approximately 10% of adult amylase activity in pancreatic homogenates but had no amylase activity in the duodenal secretions. This observation raises the question of the lack of secretion of amylase from the pancreas despite its presence in the acinar cells of the pancreas. Klumpp and Neale [15] and Shwachman and Leubner [16] have shown that α-amylase activity in the duodenal fluid of infants up to the age of 6 months remains low or nonexistent. Zoppi et al. [17, 18] have reported essentially the same finding. Delachaume-Salem and Sarles [19] have been unable to demonstrate any significant amylase activity in infants weighing less than 8 kg. Infants weighing between 8 and 12 kg have approximately half the amylase activity of that seen in infants greater than 12 kg [19]. Zoppi et al. [17, 18] studied premature neonates of 32-34 weeks of gestation. He found virtually no α-amylase activity in these children during the first month of life. In our own laboratory we have studied 20 infants in whom no pancreatic amylase activity was detected in the first 3 months of life, either in resting duodenal drainage or in response to pancreozymin-secretin stimulation.*

III. Fat Digestibility and the Development of Pancreatic Lipase

Pancreatic lipase activity is detected in 16-week fetuses, and there are increases in activity up to 28 weeks of gestation [20]. Lipase activity in the full-term

*Unpublished data.

newborn is no more than 10% of that in older children [18]. The infant absorbs lipids inefficiently. The preterm infant of 32-34 weeks of gestation absorbs only 65-75% lipid intake of human milk. The full-term infant may absorb up to 85% lipid intake of human milk, but the adult coefficient of absorption is not achieved before 4-6 months of age [21].

The fat of cow's milk is absorbed in infants to a lesser degree than the fat of human milk. Full-term infants absorb only 60-70% of cow's-milk fat (adults 95%) [21], and premature infants at less than 34 weeks of gestation absorb only 45-60% of butterfat [22]. The fact that the digestibility of the fat of human milk is superior to that of cow's milk was explained recently by the discovery of the existence of lipases in human milk. Human milk contains at least two lipases. One lipase is stimulated by serum and inhibited by bile salts, while the other is stimulated by bile salts [23].

It has been suggested that the lipolytic process begins in the stomach, where triglycerides are hydrolyzed—primarily to diglycerides and fatty acids—by a pharyngeal lipase [24, 25]. Further hydrolysis to monoglycerides and fatty acids occurs by pancreatic lipase. Pancreatic lipase is a water-soluble enzyme which acts on the triglyceride emulsion particle only at the oil-water interface [24]. Maximum lipase activity occurs in the presence of bile salts and a polypeptide factor secreted by the pancreas and termed colipase. Pancreatic lipase is specific for the 1 and 3 ester linkages of the triglyceride molecule and is affected by the chain length of the fatty acid and by its solubility within the aqueous environment of the duodenal fluid.

In addition to the low lipase activity in the preterm infant, there is a low bile acid concentration in the intraluminal fluid. In prematures, bile acids obtained during feedings are in the range of 1-2 mmol, values at or below the critical micellar formation level for conjugated bile salts [26]. It has been demonstrated that the bile acid pool in the newborn infant is approximately one-half that in the adult, when compared on the basis of body surface area [27]. The evaluation of formulas containing high levels of saturated fatty acids, such as palmitic acid, has revealed a marked increase in fat excretion in the stools of full-term infants [28]. These findings suggest that triglyceride structure is important in lipid absorption in infants, and that saturated fatty acids are poorly absorbed. Thus, unsaturated triglycerides, such as vegetable oils, have been added to infant formulas.

It has also been observed that a high intake of saturated lipids diminishes calcium absorption in the neonate [29]. It has been postulated that saturated fatty acids, in the absence of the micellar phase, often form insoluble calcium soaps and are not absorbed. This observation is particularly important in preterm infants [22]. Another therapeutic alternative to saturated fatty acids given in the neonatal period is the use of medium-chain triglycerides. A medium-chain triglyceride readily forms triglyceride emulsions that are rapidly hydrolyzed by lipase, and are water-soluble in the absence of a micellar phase. The medium-chain triglycerides are not reesterified within the small-intestinal epithelial cell, but rather are bound to albumin and metabolized primarily in the liver. The absorption of nonpolar lipids, such as vitamins D and E and cholesterol, is poor during the neonatal period in general, and for the preterm infant in particular [30]. It is conceivable that the addition of water-soluble vitamins D and E will increase their absorption in the newborn.

IV. Proteolytic Activity and the Development of Zymogen Enzymes

Data on the digestibility of various dietary proteins in infants are lacking. Pancreatic trypsin is detectable in the lumen of the small intestine by 16 weeks of intrauterine life [12, 13]. Activity remains constant until 28 weeks of gestation when there is a marked rise [22, 23]. At term, the newborn infant possesses approximately 10% of the tryptic activity that may be identified in older children [17, 18]. Adequate tryptic activity in relation to the amount of protein ingested has been noted by the age of 1 month [16]. With the use of the pancreozymin-secretin test, a functional test of pancreatic enzyme production, the infant at 1 month of age possesses approximately 30% of the tryptic activity found in older children [17, 18]. Subsequently, tryptic activity increases and uniformly approaches the level of adult function by the age of 4 months [31-33].

Enterokinase is a small-intestinal enzyme that is present in the proximal duodenum and jejunum. Though not an enzyme of pancreatic origin, enterokinase activity is required to initiate intraluminal proteolytic activity as it serves to activate the proenzyme, trypsinogen, to the active enzyme trypsin. Further activation of the proenzymes is produced both by trypsin and enterokinase. Thus, the activity of the pancreatic proteolytic enzymes depends upon the presence of this activating enzyme within the lumen of the proximal small intestine. Interestingly, enterokinase activity is detected in fetuses from the 26th week of gestation, paralleling the appearance and development of tryptic activity in the meconium [34]. Between 26 and 30 weeks of gestation, the enterokinase activity is 6% that seen in older children [34]. At term, the enterokinase activity reaches 20% that seen in older children [34].

V. Dietary Adaptation of Pancreatic Function

How to study the effects of various dietary modifications on the pancreatic exocrine function of the infant is a subject of controversy. Many studies have been performed, using animal models or adult human subjects, and the applicability of such findings to the pediatric patient is questionable. Two hypotheses have been advanced concerning the mechanism of exocrine pancreatic adaptation to diet. Pavlov has described rapid and selective adaptive changes in the amount of individual pancreatic enzymes [35]. An alternative hypothesis advanced by Babkin [36] suggested a parallel secretion of pancreatic enzymes without short-term evidence of change related to diet. Recently, a topographic variation of exocrine pancreatic secretory function has been reported. Present evidence suggests that, in the human adult, enzyme secretion by the pancreas occurs basically in a nonparallel fashion, perhaps explained by such a topographic variation in enzyme secretion. Modulation in the synthesis of individual pancreatic enzymes appears to require prolonged dietary changes of days to weeks [4, 37-40].

Animal studies have shown that a diet containing excess carbohydrate results in a high content of pancreatic amylase. Dietary carbohydrates in the form of starch, sucrose, and glucose increase pancreatic intracellular levels of amylase and lower lipase, while unsaturated fatty acids increase the levels of lipase [24]. A high-protein diet results in a high content of proteases [37-41]. The response to a protein-rich diet is more complex, since the feeding of casein increases the synthesis of amylase more than that of trypsinogen or chymotrypsinogen. On the other hand, whole-egg protein increases the synthesis of chymotrypsin more than amylase [39]. Supplements of methionine increase the pancreatic content of lipase and proteases, while phenylalanine and isoleucine increase the pancreatic content of proteases only. Lysine deficiency in the rat reduces the pancreatic content of amylase and chymotrypsinogen [42]. Methionine- and leucine-deficient diets decrease pancreatic lipase and proteases much more than amylase [43]. A diet containing a trypsin inhibitor, such as is found in soybean flour, is associated with increased synthesis of trypsinogen and chymotrypsinogen and depressed synthesis of amylase [44, 45]. On the other hand, the feeding of egg-white trypsin inhibitor to rats increases chymotrypsinogen and amylase, but not trypsinogen [46]. Another trypsin inhibitor, *p*-aminobenzaminidine, increases amylase, trypsinogen, and chymotrypsinogen in rats during the first 4 weeks of diet, thereafter reducing only the amylase content [47].

Human studies in adults have suggested an influence on secreted pancreatic enzymes by variations in experimental dietary stimulation as well as by disease states [17, 48]. Feeding of starch in prematures increased the amylase output by a factor of 10, but the amylase activity induced was very low. No follow-up of amylase activity at later ages was recorded [18]. Data* derived from our laboratory have failed to confirm this. A high-protein diet in infants increased the levels of trypsin and chymotrypsin [18], while a high-fat diet had no effect on lipase [18].

VI. Conclusions

Although pancreatic zymogen granules are seen in fetal life at 5 months of gestation, pancreatic function in the newborn is significantly diminished when compared to that in the mature child and adult.

*Unpublished communication.

It is found that α-amylase activity is absent until the infant is at least 3 months of age, and this may bear important clinical significance—as certain infants prematurely fed starch may develop diarrhea and malnutrition. The specific effects of modified starches on neonatal absorptive gastrointestinal function remain unknown, despite their extensive use in infant-food processing.

Neonatal lipase activity is present in the newborn period although full-term infants display only 10% of adult lipase activity. There is a subsequent "functional" steatorrhea, which is more marked in prematures and is compounded by low bile acid concentrations in intraluminal fluid. Important clinical correlations are related to deficiencies of absorption of fat-soluble vitamins and calcium.

Trypsin activity also shows a functional deficiency in the neonate. However, the clinical significance remains unknown due to a paucity of studies concerning protein digestibility.

The response of the neonatal exocrine pancreas to challenge with various nutrients remains incompletely defined. Thus, it remains decidedly unclear as to what constitutes the ideal infant feeding regimen.

References

1. E. Lebenthal. The developmental aspects of pancreatic exocrine function. In *Digestive Diseases in Children* (E. Lebenthal, Ed.). Grune & Stratton, New York, 1978, pp. 489-498.
2. E. Lebenthal. Pancreatic function and disease in infancy and childhood. *Adv. Pediatr. 25,* 223-261 (1978).
3. T. A. Anderson, S. J. Fomon, and L. J. Filer. Carbohydrate tolerance studies with 3 day old infants. *J. Lab. Clin. Med. 79,* 31-37 (1972).
4. B. DeVizia, F. Ciccimarra, N. DeCicco, and S. Auricchio. Digestibility of starches in infants and children. *J. Pediatr. 86,* 50-55 (1975).
5. C. B. Lilibridge and P. L. Townes. Physiologic deficiency of pancreatic amylase in infancy: A factor in iatrogenic diarrhea. *J. Pediatr. 82,* 279-282 (1973).
6. S. Auricchio, D. Della Pietra, and A. Vegnente. Studies on intestinal digestion of starch in man. II. Intestinal hydrolysis of amylopectin in infants and children. *Pediatrics 39,* 853-862 (1967).
7. *Safety and Suitability of Modified Food Starches for Use in Baby Food.* Subcommittee on the Evaluation of the Safety of Modified Starches in Infant Foods. Committee on Nutrition, American Academy of Pediatrics, Houston, Texas, 1977.
8. *Safety and Suitability of Modified Starches for Use in Baby Food.* Subcommittee on Safety and Suitability of MFS and Other Substances in Baby Foods, National Research Council, National Academy of Sciences, Washington, D.C., 1970.

9. S. J. Fomon. Voluntary food intake and its regulation. In *Infant Nutrition* (S. J. Fomon, Ed.). Saunders, Philadelphia, 1974, pp. 20-33.
10. B. J. Allan, N. I. Zager, and P. J. Keller. Human pancreatic proteins: Amylase, proelastase and trypsinogen. *Arch. Biochem. Biophys. 136,* 529-540 (1970).
11. H. Rosenmund and M. J. Kaczmorek. Isolation and characterization of isoenzymes of human salivary and pancreatic alpha amylase. *Clin. Chim. Acta 71,* 185-189 (1976).
12. M. F. L. Keene and E. E. Hewer. Digestive enzymes in the human fetus. *Lancet 1,* 767-769 (1929).
13. R. O. Wolf and L. M. Taussig. Human amniotic fluid isoamylases. *Obstet. Gynecol. 41,* 337-342 (1973).
14. S. Auricchio, A. Rubino, and G. Murset. Intestinal glycosidase activities in the human embryo, fetus and newborn. *Pediatrics 35,* 944-954 (1965).
15. T. G. Klumpp and A. V. Neale. The gastric and duodenal contents of normal infants and children. *Am. J. Dis. Child. 40,* 1215-1229 (1930).
16. H. Shwachman and H. Leubner. Mucoviscidosis. *Adv. Pediatr. 7,* 249-323 (1955).
17. G. Zoppi, D. H. Shmerling, D. Gaburro and A. Prader. The electrolyte and protein contents and outputs in duodenal juice after pancreozymin and secretin stimulation in normal children and children with cystic fibrosis. *Acta Paediatr. Scand. 59,* 692-696 (1970).
18. G. Zoppi, G. Andreotti, F. Pajno-Ferrara, D. M. Njai, and D. Gaburro. Exocrine pancreas function in premature and full term neonates. *Pediatr. Res. 6,* 880-886 (1972).
19. E. Delachaume-Salem and H. Sarles. Évolution en fonction de l'age de la sécrétion pancréatique humaine normale. *Biol. Gastroenterol. (Paris) 2,* 135-146 (1970).
20. T. Tachibana. Physiological investigation of fetus. 4. Lipase in pancreas. *Jpn. J. Obstet. Gynecol. 11,* 92-99 (1928).
21. S. J. Fomon, E. E. Ziegler, and L. N. Thomas. Excretion of fat by normal full term infants fed various milks and formulas. *Am. J. Clin. Nutr. 28,* 1299-1313 (1970).
22. L. Katz and J. R. Hamilton. Fat absorption in infants of birthweight less than 1300 grams. *J. Pediatr. 85,* 608-614 (1974).
23. O. Hernell and T. Olivercrona. Human milk lipases II. Bile salt-stimulated lipase. *Biochim. Biophys. Acta 369,* 234-244 (1974).
24. G. Benzonana and P. Desnuelle. Etude cinétique de l'action de la lipase pancréatique sur des triglycerides an emulsion: Essai d'une enzymologice en milieu hétérogené. *Biochim. Biophys. Acta 105,* 121-136 (1965).
25. A. Norman, B. Strandvik, and O. Ojamae. Bile acids and pancreatic enzymes during absorption in the newborn. *Acta Paediatr. Scand. 61,* 571-576 (1972).
26. E. Singer, G. M. Murphy, S. Edkins, and C. M. Anderson. Role of bile salts in fat malabsorption of premature infants. *Arch. Dis. Child. 49,* 174-180 (1974).

27. J. B. Watkins, D. Ingall, P. Szczepanik, P. D. Klein, and R. Lester. Bile salt metabolism in the newborn infant: Measurement of pool size and synthesis by stable isotope technique. *N. Engl. J. Med. 288,* 431-434 (1973).
28. L. S. Filer, F. H. Mattson, and S. J. Fomon. Triglyceride configuration and fat absorption by the human infant. *J. Nutr. 99,* 293-298 (1969).
29. M. L. Williams, C. S. Rose, G. Morrow, S. E. Sloan, and L. A. Barness. Calcium and fat absorption in the neonatal period. *Am. J. Clin. Nutr. 23,* 1322-1330 (1970).
30. S. Gross and D. K. Melnorn. Vitamin E dependent anemia in the premature infant. *J. Pediatr. 85,* 753-759 (1974).
31. T. Tachibana. Physiological investigation of the fetus. I. On the trypsinogen in the pancreas. *Jpn. J. Obstet. Gynecol. 10,* 27-32 (1927).
32. J. Lieberman. Proteolytic enzyme activity in fetal pancreas and meconium. *Gastroenterology 50,* 183-190 (1966).
33. B. Werner. Peptic and tryptic capacity of the digestive glands in newborns. *Acta Paediatr. 35,* 1-80 (1948).
34. I. Antonowicz and E. Lebenthal. Developmental pattern of small intestinal enterokinase and disaccharidase activities in the human fetus. *Gastroenterology 72,* 1299-1303 (1977).
35. J. P. Pavlov. *Die arbeit der verdeuungsdrusen* (translated by A. Walther). Springer-Verlag (Bergmann), Weisbaden, 1898, pp. 48-55.
36. B. P. Babkin. Parallel concentrations of trypsin, lipase and amylase. In *Secretory Mechanisms of the Digestive Glands,* 2d Ed. Harper & Rowe (Med. Dept.), Hagerstown, Md., 1950, pp. 54-58.
37. A. Ben Abdeljlil, A. M. Visani, and P. Desnuelle. Adaptation of the exocrine secretion of rat pancreas to the composition of the diet. *Biochem. Biophys. Res. Commun. 10,* 112-116 (1963).
38. F. Howard and J. Yudkin. Effect of dietary change upon the amylase and trypsin activities of the rat pancreas. *Br. J. Nutr. 17,* 281-294 (1963).
39. J. T. Snook. Dietary regulation of pancreatic enzyme synthesis, secretion and inactivation in the rat. *J. Nutr. 87,* 297-305 (1965).
40. J. T. Snook. Dietary regulation of pancreatic enzymes in the rat with emphasis on carbohydrate. *Am. J. Physiol. 221,* 1383-1387 (1971).
41. S. S. Hong and D. F. Magee. Influence of dietary amino acids on pancreatic enzymes. *Am. J. Physiol. 191,* 71-74 (1957).
42. J. Christophe. Effects of lysine deficiency on hydrolases in the pancreas and small intestine of young rats. Abstract. *Gut 7,* 298 (1966).
43. R. L. Lyman and S. S. Wilcox. Effect of acute amino acid deficiencies on carcass composition and pancreatic function in the force fed rat. *J. Nutr. 79,* 28-36 (1963).
44. A. M. Konijn, Y. Birk, and K. Guggenheim. In vitro synthesis of pancreatic enzymes. Effects of soybean trypsin inhibitor. *Am. J. Physiol. 218,* 1113-1117 (1970).
45. A. J. Salman, G. Dal Borgo, M. H. Pubols, and J. McGinnis. Changes in pancreatic enzymes as a function of diet in the chick. *Proc. Soc. Exp. Biol. Med. 126,* 694-698 (1967).

46. S. S. Rothman and H. Wells. Selective effects of dietary egg white trypsin inhibitor on pancreatic enzyme secretion. *Am. J. Physiol. 217,* 504-507 (1969).
47. J. D. Geratz and J. P. Hurt. Regulation of pancreatic enzyme levels by trypsin inhibitors. *Am. J. Physiol. 219,* 705-711 (1970).
48. H. Shwachman, E. Lebenthal, and K. T. Khaw. Recurrent acute pancreatitis in patients with cystic fibrosis with normal pancreatic enzymes. *Pediatrics 55,* 86-95 (1975).

10
Inflammatory Bowel Disease in Children

FREDRIC DAUM and HARVEY W. AIGES / Cornell University Medical College, New York, New York, and North Shore University Hospital, Manhasset, New York

I. Introduction

In our discussion of inflammatory bowel disease (IBD), we will concern ourselves with the so-called idiopathic chronic inflammatory intestinal diseases, namely, chronic ulcerative colitis (UC) and regional enteritis or Crohn's disease. The former is primarily a mucosal process involving only the colon, while the latter results in transmural inflammation and most commonly attacks the small intestine and/or the colon. We will not deal with ulcerative proctitis, although this entity probably accounts for 10% of our patients with inflammatory bowel disease.

II. History

Although the term "simple ulcerative colitis" first appeared in the medical literature in 1875, the entity was probably first appreciated by Soranos in A.D. 117. In about A.D. 200, Aretaeos of Cappadocia described various types of diarrhea, including a noncontagious diarrhea with colonic inflammation, which was noted in adults and older children, but, interestingly, not in infants. In 1859, Wilkes, in a letter to the *Medical Times and Gazette,* described "the morbid appearance" of the intestines of Miss Banks—the first account of toxic megacolon. Again, it was Wilkes and Moxon in 1875 who, in their *Lectures on Pathological Anatomy,* coined the term "simple ulcerative colitis" [1]. Helmholtz was the first to describe ulcerative colitis in children in 1923 [2].

Although less precise descriptions date back to the 1700s, it was Crohn, Ginzburg, and Oppenheimer who (in 1932) first described patients with terminal ileitis in clinical and pathologic terms as we understand them today [3, 4]. Brown and his colleagues [56] two years later suggested that a more applicable term was regional enteritis, after they evaluated three patients who had only jejunal involvement. At the same time, Colp [57] noted that the right colon might also be involved. It was not until 1960 that Lockhart-Mummery and Morson finally distinguished Crohn's disease of the colon from inflammation due to ulcerative colitis [5, 6]. It is now appreciated that Crohn's disease may involve the entire alimentary tract including the perianal area.

III. Epidemiology

Recently, Aiges and colleagues have completed the first epidemiologic study focusing specifically on 105 families of children with inflammatory bowel disease [7]. The results of this study indicate there is an increased incidence of ulcerative colitis and Crohn's disease in families of higher socioeconomic status and a surprisingly high incidence of inflammatory bowel disease among Jewish children (62% of patients were Jewish, as compared to 33% of the control population). There was also a 25% incidence of inflammatory bowel disease among relatives of patients with inflammatory bowel disease, a higher incidence than has been reported recently in studies in families of adult patients with inflammatory bowel disease (10-14%) [8, 9]. Finally, no correlation with birth order, place of residence, or level of parental education was noted.

The discovery of a genetic marker for inflammatory bowel disease has unfortunately eluded investigators. The distribution of the ABO blood groups does not differ from expectations in ulcerative colitis or Crohn's disease, nor has the correlation between either disease and a particular HLA antigen been noted. However, ankylosing spondylitis, a familial disorder associated with the HLA-B27 histocompatibility antigen in 80-90% of cases, occurs with increased frequency in patients with inflammatory bowel disease. Adults with both inflammatory bowel disease and ankylosing spondylitis will have an incidence of HLA-B27 postivity similar to those with only ankylosing spondylitis.

At present, there is no evidence to demonstrate that patients with inflammatory bowel disease have psychological profiles different from those of control subjects, nor do they appear to experience unique psychological precipitating factors prior to the onset of illness.

IV. Etiology

Several etiologies for IBD have been proposed, but none substantiated. These have included immunologic deficiencies, food allergies, psychologic disturbances, and infection. Recently, there have been several studies suggesting that Crohn's disease, in particular, may be caused by a virus [10-13]. These studies are based on work done by Mitchell and Rees, who, in 1970, injected homogenate from the intestine of patients with Crohn's disease into the footpads of mice and subsequently noted granulomas [14, 15]. Cave and associates, in 1973, injected the filtrate from the ileum of patients with Crohn's disease intravenously and intraserosally into rabbit intestine; they also described pathology consistent with Crohn's disease [16]. More recently, Gitnick and Rosen injected the filtrate from the ileum of patients with Crohn's disease into a new tissue culture line of continuous rabbit ileum; by electron microscopy they noted virus particles consistent with a rotavirus in the tissue [17]. Gitnick et al. also noted that viral particles different from those in the experiments with Crohn's disease were seen if one performed similar experiments using tissue from patients with ulcerative colitis [18]. The question remains as to whether these viruses are the primary offenders or are merely secondary invaders.

V. Clinical Presentation

A. Observations

The clinical aspects of IBD in children have recently been reviewed in a survey of 130 children with UC and Crohn's disease, who are being cared for at North Shore University Hospital (Table 1). Fifty percent of these patients had symptoms at age 10 years or less. Of the patients, 75 had Crohn's disease and 55 UC. Of the 75 children with Crohn's disease, 30% had only ileal disease, 55% had ileal and colonic involvement, and only 15% had pathology confined to the colon. Therefore, 85% of these children had involvement of the ileum.

Abdominal pain was by far the most common symptom and often awakened the patient from sleep. Diarrhea was frequent, as were guaiac-positive stools, although the latter are more commonly seen with ulcerative colitis because the mucosa is primarily involved. Other common manifestations of inflammatory bowel disease were anorexia, weight loss, and low-grade fever. Ten percent of the patients had significant anemia with hematocrits of less than 30%. The anemia was either hypochromic, suggestive of iron deficiency, or normochromic and normocytic, commonly seen with chronic inflammatory disease. None of our patients had abnormalities of peripheral blood cells suggestive of folate or vitamin B_{12} deficiency [19]. Similarly, 10% of patients had significant hypoalbuminemia with less than 3 g% serum albumin. Commonly, these patients also had pitting edema of the lower extremities. Growth and sexual retardation are not uncommon and have been described in 20-30% of patients with IBD, particularly Crohn's disease [20]. Noteworthy is the fact that 10% of our patients with Crohn's disease were felt to have acute appendicitis when they first presented with their symptoms. This is a feature of acute ileitis well appreciated in adults [21, 22], but not emphasized in the pediatric population.

Table 1 Clinical Features of Inflammatory Bowel Disease

Symptoms or signs	Percent of patients
Abdominal pain, diarrhea, guaiac (+) stools	70-80
Anorexia, weight loss, fever	70-80
Anemia	10
Edema (hypoalbuminemia)	10
Growth and sexual retardation	20-30
Acute appendicitis	10
Carcinoma	0

Table 2 Extraintestinal Manifestations of Inflammatory Bowel Disease

Manifestation	Percent of patients
Perianal disease	30
Joints: arthralgia or arthritis	20
Rashes	7
Mouth sores	7
Uveitis	7
Episcleritis	30
Phlebitis	1
Hepatobiliary disease	<1
Ankylosing spondylitis	<1

Although carcinoma of the colon is a feared complication of UC [23-25], none of our patients thus far has encountered this problem.

Extraintestinal manifestations are a considerable problem for children with inflammatory bowel disease (Table 2). Of the 60 episodes of extraintestinal disease recorded in our patients, 55 were associated with Crohn's disease and only 5 with ulcerative colitis. Thirty percent of our children with Crohn's disease had perianal lesions [26]. These children had involvement of either the small or large bowel or both. Perianal fistulas did not appear to arise from communication with the bowel, but rather from the anal crypts. Twenty percent had either arthralgia or arthritis involving knees, ankles, and elbows [27, 28]. Rashes were seen in 7% with erythema nodosum most common. Pyoderma gangrenosum was also seen in a youngster with Crohn's disease.

Mouth sores occurred in approximately 7% of patients. Except for the fact that these sores were painless, they mimicked the lesions of aphthous stomatitis [29].

Uveitis is a complication of IBD in children, which until recently has not been well appreciated. In a previous study we were able to demonstrate a 30% incidence of subclinical uveitis in children with Crohn's disease [30]. In those children with ulcerative colitis, no uveitis was noted. Acute symptomatic uveitis would appear to be quite uncommon in this age group. Vascular lesions are uncommon in children with IBD, but we have had one patient with phlebitis and one with cutaneous polyarteritis nodosa and Crohn's disease [31]. The latter association was first reported in 1975 [32]. Clinical symptoms of hepatobiliary disease and ankylosing spondylitis were uncommon in our patient population [33].

B. Evaluation

The evaluation of IBD (Table 3) requires a thorough history and comprehensive physical examination with special attention paid to the perianal area. A complete blood count (CBC) and reticulocyte count may demonstrate an anemia and indicate whether there has been blood loss. The erythrocyte sedimentation rate would appear to be an unreliable, but sometimes useful, laboratory test. If the sedRATE is elevated, one might think of IBD rather than a irritable bowel, in which case the laboratory data are all normal. However, Werlin and Grand [34] have noted that children with fulminant colitis often have normal erythrocyte sedimentation rates. A stool culture and sensitivity and a stool for ova and parasites (O&P) should be requested for primary or superimposed infection. A low serum albumin level suggests that protein loss may be occurring from the gastrointestinal mucosa, while a low serum cholesterol usually reflects loss of bile salts in the feces because of significant ileal disease. The serum magnesium concentration may also be diminished if there is enteric protein loss and/or steatorrhea. A low serum folate level suggests that the proximal small bowel is involved, while a low serum concentration of vitamin B_{12} indicates ileal involvement.

Barium studies are an intrinsic part of the evaluation, but certain pitfalls should be appreciated. Both a barium enema and a small-bowel series are essential for a complete evaluation. In UC, in which only the colon is involved (by definition), we have found the results of barium enema examination to be normal in 25% of children with active disease. In children with Crohn's disease, the barium enema findings will be normal 50% of the time [35-37]. Once again, since the ileum is abnormal in 85% of children with Crohn's disease, one must do a small-bowel series for a proper evaluation.

In UC, it is generally agreed that the rectum is almost always abnormal by proctosigmoidoscopy and/or rectal biopsy. However, it has been less clear as to

Table 3 Evaluation of Inflammatory Bowel Disease

History
Physical examination
CBC, sedimentation rate, reticulocyte count
Stool: culture and sensitivity, O & P
Serum chemistry (albumin, cholesterol, magnesium, liver function tests)
Serum folate, vitamin B_{12}
Barium enema, small-bowel series, intravenous pyelogram
Proctosigmoidoscopy, rectal biopsy
? Colonoscopy
Ophthalmologic examination
Growth velocity, Tanner stage, bone age
72-hr fecal fat
? Serum and urine zinc, serum 25-hydroxyvitamin D

how often the rectum is diseased in Crohn's disease. Should a biopsy be done at the time of sigmoidoscopy in a child with Crohn's disease or perhaps by a Ruben tube in a patient who refuses proctosigmoidoscopy? Our experience suggests that when the colon is abnormal by X ray, but the rectum spared, proctosigmoidoscopy and/or biopsy will reveal an abnormal rectum in 70-80% of children. (These data are in contradistinction to the adult experience, in which the rectum is said to be spared in 50% of adults with more proximal colonic disease.) Even in the child with a colon that is normal radiographically, the rectum will also be abnormal 50% of the time if both proctosigmoidoscopy and biopsy are done. Therefore we feel that proctosigmoidoscopy and biopsy are essential features of the diagnostic evaluation for Crohn's disease. The indications for colonoscopy in the child with IBD are controversial. Colonoscopy should be performed when IBD is suspected, but the diagnostic evaluation is equivocal. Perhaps colonoscopy also serves to help the surgeon prior to bowel surgery for IBD.

An ophthalmologic examination, including slit lamp examination for subclinical uveitis, is also indicated. Growth velocity curves, Tanner staging for sexual maturation, and a bone age determination are all useful in assessing the patient's growth and development and potential for future growth and maturation. A 72-hr fecal fat study may suggest the diagnosis of IBD when all other studies have proved normal and may also indicate the possible etiology (steatorrhea) of growth failure.

Finally, there has been an increasing interest in mineral metabolism in IBD and its possible relationship to growth disturbance. In 1977, Nishi and his colleagues studied zinc metabolism in children with IBD [38]. The conclusions derived from this study were: (1) hypozincemia is frequent among patients with Crohn's disease; (2) hypozincemia is more likely to occur with Crohn's disease and short stature, weight deficit, and retarded sexual development; (3) not all patients with Crohn's disease and retardation of growth and development have low serum zinc levels; and (4) there were no abnormalities of taste acuity in patients with hypozincemia.

VI. Treatment

The treatment of IBD is still geared primarily toward the alleviation of symptoms and signs.

In UC, it has been clearly shown that salicylazosulfapyridine (Azulfidine) is effective in the treatment of mild active colitis and significantly diminishes the frequency of relapse [39, 40]. The dose for acute disease is arbitrary, but we usually offer about 70 mg/kg body weight per day. Recent work by Truelove and his colleagues would suggest that, in the adult, only about 2 g per day is required to prevent relapse, about half the dose for acute disease [41].

Few if any data are available to indicate whether Azulfidine should be used in a patient with acute Crohn's disease. Because Azulfidine is metabolized to its active components by bacteria in the distal small bowel and colon, perhaps children with colonic disease will respond more favorably to this drug. According to the National Cooperative Crohn's Disease Study, Azulfidine would appear to be of little or no value in decreasing the incidence of relapses in adults with Crohn's disease.

High-dose, short-term daily steroids are used to treat acute symptoms in children with both illnesses [42, 43]. Recently there have been some data to suggest that alternate-day, low-dose steroids may be helpful in maintaining remission in adolescents with Crohn's disease without interfering with their normal growth pattern [44].

Azathioprine and 6-mercaptopurine have been used in patients with Crohn's disease with variable results. The National Cooperative Crohn's Disease Study has suggested that azathioprine used during a 4-month period was of no value in Crohn's disease [45]. However, Korelitz et al., using 6-mercaptopurine in a double-blind cross-over control study, contend that long-term (1 year or longer) therapy with this medication allows steroid sparing in the patient previously steroid dependent [46]. Antispasmodics are used to alleviate cramps and diarrhea, but may precipitate toxic megacolon. Loperamide, a relatively new drug, has alleviated diarrhea in adults with IBD, but has not been evaluated in children under the age of 12. Recently, Schnape and colleagues have suggested that the diarrhea and urgency in adult patients with UC is associated with an increase in colonic fast activity [47]. The patient receiving Azulfidine should receive folate, as Azulfidine interferes with the absorption of folate and may also lead to hemolysis, with an increase in red cell turnover [48].

Elemental diets and total parenteral nutrition may be used individually or concomitantly to improve the nutritional status of children with IBD. There is also evidence to indicate that in Crohn's disease these two modalities may bring about clinical and radiographic remission by placing the bowel at relative rest [49]. However, the salutary effect of these therapies appears to be temporary, as most patients will eventually relapse. Finally, total parenteral nutrition may help in reversing growth arrest in patients with Crohn's disease [50].

In ulcerative colitis surgery may be necessary because of acute catastrophic events including massive gastrointestinal bleeding, acute fulminating colitis, and toxic megacolon. Steroid dependence and growth and sexual retardation are the most common reasons for elective resection [51]. The issue as to whether and when to operate as prophylaxis against colonic carcinoma still remains unsettled.

Actuarial data from a select population of patients indicate that, after having had ulcerative colitis for 10 years or more, one is at much higher risk for colonic carcinoma [23]. This would appear to be particularly true in the patients with universal colitis since childhood. The surgical approach depends on the patient's medical status and often consists of a subtotal colectomy with ileostomy and sigmoid mucus fistula at initial operation. Subsequently, the patient may then undergo an ileorectal anastamosis [52, 53] or removal of the sigmoid rectal stump and a Kock procedure [54]. The Kock procedure, which provides a continent reservoir ileostomy under the abdominal wall, results in a permanent ileostomy, which is usually more acceptable psychologically. In ulcerative colitis, a total colectomy with either a traditional ileostomy or a Kock procedure is curative.

On the other hand, the recurrence rate in patients with Crohn's disease who have undergone surgery approaches 95%, and therefore surgery should be considered only as a palliative alternative to medical therapy [55]. Acute indications for surgery in Crohn's disease include intestinal obstruction, free perforation, and massive gastrointestinal bleeding. Elective indications include steroid dependence, growth and sexual retardation, and the presence of an abdominal mass which may be an abscess, the result of intraabdominal fistula formation. The diverting ileostomy is an effective means of decreasing perianal complications when medical therapy has failed. When resection of the small bowel is warranted, it should be of a limited nature so as to not create a short-bowel syndrome.

VII. Prognosis

A. Ulcerative Colitis

The prognosis for patients who develop ulcerative colitis during childhood remains guarded. Although many children with ulcerative colitis are able to live relatively normal lives while receiving medical therapy, others have frequent relapses or incapacitating symptoms often requiring multiple hospitalizations. The course of their disease results in frequent absences from school and often retardation—not only in their physical, but also in their psychosocial growth and development. Moreover, the risk of adenocarcinoma of the colon, which has been noted to occur in approximately 3-5% of patients during the first 10 years of their disease, increases to 25% during the next decade, and to 50% after the patient has had the disease for 20 years. Adenocarcinoma of the colon associated with ulcerative colitis is a virulent lesion with early metastasis. The prognosis for a 5-year survival, once the pathology has been diagnosed, is less than 25%.

It is still unclear as to what diagnostic studies should be performed in patients with chronic ulcerative colitis who are at risk for developing adenocarcinoma of the colon. At present, proctosigmoidoscopy, multiple rectal biopsies, colonic washings, barium enema, and colonoscopy have all been suggested as diagnostic studies in these patients. Although the pediatrician infrequently manages patients with ulcerative colitis for more than a 10-year period, it is important that he educate and advise patients and their families—keeping in mind that panproctocolectomy with permanent ileostomy is a curative procedure.

B. Crohn's Disease

Although the mortality in Crohn's disease appears to be less than in ulcerative colitis, morbidity is significant. Patients may have a chronic, indolent, unremitting course with frequent acute exacerbations of their symptoms. Complications such as growth failure, sexual retardation, abscess formation, fistulization, and malabsorption are common; and although surgical intervention may improve a patient's quality of life, the recurrence rate in this disease following surgery approaches 95%.

VIII. Summary

Both ulcerative colitis and Crohn's disease are chronic illnesses with periods of clinical remission and exacerbation. The two diseases share many similarities, but long-term management and prognosis may be different. However, neither illness has specifically unique features, and distinguishing between them requires careful consideration of the clinical presentation, histopathology, and radiographic data.

References

1. S. Wilkes and W. Moxon. *Lectures on Pathological Anatomy,* 2d Ed. Churchill, London, 1875.
2. H. F. Helmholtz. Chronic ulcerative colitis in childhood. *Am. J. Dis. Child. 26,* 418-430 (1923).
3. B. B. Crohn, L. Ginzburg, and G. D. Oppenheimer. Regional ileitis. *JAMA 99,* 1323-1329 (1932).
4. B. B. Crohn and H. D. Janowitz. Reflections on regional enteritis twenty years later. *JAMA 156,* 1221-1231 (1965).
5. H. Lockhart-Mummery and B. Morson. Crohn's disease of the large intestine and its distinction for ulcerative colitis. *Gut 1,* 87-105 (1960).
6. H. E. Lockhart-Mummery and B. C. Morson. Crohn's disease of the large intestine. *Gut 5,* 493-509 (1964).
7. H. W. Aiges, J. Portnoy, F. Daum, and M. Silverberg. Families of adolescents with inflammatory bowel disease: A demographic analysis. *Pediatr. Res. 12,* 364 (1978).
8. J. B. Kirsner and J. A. Spencer. Family occurrences of ulcerative colitis, regional enteritis and ileocolitis. *Ann. Intern. Med. 59,* 133-144 (1963).
9. M. Monk, A. I. Mendeloff, C. I. Siegel, and A. Lilienfeld. An epidemological study of ulcerative colitis and regional enteritis among adults in Baltimore. *Gastroenterology 56,* 847-857 (1969).
10. R. N. Taub, D. Sacher, and L. Siltzbach. Transmission of ileitis and sarcoid-granuloma to mice. *Trans. Assoc. Am. Physycians 87,* 219-222 (1974).
11. R. V. Heatley, P. M. Bolton, E. Owen, W. J. Williams, and L. E. Hughes. A search for a transmissible agent in Crohn's disease. *Gut 16,* 528-532 (1975).
12. D. R. Cave, D. N. Mitchell, and B. N. Brooke. Experimental animal studies of the etiology and pathogenesis of Crohn's disease. *Gastroenterology 69,* 618-624 (1975).
13. D. R. Cave, D. N. Mitchell, and B. N. Brooke. Evidence of an agent transmissible from ulcerative colitis tissue. *Lancet 1,* 1311 (1976).
14. D. N. Mitchell and R. J. W. Rees. Agent transmissible from Crohn's disease tissue. *Lancet 2,* 168-171 (1970).
15. D. N. Mitchell and R. J. W. Rees. Further observations on the transmissibility of Crohn's disease. *Ann. N.Y. Acad. Sci. 278,* 546-559 (1976).
16. D. R. Cave, D. N. Mitchell, S. P. Kane, and B. N. Brooke. Further evidence of a transmissible agent in Crohn's disease. *Lancet 2,* 1120-1122 (1973).
17. G. L. Gitnick and V. J. Rosen. Electron microscopic studies of viral agents in Crohn's disease. *Lancet 2,* 217-219 (1976).

18. G. L. Gitnick, M. H. Arthur, and I. Shibata. Cultivation of viral agents from Crohn's disease: A new sensitive system. *Lancet 2,* 215-217 (1976).
19. F. Steinberg. The megaloblastic anemia of regional enteritis. *N. Engl. J. Med. 264,* 186-188 (1961).
20. T. D. McCaffrey, K. Nasor, A. M. Lawrence, and J. B. Kirsner. Severe growth retardation in children with inflammatory bowel disease. *Pediatrics 45,* 386-393 (1970).
21. S. W. B. Essen, J. Anderson, J. M. D. Galloway, J. D. B. Miller, and J. Kyle. Crohn's disease initially confirmed to the appendix. *Gastroenterology 60,* 853-857 (1971).
22. R. M. Hollings. Crohn's disease of the appendix. *Med. J. Aust. 1,* 639-641 (1969).
23. G. J. Devroede, S. F. Taylor, W. G. Sauer, R. J. Jackman, and G. B. Stickler. Cancer risk and life expectancy of children with ulcerative colitis. *N. Engl. J. Med. 285,* 17-21 (1971).
24. R. G. Farmer, W. A. Hawk, and R. B. Turnbull. Carcinoma associated with mucosal ulcerative colitis and with transmural colitis and enteritis. *Cancer 28,* 289-292 (1971).
25. D. D. Weedon, R. G. Shorter, D. M. Ilstrup, K. A. Huizenga, and W. F. Taylor. Crohn's disease and cancer. *N. Engl. J. Med. 289,* 1099-1103 (1973).
26. H. E. Lockhart-Mummery. Anal lesions of Crohn's disease. *Clin. Gastroenterol. 1,* 377-382 (1972).
27. R. Wright, K. Lumsden, M. G. Luntz, D. Sevel, and S. C. Truelove. Abnormalities of the sacroiliac joints and uveitis in ulcerative colitis. *Q. J. Med. 34,* 229-236 (1965).
28. D. A. Brewerton, M. Caffrey, A. Nicholls, D. Walters, and D. C. O. James. HL-A 27 and arthropathies associated with ulcerative colitis and psoriasis. *Lancet 1,* 956-957 (1974).
29. T. P. Dudeney. Crohn's disease of the mouth. *Proc. R. Soc. Med. 62,* 1237 (1969).
30. F. Daum, H. B. Gould, D. Gold, A. H. Friedman, P. Zucker, and M. I. Cohen. Asymptomatic transient uveitis in children with inflammatory bowel disease. *Am. J. Dis. Child. 133,* 170-172 (1979).
31. E. I. Kahn, F. Daum, H. W. Aiges, and M. Silverberg. Cutaneous polyarteritis nodosa associated with Crohn's disease. *Dis. Colon Rectum* (1979). In press.
32. G. O. Solley, R. F. Winkelmann, and R. A. Rovelstad. Correlation between regional enterocolitis and cutaneous polyarteritis nodosa. *Gastroenterology 69,* 235-239 (1975).
33. S. Cohen, M. Kaplan, L. Gottleib, and J. Patterson. Liver disease and gallstones in regional enteritis. *Gastroenterology 60,* 237-245 (1971).
34. S. L. Werlin and R. J. Grand. Severe colitis in children and adolescents. *Gastroenterology 73,* 828-832 (1977).
35. F. M. Gutman. Granulomatous enterocolitis in children and adolescents. *J. Pediatr. Surg. 9,* 115-121 (1974).

36. T. H. Ehrenpreis, J. Gierup, and R. Lagercrantz. Chronic regional enterocolitis in children and adolescents. *Acta Paediatr. Scand. 60,* 209-215 (1971).
37. R. C. Miller and E. Larsen. Regional enteritis in infancy. *Am. J. Dis. Child. 122,* 301-311 (1971).
38. Y. Nishi, F. Lifshitz, M. A. Bayne, F. Daum, M. Silverberg, and H. W. Aiges. Zinc status and its relation to growth retardation in children with chronic inflammatory bowel disease. *Am. J. Clin. Nutr.* (1979). In press.
39. A. P. Dick, M. J. Grayson, R. G. Carpenter, and A. Petrie. Controlled trial of sulphasalazine in treatment of ulcerative colitis. *Gut 5,* 437-441 (1964).
40. J. E. Lennard-Jones, A. M. Connell, J. H. Baron, and F. A. Jones. Controlled trial of sulphasalazine in maintenance therapy for ulcerative colitis. *Lancet 1,* 185-188 (1965).
41. A. Dissanayake and S. Truelove. A controlled therapeutic trial of long term maintenance treatment of ulcerative colitis with sulphasalazine. *Gut 14,* 923-926 (1973).
42. S. C. Truelove and L. J. Witts. Cortisone and cortiocotropine in ulcerative colitis. *Br. Med. J. 1,* 387-394 (1959).
43. J. E. Lennard-Jones, J. J. Misiewicz, A. M. Connel, J. H. Baron, and F. A. Jones. Prednisone as maintenance treatment for ulcerative colitis in remission. *Lancet 1,* 188-189 (1965).
44. P. F. Whittington, H. V. Barnes, and T. M. Bayless. Medical management of Crohn's disease in adolescence. *Gastroenterology 72,* 1338-1344 (1977).
45. J. W. Singleton. The national cooperative Crohn's disease study. Results of drug treatment. *Gastroenterology 72,* 1133 (1977).
46. B. I. Korelitz, N. Wisch, J. L. Glass, and D. H. Present. Long term response of Crohn's disease to treatment with 6-mercaptopurine. *Gastroenterology 74,* 1130 (1978).
47. W. J. Schnape, S. A. Matarazzo, and S. Cohen. Abnormal colonic myoelectric and motor responses to eating in ulcerative colitis. *Gastroenterology 74,* 1097 (1978).
48. R. E. Pounder, E. R. Craven, J. S. Henthorn, and J. M. Bannatyre. Red cell abnormalities associated with sulphasalazine maintenance therapy for ulcerative colitis. *Gut 16,* 181-185 (1975).
49. J. E. Fischer, G. S. Foster, R. M. Abel, W. M. Abbott, and J. A. Ryan. Hyperalimentation as primary therapy for inflammatory bowel disease. *Am. J. Surg. 125,* 165-175 (1973).
50. C. Vogel, T. Corwin, and A. Bave. Intravenous hyperalimentation in the treatment of inflammatory disease of the bowel. *Arch. Surg. 108,* 460-467 (1974).
51. T. H. Ehrenpreis. Surgical treatment of ulcerative colitis in childhood. *Arch. Dis. Child. 41,* 137-142 (1966).
52. S. O. Aylett. Three hundred cases of ulcerative colitis treated by total

colectomy and ileorectal anastomosis. *Br. Med. J. 1,* 1001-1005 (1966).

53. H. N. Nixon. Ileorectal anastomosis for inflammatory bowel disease in children. *Arch. Fr. Mal. App. Dig. 63*, 590-596 (1974).
54. N. G. Kock. Ileostomy without external appliance. *Am. Surg. 173,* 515-520 (1971).
55. A. J. Greenstein, D. B. Sacher, B. S. Pasternack, and H. D. Janowitz. Reoperation and recurrence in Crohn's colitis and ileocolitis. *N. Engl. J. Med. 293,* 685-690 (1975).
56. P. W. Brown, J. A. Bargen, and H. M. Weber. Chronic inflammatory lesions of small intestine (regional enteritis). *Am. J. Dig. Dis. Nutr. 1,* 426-431 (1934).
57. R. Colp. A case of nonspecific granuloma of terminal ileum and cecum. *Surg. Clin. N. Amer. 14,* 443-449 (1934).

11 Surgical Treatment of Inflammatory Bowel Disease in Children

KEITH M. SCHNEIDER and DAVID L. SCHWARTZ / Albert Einstein College of Medicine, Bronx, New York, and North Shore University Hospital, Manhasset, New York

JERROLD M. BECKER / State University of New York at Stony Brook Health Science Center, Stony Brook, New York, and Long Island Jewish Hospital Medical Center, New Hyde Park, New York

HENRY B. SO / Cornell University Medical College, New York, New York, and North Shore University Hospital, Manhasset, New York

I. Introduction and Background

Inflammatory bowel disease (IBD) in children includes ulcerative colitis and granulomatous disease of the small bowel and/or large intestine (Crohn's disease). A significant increase has been noted in the incidence of these diseases throughout the world. The highest incidence remains in the Western world, but cases are being reported more frequently in developing nations. The most striking change in incidence has been in granulomatous intestinal disease. Within the last two decades there have been reports of a doubling to quadrupling in frequency; the increase in ulcerative colitis has been more modest [1, 2].

Apporximately 20% of all patients with IBD will have their disease onset prior to 20 years of age [3]. About 3000 American children under 15 years of age will develop one of these two diseases each year. The literature does not substantiate a sex preponderance; however our own operative experience with 69 of these patients shows a 2:1 female preponderance in the 29 patients with ulcerative colitis and a 2:1 male preponderance in the 40 patients with granulomatous intestinal disease. A familial incidence is recorded in up to 15% [4] of all patients, but is more frequent in children. "Mixed disease," meaning ulcerative colitis in one family member and Crohn's disease in another is not uncommon. There have been nine sets of twins with IBD [5]. A striking similarity in age of onset and sites of involvement has been noted.

The etiology remains a mystery. There is no evidence to support a purely infectious origin [6]. The evidence implicating psychologic factors in the initiation of disease is unclear. Surgeons generally attribute psychologic stigmata in these patients to inanition, pain, and the inability to stray far from toilet facilities. The loss of these stigmata after successful therapy seems to substantiate this view. Nonetheless there is some evidence that a "premorbid" personality [7] may exist and antedate the disease onset. Our experience seems to substantiate such a concept, at least in some children; we see a typically egocentric, compulsively neat, dependent, and demanding child more frequently in IBD than in other illnesses requiring surgical intervention. There is little doubt that psychologic factors can provoke relapses and perhaps induce chronicity, but their ability to initiate the disease remains unproved.

The most attractive theory at the present time to explain the etiology of IBD is by an immune response in a hypersensitive patient to some enterobacterial antigen. In order to produce such a response the mucosal barrier to the penetration of antigen must be damaged; perhaps by an invasive organism (e.g., *Shigella, Yersinia*), drug (e.g., lincomycin, clindamycin), endotoxin, or other stimulus.

II. Ulcerative Colitis

Ulcerative colitis is a mucosal disease that generally begins in the rectum with nonspecific crypt abscesses and ulceration and advances proximally. A dilated ileocecal valve in "universal" (total) colitis results in a clinically insignificant "backwash" ileitis that extends no more than 10 cm into the terminal ileum. The onset of the disease is usually insidious; bloody diarrhea, tenesmus, and crampy abdominal pain are characteristic. In 5-10% of children however, the onset can be explosive, with fulminating disease, toxic megacolon, or massive hemorrhage [8]. In children this is more frequent than it is reported to be in adults. Fulminating disease does not require the presence of toxic megacolon; perforation can occur in its absence. Children are also more likely to have total involvement of the colon as well as a chronic, continuous course rather than an intermittent one.

Extraintestinal manifestations of the disease occur in up to 50% of pediatric patients [9]. These include growth retardation, delay in sexual maturation, "colitic" arthritis, uveitis, liver disease (e.g., fatty liver, pericholangitis), erythema nodosum, pyoderma gangrenosum, and nephrolithiasis. These manifestations may antedate bowel symptoms by several years and be responsible for significant delay in diagnosis.

Medical therapy of ulcerative colitis may be disappointing. The optimism engendered by the introduction of corticosteroids has diminished. It is unlikely that they increase the interval between disease onset and possible surgery [10]. Problems associated with their use include cushingoid appearance, osteoporosis, and accentuation of the delay in growth and maturation attributable to the primary disease. Steroids are, however, extremely valuable in the management of fulminating disease with or without toxic megacolon. Their use in combination with antibiotics and gastrointestinal decompression has allowed children to overcome such episodes, reserving surgery until their general condition has improved. Prior to the introduction of corticosteroids, more than 70% of children came to surgery because of one of the acute manifestations of the disease.

A. Indications for Surgery

Approximately 30-50% of children with ulcerative colitis may require surgery [12]. Variations in different clinics probably reflect both case selection and the differing philosophies of individual medical-surgical teams.

The results of chronic invalidism are now the most common indications for surgery. These include physical and sexual retardation, risk of malignancy, intractability, and the extraintestinal manifestations previously noted. Severe perianal disease, colonic stricture, and rectoperineal and rectovaginal fistulas are more commonly seen in granulomatous intestinal disease.

These indications differ from those in the adult only because of the remarkable retardation of growth seen in many of these children. Unless the progress of the disease is halted by medical or surgical means prior to puberty, as evidenced by epiphyseal closure, this growth deficit can be permanent. Colectomy prior to these events usually results in a resumption of normal growth and development. The diagnosis of growth delay may be subtle; standard pediatric developments charts can be misleading. Tanner's growth velocity curves and the measurement of serum follicle-stimulating hormone (FSH) and luteinizing hormone (LH) levels are important in documenting such delay and in appreciating postoperative "catch-up" growth spurts.

The risk of malignancy in ulcerative colitis has been well documented; the degree of such risk however, is still not generally appreciated. Carcinoma of the colon in such patients has a low salvage rate (24%) [13] because of the following factors: (1) these lesions are usually anaplastic; (2) diagnosis is delayed because of confusion with the symptoms of colitis; and (3) these tumors have an atypically flat radiographic appearance. Carcinoembryonic antigen levels have not been useful, since they can be elevated in patients with ulcerative colitis without carcinoma.

The risk of malignancy increases dramatically after 10 years of disease. For each ensuing decade 20% of these patients will develop a neoplasm [13]. Clinical quiescence offers no assurance of safety; to the contrary, most malignancies have occurred in youngsters with mild but prolonged disease. The risk for development of a carcinoma during the first 10 years of disease is approximately 3% [14]. Thus it is lower than in subsequent decades, but cannot be considered a "grace period." Any stricture occurring in ulcerative colitis, as opposed to granulomatous intestinal disease, must be considered malignant until disproved by colonic biopsy.

Intractability is the most frequent indication for surgery and the most difficult to quantitate and justify to our pediatric and gastroenterologic colleagues. It includes both intestinal and extraintestinal manifestations, the latter commonly being the major clinical determinant. Ehrenpreis and his associates [15] consider 1 year of total disability or 5 years of intermittent disability as adequate indication for surgery. The authors of this chapter believe that any child who has stigmata of the disease after 2 years of adequate therapy or who cannot be weaned from corticosteroid therapy is a surgical candidate.

B. Preparation for Surgery

Preparation for surgery includes adjustments of blood volume, albumin, prothrombin, and electrolytes. Total parenteral nutrition has been invaluable in the cachectic child. Adequate steroid support is mandatory in any patient who has received these drugs within a 3-year period prior to surgery. In uncomplicated cases steroid therapy is rapidly tapered within 7-10 days. A longer period is required for those patients with a significant postoperative complication. Because of inadequately explained seizures in three of our patients during the postoperative period, an electroencephalogram is now part of the preoperative work-up.

The psychologic preparation of these patients is equally important. This includes a frank but optimistic explanation of the operative procedure and its sequelae. If a standard ileostomy or a continent ileostomy is contemplated, the child is introduced to another youngster who has previously undergone a similar procedure. Most of our postoperative patients are outgoing and cheerfully participate in this program.

Prior to surgery an infraumbilical, transrectus site for placement of the stoma is chosen and indelibly marked. This is done with the patient in a sitting position, using the same ileostomy faceplate that will be used postoperatively. The sitting position is important to prevent displacement of the faceplate by the flexed thigh, with resultant injury to the stoma. The continent ileostomy can be placed lower because no appliance is required; it is located just above the pubic escutcheon in the right lower quadrant.

C. Surgical Procedure

The treatment of choice for the elective patient with ulcerative colitis is a one-stage proctocolectomy and ileostomy. The authors believe this procedure should be reserved for those patients with severe rectal disease but in good general condition. The poorer-risk patient is treated with a first-stage ileostomy and subtotal colectomy. Abdominoperineal resection of the rectum is reserved for a later date. Resection of the colon and rectum prior to the development of irreversible complications seems to cure ulcerative colitis. These patients have virtually the same life expectancy as a sample of the general population of the same age [13]. The operative mortality should be less than 5% in all patients and considerably less in the elective child. In 52 operations on 29 children, our only mortality occurred in a moribund 6-year-old boy who died within 8 hr of admission, despite an emergency cecostomy under local anesthesia.

Modern ileostomy techniques have almost eliminated such problems as prolapse, retraction, and stricture. The mucosa-lined stoma, as advocated by Brooke [16], has resulted in the elimination of the more severe forms of ileostomy dysfunction. Ileostomy appliances are now simple and effective.

Ileoproctostomy with preservation of the rectum is an alternative procedure that the authors have advocated in certain clinical settings. The adolescent without significant growth retardation, and with a short history of disease and minimal rectal involvement, is the ideal candidate for this procedure. Despite the fact that most of these patients will eventually require removal of the rectum, some can be maintained through the dating, courtship, and marriage period before surgery is required. The subject of rectal salvage remains controversial; the advantages of such a procedure may be counterbalanced by the need to maintain constant surveillance of the retained rectum by rectal biopsy and washings. Furthermore, less than optimum growth spurts are not uncommon. The authors have performed this procedure in 11 patients. Six have already required rectal resection.

The continent ileostomy [17] (Kock procedure) is an important addition to the surgeon's armamentarium. An intraabdominal reservoir is constructed with an intussusception in the efferent limb. The intussusception functions as a "one-way valve." No external appliance is required; patients catheterize their pouches three to five times daily with a relatively soft, large-bore plastic tube.

The authors have created such pouches in eight children, the youngest being 9 years of age. One patient required operative revision because of an inability to introduce the catheter easily. This was the consequence of an enlarging pouch being inadequately anchored to the anterior abdominal wall. All of our patients are now continent. They (and their parents) feel that this procedure has improved the quality of their lives.

Technical details in the performance of a continent ileostomy are vital to success. Lack of attention to them will result in an unacceptably high percentage of failures. Any surgical team embarking on such a program would be well advised to perfect their technique in the dog laboratory.

Ileoanostomy following colectomy and rectal mucosal excision ("pull-through" procedure) as described by Ravitch [18] has recently been enthusiastically endorsed by Martin et al. [19]. It would appear that continence can be achieved, but at the cost of a long period of disability resulting from the frequency of bowel movements and occasional nocturnal incontinence. This appears to subside within a year following closure of a diverting ileostomy. The "coring out" procedure requires a rectal mucosa that appears to be almost normal on gross inspection—total parenteral nutrition or a preliminary subtotal colectomy having been required to achieve this degree of healing. Further experience with this operative approach is required, but it appears to deserve a thorough clinical trial.

The management of toxic megacolon remains a difficult problem. Most, but not all, such children will require urgent surgery. Turnbull's "blowhole" technique of ileostomy and one or two colostomies have resulted in improved salvage [20]. Most patients will require secondary surgery for resection of the retained colon. The authors prefer a first-stage ileostomy and subtotal colectomy in such clinical situations, but would not hesitate to resort to venting in the critically ill child.

Postoperative problems are not uncommon. In particular, small-intestinal obstruction has not been eliminated. In most patients the obstruction responds to the passage of a long intestinal tube; on occasion, lysis of adhesions is required. Preoperative passage of intestinal tubes may decrease the incidence of early postoperative obstruction.

III. Granulomatous Intestinal Disease

Granulomatous intestinal disease (Crohn's disease) is a submucosal process that progresses transmurally to involve the entire wall of the bowel. It can involve any part of the gastrointestinal tract from the mouth distally. In approximately 50% of cases both small and large intestine will be involved. Approximately 10-15% of cases will be confined to the large intestine—creating diagnostic confusion with ulcerative colitis. The remainder are limited to the small intestine. Duodenal and jejunal involvemnt are relatively uncommon. Skip lesions occur in 15% of patients, while granulomas can be found in about 50%. Longitudinal ulcers and transverse fissures give rise to the typical "cobblestone" appearance of the mucosa. It is the slow penetration of these ulcers that give rise to the fistulas, sinuses, and abscesses that are the hallmarks of this disease. Sparing of the rectum is common, particularly on gross inspection, and right-sided colonic involvement is more common than left-sided disease.

Children with Crohn's disease have a more variable presentation than those with ulcerative colitis. Five percent are first seen with signs mimicking acute appendicitis. Perianal abscesses or fistulas are frequent presenting symptoms, and approximately 75% of the children will eventually have this problem. Other methods of presentation include: (1) fever of unknown origin, (2) protein-losing enteropathy, and (3) anemia without obvious gastrointestinal symptoms. As with ulcerative colitis, extraintestinal manifestations occur in 50% of patients, and these symptoms may precede the onset of bowel symptoms by many years [9]. A delay in diagnosis of 3-4 years is not infrequent. Unlike ulcerative colitis, in which remissions and relapses are clear-cut, Crohn's disease results in gradual but progressive deterioration.

Specific clinical manifestations are related to the site and extent of involvement. Abdominal cramps, diarrhea, and malabsorption are the result of small-intestinal disease. Colorectal disease produces bloody diarrhea, while gastroduodenal involvement is suggested by signs of pyloric obstruction and/or peptic ulcer.

Acute ileitis is probably not granulomatous intestinal disease. The clinical picture usually cannot be differentiated from acute appendicitis. It resolves rapidly without recurrence in the majority of patients. Yersinia infection has been implicated in some of these patients; culture of mesenteric nodes and/or blood agglutination studies are confirmatory. Surgery should be limited to appendectomy.

Indications for surgery are similar to those for ulcerative colitis. However, the risk of malignancy, while increased [21], is lower than in ulcerative colitis and does not support a policy of prophylactic resection. Internal fistulas, abscesses, intestinal strictures, and hydronephrosis secondary to retroperitoneal inflammation are indications found almost exclusively in granulomatous intestinal disease.

Medical therapy, including steroids, Azulfidine, immunosuppressives, antibiotics, rest, antispasmodics, vitamins, elemental diets, and total parenteral nutrition can usually give long periods of relatively good health and vigor before surgery is required. Eventually about 70% may require operative treatment [22].

The surgical treatment of granulomatous intestinal disease is local resection of the diseased bowel and end-to-end anastamosis. In more complicated cases (e.g., intraabdominal fistuals, abscesses, or severe cachexia) the authors prefer a diverting ileostomy. Bypass ileotransverse colostomy with exclusion is avoided because of a higher recurrence rate and the potential development of carcinoma in the bypassed segment. In the authors' experience the diverting ileostomy will almost invariably result in subsidence of the inflammation; secondary resection is performed within 12-16 weeks. Patients with severe perianal disease are candidates for resection and ileostomy, to divert the fecal stream and allow for characteristically slow healing [23]. An operative mortality of 2-3% is representative of results throughout the world. In our personal experience of 46 operations on 40 children there have been no early or late mortalities.

The recurrence rate following surgery for Crohn's disease is high. Actuarial studies indicate eventual recurrence in 80-90% of patients [24]. It appears that early recurrence is more common in the young. Despite the foregoing however, long periods of good health and catch-up growth generally occur before recurrences become clinically significant.

IV. Conclusions

Dramatic improvement is the almost invariable result of surgery for IBD. The development of secondary sexual characteristics and general body growth are a very satisfying feature of surgical therapy.

In ulcerative colitis, medical therapy has led to a mortality of 40% after 20 years of disease [13]. This is contrasted with an almost normal life expectancy following surgery. Ileostomy life cannot be compared with the security of normal bowel function; *it must be compared to life with ulcerative colitis.* Our patients uniformly regret the usual delay that occurred before surgery was performed. Children quickly learn to care for both the conventional ileostomy and the continent ileostomy. They no longer require medication and they can participate in most athletics. We are gratified by the excellent results that have been achieved in the surgery of ulcerative colitis.

In granulomatous intestinal disease a mortality of 10% after 15 years of disease has been reported [21]. Surgery decreases this mortality rate by a smaller degree than it reduces the mortality rate in ulcerative colitis. Nonetheless, operative intervention that is appropriately conceived and timed will usually result in improved health, vigor, and quality of life for prolonged periods.

References

1. J. Kyle and D. Blair. Epidemiology of regional enteritis in northeast Scotland. *Br. J. Surg. 52,* 215-217 (1965).
2. J. Myren, E. Gjone, J. N. Hertzberg, O. Rygvold, L. S. Semb, and B. Fretheim. Epidemiology of ulcerative colitis and regional enteritis (Crohn's disease) in Norway. *Scand. J. Gastroenterol. 6,* 511-514 (1971).
3. J. C. Goligher, H. L. Duthie, and H. H. Nixon. *Surgery of the Anus, Rectum and Colon,* 3 Ed. London, Baillière Tindall, Chap. 21, pp. 843-1012.

4. H. C. Singer, J. G. D. Anderson, H. Frischer, and J. B. Kirsner. Familial aspects of inflammatory bowel disease. *Gastroenterology 61,* 423-430 (1971).
5. J. F. Fielding. In *Recent Advances in Gastroenterology,* 2d Ed. (J. Badenoch and B. N. Brooke, Eds.). Williams & Wilkins, Baltimore, 1973, pp. 276-284.
6. S. L. Gorbach. In *Inflammatory Bowel Disease* (J. B. Kirsner and R. G. Shorter, Eds.). Lea & Febiger, Philadelphia, 1975, Chap. 4, pp. 47-59.
7. A. W. MacMahon, P. Schmitt, J. F. Patterson, and E. Rothman. Personality differences between inflammatory bowel disease patients and their healthy siblings. *Psychosom. Med. 35,* 91-103 (1973).
8. O. Broberger and R. Lagercrantz. Ulcerative colitis in childhood and adolescence. *Adv. Pediatr. 14,* 9-54 (1966).
9. R. Lagercrantz, J. Winberg, and R. Zeiterstrom. Extra-colonic manifestations in chronic ulcerative colitis. *Acta Paediatr. 47,* 675-687 (1958).
10. S. C. Truelove and L. J. Witts. Cortisone in ulcerative colitis. Final report on a therapeutic trial. *Br. Med. J. 1,* 387-394 (1959).
11. K. M. Schneider, J. M. Becker, B. I. Korelitz, I. H. Krasna, and A. Kark. The surgical treatment of ulcerative colitis in childhood. *J. Pediatr. Surg. 3,* 12-18 (1968).
12. T. H. Ehrenpreis, J. Gierup, and R. Lagercrantz. Chronic regional entercolitis (M. B. Crohn) in children and adolescents. *Acta Paediatr. Scand. 60,* 209-215 (1971).
13. G. J. Devroede, M. D. Dockerty, and W. G. Sauer. Cancer of the colon in patients with ulcerative colitis since childhood. *Can. J. Surg. 15,* 369-374 (1972).
14. G. J. Devroede, W. F. Taylor, W. Sauer, R. Jackman, and G. Stickler. Cancer risk and life expectancy of children with ulcerative colitis. *N. Engl. J. Med. 285,* 17-21 (1971).
15. T. H. Ehrenpreis. Ulcerative colitis. In *Pediatric Surgery,* 2d Ed. (W. T. Mustard, M. Ravitch, K. Welch, and W. Snider, Eds.). Year Book Med. Pub., Inc., 1969, pp. 940-948.
16. B. N. Brooke. The management of an ileostomy including its complications. *Lancet 2,* 102-104 (1952).
17. N. G. Kock. Ileostomy without external appliances. *Ann. Surg. 173,* 545-550 (1971).
18. M. M. Ravitch. Anal ileostomy with sphincter preservation in patients requiring total colectomy for benign conditions. *Surgery 24,* 170-187 (1948).
19. L. W. Martin, C. Lecoultre, and W. K. Schubert. Total colectomy and mucosal protectomy with preservation of continence in ulcerative colitis. *Ann. Surg. 186,* 477-480 (1977).
20. R. B. Turnbull, F. L. Weakley, W. A. Hawk, and P. Schofield. Choice of operation for the toxic megacolon phase of non-specific ulcerative colitis. *Surg. Clin. North Am. 50,* 1151-1169 (1970).

21. D. D. Weedon, R. G. Shorter, and D. M. Illstrup. Crohn's disease and cancer. *N. Engl. J. Med. 289,* 1099-1103 (1973).
22. J. Kyle. *Crohn's Disease.* Appleton-Century Crofts, New York, 1972, Chap. 8, pp. 149-163.
23. B. P. Colcock and J. H. Vansant. Surgical treatment of regional enteritis. *N. Engl. J. Med. 262,* 435-439 (1960).
24. A. J. Greenstein, D. B. Sachar, B. S. Pasternack, and H. D. Janowitz. Reoperation and recurrence in Crohn's colitis and ileocolitis. *N. Engl. J. Med. 293,* 685-690 (1975).

12 Nonabsorbable Resins in the Management of Gastrointestinal Disease

MOSHE BERANT / Cornell University Medical College, New York, New York, and North Shore University Hospital, Manhasset, New York

I. Introduction: General Properties

Cholestyramine is the chloride salt of a quaternary ammonium anionic exchange resin in which the basic group is attached to a styrene-divinylbenzene copolymer. It is insoluble in water and is not absorbed in the gut, as demonstrated by studies performed with ^{14}C-labeled cholestyramine [1]. The molecular weight of the resin is about one million. Cholestyramine is capable of binding a variety of anions, but the most characteristic property of the resin for its clinical use is the strong affinity for bile acid anions [2] and for long-chain fatty acid anions [3]. Each gram of cholestyramine resin is capable of binding about 910 mg sodium cholate. The relative in vitro capacity of various types of fiber for bile salt binding was investigated, and it was found that while lignin bound 30%, alfalfa 16%, bran 9%, and cellulose only negligible amounts, cholestyramine sequestered 81% of the bile salts [4]. A similar trend was observed when bile salt binding capacity of diverse fibers was studied in humans: fecal excretion of bile salts was greatest in subjects who received oral cholestyramine [2].

Bile salts are bound to the resin in the monomer rather than in the micellar form [5]. A carboxyl group on the side chain of the bile salt provides the anionic site for binding, while on cholestyramine the quaternary ammonium groups, after release of the chloride, provide the cationic site [6]. Thus, chloride is exchanged for the bile salt anion. Bile salt structure appears to be

Present Affiliation:
Rambam Medical Center, Haifa Israel

important in the determination of the bile salt's affinity for cholestyramine, by conferring to the bile salt ionic and/or steric factors which participate in the binding process. Taurine-conjugated bile salts have a higher affinity for cholestyramine than the glycine conjugates [6] because the relatively stronger acidic sulfonic group of taurine conjugates attracts the fixed quaternary ammonium groups on the resin better than the less acidic carboxyl group of glycine conjugates. Furthermore, it is assumed that the longer taurine side chain lends the bile salt a molecular configuration which brings its carboxyl group more easily in contact with the active groups on the resin. Bile salts, as well as fatty acids, seem to combine with cholestyramine in proportion to their degree of hydrophobic character. The hydrophobic dihydroxy bile salts, such as deoxycholate, are more firmly bound by cholestyramine than the relatively more hydrophilic trihydroxy bile salts, such as cholate [7]. Similarly, the hydrophobic long-chain fatty acids are strongly bound by the resin while the hydrophilic medium-chain fatty acids are practically unaffected [8].

Because of its sequestering properties, the administration of cholestyramine is likely to be of benefit principally in the management of clinical disorders which result from derangements in the quantity, quality, or localization of bile salts in the gastrointestinal tract. Bile salts are released into the duodenum as conjugates with glycine and taurine. These primary bile salts interact with the products of lipid digestion in the small intestine to form micelles, which allow the solubilization, transport, and absorption of mono- and diglycerides and fatty acids. During their transit distally toward the ileum, the bile salts are 7α-dehydroxylated, and a certain proportion are also deconjugated by the anaerobic bacteria which normally reside in the lower ileum and in the large intestine. The major site of bile salt reabsorption is the distal ileum; the integrity of this anatomic portion of the gut is essential for the adequate clearance of bile salts from the bowel, for their enterohepatic circulation, and for the maintenance of the body's bile acid pool. Aberrations in bile salt metabolism may result in products which are injurious to normal gastrointestinal function, as described below.

II. Pathophysiology and Experimental Observations

Experimental work with animals and with humans has demonstrated that an infusion of deconjugated bile salts into the large intestine evokes a variety of alterations: there may be a cathartic effect, with increased colonic motility [9] and a derangement in glucose, water, and electrolyte transport [10, 11], as well as activation of adenylate cyclase in colonic epithelial cells, with a rise in cyclic AMP (cAMP) and consequent electrolyte and water secretion [12, 13].

In the small intestine, the jejunum is the portion which is the most sensitive to the deleterious effects of deconjugated bile salts [14]. Exposure of the jejunal mucosa of rats to deconjugated bile salts results in a depression of the epithelial enzyme, (Na^+-K^+)-ATPase, with a consequent impairment in glucose and sodium transport. These derangements have been demonstrated both by the feeding of deconjugated bile salts to rats [15] and by the in vivo perfusion of the rat jejunum with deconjugated bile salts [16]. Perfusion studies have also shown that deconjugated bile salts cause disruption of the jejunal mucosal barrier to the absorption of potentially antigenic macromolecules [17]. Deconjugation of bile salts in the upper small intestine may also impair fat absorption [18]. The formation of micelles for the proper solubilization, transport, and absorption of fats demands an adequate proportion of conjugated bile salts. Therefore, if the extent of deconjugation of the bile salts is carried beyond the levels which would enable micelle formation (critical micellar concentration), long-chain fatty acids will fail to be incorporated into micelles and will accumulate in the small-intestinal lumen [18].

Free fatty acids themselves are damaging to intestinal mucosa, and their hydroxylation by bacteria adds to their potential for injury [19]. When applied to intestinal mucosa, free fatty acids cause electrolyte and water secretion [20-23]; in the colon, hydroxy fatty acids activate adenyl cyclase, accounting for their secretory effect on water and sodium [24].

The majority of studies concerning the ill effects of the products of bacterial overgrowth in the upper small bowel have been conducted as "acute" experiments, by exposing the small-intestinal mucosa to artificially high concentrations of deconjugated bile salts and of free fatty acids. Therefore, the results obtained from these studies may not always reflect the consequences of bacterial colonization of the upper gut in a true-to-life situation, as in malnutrition and diarrheal disease.

We have recently studied the effects of cholestyramine on the alterations induced by colonization with fecal and colonic bacteria in the upper small intestine in rats [25]. Bacterial colonization of the jejunum was achieved, in male Wistar rats weighing 70-90 g, by inhibition of normal peristalsis with injections of an autonomic ganglionic blocking agent—mecamylamine hydrochloride—for 3 days. The counts of anaerobic bacteria—bacteroides, clostridia, and lactobacilli—were found to be higher by three orders of magnitude in the jejunal fluid of the mecamylamine-treated rats than in the controls.

The rats with the higher anaerobic population in the upper gut had significantly higher intraluminal concentrations of free fatty acids and deconjugated bile salts than the controls, and demonstrated jejunal transport derangements. In vivo perfusion of a jejunal segment showed a striking difference in the jejunal transport of sodium: the rats with the high jejunal anaerobic flora had marked Na^+ secretion into the jejunal lumen, whereas the control rats had Na^+ absorption. The deranged Na^+ absorption could not be ascribed to a depression of mucosal (Na^+-K^+)-ATPase, since the levels of this enzyme were similar in the jejunal mucosa of the experimental and the control rats. On the other hand, the Na^+ secretion in the mecamylamine-treated rats was correlated with a jejunal mucosal cAMP which was increased threefold over that of the controls. A rise in mucosal cAMP is known to mediate jejunal Na^+ secretion [26], and appears to be the mechanism implicated in the jejunal Na^+ secretion observed in the mecamylamine-treated rats.

The possibility of enterotoxin (elaborated by the colonizing bacteria in the small-intestinal contents) inducing the rise in mucosal cAMP was examined, but no enterotoxin could be detected in the luminal fluid. The feeding of cholestyramine to mecamylamine-treated rats blunted the derangements of intestinal function which were induced by bacterial colonization of the upper small bowel. Cholestyramine (4%), in the diet fed to rats for the 3-day period during which bacterial overgrowth in the jejunum was induced by means of mecamylamine, resulted in low luminal concentrations of free fatty acids and undetectable levels of deconjugated bile salts. Furthermore, the jejunal mucosal cAMP concentrations were like those of the normal controls, and there was Na^+ absorption in the jejunum. Thus, the rise in mucosal cAMP and the consequent Na^+ secretion appear to be related to the intraluminal accumulation of free fatty acids and deconjugated bile salts resulting from bacterial metabolism.

III. Clinical Applications of Cholestyramine

A. Cholerheic (Cholegenic) Enteropathy

The term cholerheic (cholegenic) enteropathy is applied to the clinical entity which results from the effect of bile salts on the colon. Patients who have a diseased ileum, or who have undergone resection or bypass of the distal ileum, tend to suffer from troublesome diarrhea, abdominal cramps, tenesmus, and also steatorrhea. Since the distal ileum is the main site for reabsorption of bile salts, it has been assumed that these symptoms are caused by exaggerated amounts of bile salts—mostly deconjugated—reaching the large bowel. These patients excrete large amounts of bile salts in their stools, and cholestyramine has dramatic effects in the management of this bile salt-induced diarrhea [27-30]. There are additional clinical situations, besides ileal disease or resection, in which cholerheic enteropathy is involved, and therapy with cholestyramine has given satisfactory results.

B. Postvagotomy Syndrome

About 1-2% of patients who have undergone truncal vagotomy suffer from troublesome continuous diarrhea, abdominal cramps, and tenesmus, and have increased amounts of deconjugated bile salts in their stools [31, 32]. The theory behind these features is that the denervation causes a relaxation of the ileocecal valve, resulting in the onrush of ileal contents into the colon. The exaggerated amounts of bile salts propelled into the colon then exert their damaging effect. Several studies, including double-blind trials, indicate that cholestyramine is of definite value in the management of these patients [32-35]. It has been proposed that *diabetic diarrhea,* caused by gastrointestinal diabetic neuropathy, is induced similarly to the postvagotomy syndrome—namely, by cholerheic enteropathy—and that cholestyramine might be indicated [36].

C. Radiation Enteritis

Radiation therapy to the abdomen is frequently complicated by profuse diarrhea. Irradiation of the abdomen of rats with 1250 rad caused severe diarrhea and 100% mortality within 4-6 days. Further experiemnts showed that the diarrhea and the mortality could be prevented if the bile flow into the intestine was diverted [37, 38]. The administration of cholestyramine was found to have a protective effect, similar to that of the diversion of bile from the intestinal lumen [39].

D. "Bile Salt Gastritis"

Endoscopic observations have confirmed earlier reports that duodenogastric reflux is important in the pathogenesis of erosive gastritis and gastric ulcer [40]. In vitro and in vivo experiments demonstrate that bile salts can provoke extensive damage to gastric mucosa when local hyperacidity prevails [40, 41]. Consequently, a bile salt binding agent, i.e., cholestyramine, has been employed in the treatment of gastritis and gastric ulcer, but with conflicting results [41-44]. An understanding of the conflicting data may be obtained by consideration of the conditions that prevail in the stomach. In the small intestine the alkaline environment is above the pK_a of the bile salts, which are thus in an ionized state and are therefore amenable to anion exchanging with—and binding to—cholestyramine. In the stomach, on the other hand, the acidic pH is lower than the pK_a of the bile salts; these are therefore nonionized, and cholestyramine becomes ineffective. It is therefore not surprising that cholestyramine has a good effect on "bile salt gastritis" when antacids are given concomitantly [42].

E. Bacterial Overgrowth in the Small Bowel ("Contaminated Small-Gut Syndrome")

The upper small intestine, which normally is practically devoid of bacteria, may become colonized with fecal and colonic flora. Such bacterial overgrowth, causing malabsorption and diarrhea—the "contaminated small-gut syndrome" [45]—is encountered in (among others) malnourished children who live in a poor and insanitary environment [46], in disturbances of small-intestinal motility and drainage as in the blind-loop syndrome [47, 48], and in elderly individuals [49]. Also patients with regional ileitis [50] and with jejunoileal bypass [51, 52] have a propensity for contaminated small-gut syndrome. The anaerobic bacteria which participate in the colonization of the upper small bowel are capable of deconjugating bile salts [53], thereby contributing to the accumulation of an agent which is injurious to small-intestinal mucosa. The sequestration of the damaging deconjugated bile salts with cholestyramine may be a temporizing therapeutic approach. The patient with the contaminated upper gut, whether or not actually having overt diarrhea, is in a precarious state of balance, since fluid-electrolyte malnutrition is often a prelude or an aggravating factor in protein-energy malnutrition. Consideration of the pathophysiologic processes involved in the contaminated small-gut situation suggests that cholestyramine may be a useful therapeutic adjunct in the management of these patients.

F. Chronic, Nonspecific Diarrheal Disease

Balistreri et al. [54] reported infants with chronic diarrhea in whom increased fecal excretion of deconjugated bile salts was found. These infants responded well to treatment with cholestyramine, suggesting that their diarrhea had probably been perpetuated by the cholerheic mechanism, as ileal dysfunction could also be demonstrated. Cholestyramine has also been successfully used in the treatment of pseudomembranous colitis [55] and in intractable diarrhea following surgical correction of gastrointestinal tract disease in neonates [56].

Several reports indicate that cholestyramine is beneficial in the management of protracted infantile diarrhea [57, 58]. However, the uncritical use of cholestyramine as a panacea for diarrheal disease has led to its being discredited. In a controlled study of 120 infants with diarrhea, cholestyramine proved to be of value only in those infants whose diarrhea was of a long-term or recurrent nature, and whose nutritional state was unsatisfactory—that is, in infants who were the likely candidates for a contaminated upper small intestine.* Evidently, as is also true for any drug, the benefit from treatment with cholestyramine becomes apparent only when it is used in the appropriate patient population and with the proper indication.

G. Cholestatic Syndromes

Intrahepatic cholestasis in early infancy may result from anatomic or functional causes. The most frequent anatomic factors are related to the so-called "neonatal

*M. Berant and Y. Wagner, unpublished data.

hepatitis syndrome," which is associated with bile stasis. The rise in serum bile acids may impair hepatocellular bile acid metabolism and further derange the excretion of bile salts [59]. Thus, cholestasis per se, whatever its origin, can initiate a vicious cycle, because the accumulation of bile acids in the hepatic cell causes a self-depression of hepatocellular bile salt clearance, with further impairment of bile flow [59, 60]. During cholestasis there is an increase in monohydroxy bile salts, and one of them, 3β-hydroxy-5-cholenoate, bears the name "cholestatic acid" for good reasons [59].

The administration of cholestyramine in cholestasis results in an increased flow of bile, provided that there are at least remnants of patent bile ducts [59, 61, 62]. As a result of the trapping of bile salts in the small-intestinal lumen, their enterohepatic recirculation is broken. The resultant reduction in serum bile acid levels relieves the liver of its toxic burden and thereby enables a better processing—metabolism and transport—of the bile salt load. The reduction in serum bile salts by the administration of cholestyramine also results in improvement of the severe pruritus which frequently accompanies cholestasis [59, 61].

H. Hypercholesterolemia

Cholestyramine leads to a reduction in serum cholesterol levels via its influence on both endogenous and exogenous cholesterol metabolism.

1. Endogenous. Cholesterol is a precursor in bile acid synthesis. Trapping of bile salts by cholestyramine within the small intestine reduces bile acid concentrations in serum. This, in turn, activates increased bile acid synthesis in the liver—thereby consuming serum cholesterol and lowering serum cholesterol levels [63].

2. Exogenous. Dietary cholesterol is insoluble in water and is carried in the core of micelles to the jejunal mucosa for its absorption. Cholestyramine interferes with micelle formation and disturbs the mechanism for the absorption of cholesterol. By virtue of its cholesterol-lowering effects, cholestyramine is considered as a major drug to be employed in the management of familial hypercholesterolemia type 2 in childhood [64, 65].

I. Poisoning

Much popular attention has recently been given to the successful treatment with cholestyramine of industrial intoxication with chlordecone (Kepone), an organochloride pesticide. Kepone is secreted into the bile and is reabsorbed into the circulation from the gut. Cholestyramine intercepts Kepone in the intestinal lumen, and the poison is eliminated in the stools. A trap is established, and the gradient thus formed enables the gradual withdrawal of the toxic substance from the tissues. This course of events has been demonstrated to occur also in animal experiments [66]. It appears that cholestyramine can be of value for removing from the body toxic substances which undergo enterohepatic circulation.

IV. Side Effects and Complications of Cholestyramine

The use of cholestyramine is a difficult form of therapy because of the low palatability of the drug. However, when diluted in orange juice or apple sauce, or when suspended in water, cholestyramine is quite well accepted. Along with the drug at least a 4:1 volume of fluid must be ingested in order to provide an adequate liquid environment for the anion exchange to take place, and in order to prevent the formation of an obstructing bezoar. Intestinal obstruction is a possible complication, especially in cystic fibrosis [67]. Hyperchloremia and metabolic acidosis may occur during long-term treatment with cholestyramine as a result of the exchange of bile salt anions and other anions for the chloride anion on the resin [68]. This side effect can be easily corrected with the administration of sodium bicarbonate. There are other undesirable side effects [69]. Administration of cholestyramine in high doses may cause streatorrhea. A daily dose of 30 g resin to an adult will cause streatorrhea within 3 weeks as a consequence of sequestration of bile salts and fatty acids in the intestine and the exhaustion of the body's bile acid pool. Bile salt trapping may also lead to a deficiency of fat-soluble vitamins, which are dependent on the availability of bile salts for their absorption. Folate malabsorption and deficiency are also liable to occur, as dietary folate consists mainly of polyglutamates, which are anionic and may therefore be bound to cholestyramine. Cholestyramine can interfere with the absorption of a wide range of drugs [70], especially ionic drugs like warfarin, phenylbutazone, thiazides, and phenobarbital. In addition, cholestyramine interferes with the absorption of thyroxine, L-thyroxine, and also digitoxin. These interactions must be taken into consideration when patients receiving these drugs also need cholestyramine.

The influence of cholestyramine on intestinal absorptive function has been studied mainly by follow-up of children on long-term therapy, up to 36 months, for treatment of familial hypercholesterolemia type 2 [65, 71]. Most of the patients with a normal dietary fat intake had a fecal fat excretion of over 5 g per day, but none had diarrhea, and all grew normally. As expected, levels of vitamins A, D, E, and K and red cell folate concentrations tended to fall in all the patients; but proper supplementation of these substances prevented the development of deficiency states.

V. Conclusion

Cholestyramine is a valuable therapeutic factor in the management of gastrointestinal disease states, but it must be applied judiciously, and only in those cases where an understanding of the mode of action of the resin and an understanding of the pathophysiology of the underlying disease process indicate that the administration of the drug is warranted.

References

1. D. G. Gallo and A. L. Sheffner. The disposition of orally administered cholestyramine-C^{14}. *Proc. Soc. Exp. Biol. Med. 120,* 91-92 (1965).
2. M. M. Stanley, D. Paul, D. Gacke, and J. Murphy. Effects of cholestyramine, metamucil, and cellulose on fecal bile salt excretion in man. *Gastroenterology 65,* 889-894 (1973).
3. L. M. Hagerman, D. A. Julow, and D. L. Schneider. In vitro binding of mixed micellar solutions of fatty acids and bile salts by cholestyramine. *Proc. Soc. Exp. Biol. Med. 143,* 89-92 (1973).
4. J. A. Story and D. Kritchevsky. Comparison of the binding of various bile acids and bile salts in vitro by several types of fiber. *J. Nutr. 106,* 1292-1294 (1976).
5. L. M. Hagerman, D. A. Cook, and D. L. Schneider. Effect of cholestyramine particle size on in vitro binding of conjugated bile salts. *Proc. Soc. Exp. Biol. Med. 139,* 248-253 (1972).
6. W. H. Johns and T. R. Bates. Qualification of the binding tendencies of cholestyramine. I. Effect of structure and added electrolytes on the binding of unconjugated and conjugated bile-salt anions. *J. Pharm. Sci. 58,* 179-183 (1969).
7. A. F. Hofmann and D. M. Small. Detergent properties of bile salts: Correlation with physiological function. *Annu. Rev. Med. 18,* 333-376 (1976).
8. R. W. Harkins, L. M. Hagerman, and H. P. Sarett. Absorption of dietary fats by the rat in cholestyramine-induced steatorrhea. *J. Nutr. 87,* 85-92 (1965).
9. W. O. Kirwan, A. N. Smith, W. D. Mitchell, J. D. Falconer, and M. A. Eastwood. Bile acids and colonic motility in the rabbit and the human. *Gut 16,* 894-902 (1975).
10. D. L. Wingate, E. Krag, H. S. Mekhjian, and S. F. Phillips. Relationships between ion and water movement in the human jejunum, ileum and colon during perfusion with bile acids. *Clin. Sci. Mol. Med. 45,* 593-606 (1973).
11. D. R. Saunders, J. R. Hedges, J. Sillery, L. Esther, K. Matsumura, and C. E. Rubin. Morphological and functional effects of bile salts on rat colon. *Gastroenterology 68,* 1236-1245 (1975).
12. D. R. Conley, M. J. Coyne, G. G. Bonorris, A. Chung, and L. J. Schoenfield. Bile acid stimulation of colonic adenylate cyclase and secretion in the rabbit. *Am. J. Dig. Dis. 21,* 453-458 (1976).
13. M. Taub, G. Bonorris, A. Chung, M. J. Coyne, and L. J. Schoenfield. Effect of propranolol on bile acid- and cholera enterotoxin-stimulated cAMP and secretion in rabbit intestine. *Gastroenterology 72,* 101-105 (1977).
14. G. E. Sladen and J. T. Harries. Studies on the effects of unconjugated

dihydroxy bile salts on rat small intestinal function in vivo. *Biochim. Biophys. Acta 288,* 443-456 (1972).

15. M. Gracey, J. Papadimitriou, V. Burke, J. Thomas, and G. Bower. Effects on small-intestinal function and structure induced by feeding a deconjugated bile salt. *Gut 14,* 519-528 (1973).
16. E. Guiraldes, S. P. Lamabadusuriya, J. E. J. Oyesiku, A. E. Whitfield, and J. T. Harries. A comparative study on the effects of different bile salts on mucosal ATPase and transport in the rat jejunum in vivo. *Biochim. Biophys. Acta 389,* 495-505 (1975).
17. U. Fagundes-Neto, S. Teichbert, M. A. Bayne, B. Morton, and F. Lifshitz. Bile salt enhanced jejunal macromolecular absorption. *Fed. Proc. 37,* 699 (1978).
18. R. E. Schneider and F. E. Viteri. Luminal events of lipid absorption in protein-calorie malnourished children; relationship with nutritional recovery and diarrhea. 1. Capacity of the duodenal content to achieve micellar solubilization of lipids. *Am. J. Clin. Nutr. 27,* 777-787 (1974).
19. S. Tabaqchali. The pathophysiological role of small intestinal bacterial flora. *Scand. J. Gastroenterol. (Suppl.) 6,* 139-163 (1970).
20. H. V. Ammon and S. F. Phillips. Inhibition of ileal water absorption by intraluminal fatty acids. *J. Clin. Invest. 53,* 205-210 (1974).
21. W. S. Cline, V. Lorenzsonn, L. Benz, P. Bass, and W. A. Olsen. The effects of sodium ricinoleate on small intestinal function and structure. *J. Clin. Invest. 58,* 380-390 (1976).
22. H. V. Ammon and S. F. Phillips. Inhibition of colonic water and electrolyte absorption by fatty acids in man. *Gastroenterology 65,* 744-749 (1973).
23. P. Bright-Asare and H. J. Binder. Stimulation of colonic secretion of water and electrolytes by hydroxy fatty acids. *Gastroenterology 64,* 81-88 (1973).
24. H. J. Binder. Cyclic adenosine monophosphate controls bile salt and hydroxy fatty acid-induced colonic electrolyte secretion. *J. Clin. Invest. 53(A),* 7-8 (1974).
25. M. Berant, M. A. Bayne, R. A. Wapnir, and F. Lifshitz. Cholestyramine inhibition of jejunal Na^+ secretion in small bowel bacterial colonization. *Pediatr. Res. 12,* 430 (1978).
26. S. G. Schultz, R. A. Frizell, and H. N. Nellans. Ion transport by mammalian small intestine. *Annu. Rev. Physiol. 36,* 51-91 (1974).
27. A. F. Hofmann. The syndrome of ileal disease and the broken enterohepatic circulation: Cholerheic enteropathy. *Gastroenterology 52,* 752-797 (1967).
28. G. G. Rowe. Control of diarrhea by cholestyramine administration. *Am. J. Med. Sci. 255,* 84-88 (1968).
29. A. F. Hofmann. Bile acid malabsorption caused by ileal resection. *Arch. Intern. Med. 130,* 597-605 (1972).

30. W. G. Thompson. Treatment of cholerheic diarrhea with cholestyramine and a hydrophilic colloid. *Dis. Conol. Rectum 18,* 304-307 (1975).
31. J. G. Allan, V. P. Gerskowitch, and R. I. Russell. The role of bile acids in the pathogenesis of postvagotomy diarrhea. *Br. J. Surg. 61,* 516-518 (1974).
32. J. G. Allan and R. I. Russell. Cholestyramine in treatment of postvagotomy diarrhea—Double-blind controlled trial. *Br. Med. J. 1,* 674-676 (1977).
33. J. A. Ayulo. Cholestyramine in postvagotomy syndrome. *Am. J. Gastroenterol. 57,* 207-225 (1972).
34. J. H. B. Scarpello and G. E. Sladen. Post-vagotomy diarrhea. *Lancet 1,* 646-647 (1977).
35. T. V. Taylor, M. E. Lambert, and H. B. Torrance. Valuc of bile-acid binding agents in post-vagotomy diarrhea. *Lancet 1,* 635-636 (1978).
36. J. R. Condon, M. I. Suleman, Y. S. Fan, and M. D. McKeown. Cholestyramine and diabetic and post-vagotomy diarrhea. *Br. Med. J. 1,* 519 (1974).
37. M. F. Sullivan. Dependence of radiation diarrhea on the presence of bile in the intestine. *Nature 195,* 1217-1218 (1962).
38. J. O. Archambeau, M. Maetz, and J. E. Jesseph. The effects of bile diversion and pancreatic duct ligation on the gastrointestinal syndrome in dogs receiving 1500 rads whole body irradiation. Abstract. *Radiat. Res. 25,* 173 (1965).
39. R. N. Berk and D. G. Seay. Cholerheic enteropathy as a cause of diarrhea and death in radiation enteritis and its prevention with cholestyramine. *Radiology 104,* 153-156 (1972).
40. R. A. Rovelstad. The incompetent pyloric sphincter. Bile and mucosal ulceration. *Am. J. Dig. Dis. 21,* 165-173 (1976).
41. W. P. Ritchie, Jr. and E. W. Shearburn. Influence of isoproterenol and cholestyramine on acute gastric mucosal ulcerogenesis. *Gastroenterology 73,* 62-65 (1977).
42. N. S. Mann. Bile-induced acute erosive gastritis. Its prevention by antacid, cholestyramine and prostaglandin E_2. *Am. J. Dig. Dis. 21,* 89-92 (1976).
43. H. Meshkinpour, J. Elashoff, H. Stewart III, and R. A. L. Sturdevant. Effect of cholestyramine on the symptoms of reflux gastritis. A randomized double blind, crossover study. *Gastroenterology 73,* 441-443 (1977).
44. G. L. Eastwood. Failure of cholestyramine to prevent bile salt injury to mouse gastric mucosa. *Gastroenterology 68,* 466-472 (1975).
45. M. Gracey. Intestinal absorption in the 'contaminated small-bowel syndrome'. *Gut 12,* 403-410 (1971).
46. M. Gracey, J. Suharjono, W. Sunoto, and D. E. Stone. Microbial contamination of the gut: Another feature of malnutrition. *Am. J. Clin. Nutr. 26,* 1170-1174 (1973).

47. Y. S. Kim, N. Spritz, M. Blum, J. Terz, and P. Sherlock. The role of altered bile acid metabolism in the steatorrhea of experimental blind loop. *J. Clin. Invest. 45,* 956-962 (1966).
48. D. E. Polter, J. D. Boyle, L. G. Miller, and S. M. Finegold. Anaerobic bacteria as cause of the blind loop syndrome. *Gastroenterology 54,* 1148-1154 (1968).
49. S. H. Roberts, O. James, and E. H. Jarvis. Bacterial overgrowth syndrome without "blind loop": A cause for malnutrition in the elderly. *Lancet 2,* 1193-1195 (1977).
50. R. Prizont, T. Hersh, and M. H. Floch. Jejunal bacterial flora in chronic small bowel disease. *Am. J. Clin. Nutr. 23,* 1602-1607 (1970).
51. E. J. Drenick, M. E. Ament, S. M. Finegold, P. Corrodi, and E. Passaro. Bypass enteropathy. *JAMA 236,* 269-272 (1976).
52. P. Corrodi, P. A. Wideman, V. L. Sutter, E. J. Drenick, E. Passaro, and S. M. Finegold. Bacterial flora of the small bowel before and after bypass procedure for morbid obesity. *J. Infect. Dis. 137,* 1-6 (1978).
53. T. Midtvedt. Microbial bile acid transformation. *Am. J. Clin. Nutr. 27,* 1341-1347 (1974).
54. W. F. Balistreri, J. C. Partin, and W. K. Schubert. Bile acid malabsorption–A consequence of terminal ileal dysfunction in protracted diarrhea of infancy. *J. Pediatr. 89,* 21-28 (1977).
55. F. Sinatra, W. L. Buntain, C. H. Mitchell, and P. Sunshine. Cholestyramine treatment of pseudomembranous colitis. *J. Pediatr. 88,* 304-306 (1976).
56. H. S. Nagaraj, L. Cook, T. G. Canty, and G. Haight. Oral cholestyramine and paregoric therapy for intractable diarrhea following surgical correction of catastrophic disease of the GI tract in neonates. *J. Pediatr. Surg. 11,* 795-801 (1976).
57. M. A. Tamer, T. R. Santora, and D. H. Sandberg. Cholestyramine therapy for intractable diarrhea. *Pediatrics 53,* 217-220 (1974).
58. M. Berant, Y. Wagner, and N. Cohen. Cholestyramine in the management of infantile diarrhea. *J. Pediatr. 88,* 153-154 (1976).
59. N. B. Javitt. Cholestasis in infancy. *Gastroenterology 70,* 1172-1181 (1976).
60. J. L. Boyer. Bile secretion and the pathogenesis of cholestasis. Viewpoints on digestive diseases. *10,* 1-4 (1978).
61. H. L. Sharp, J. B. Carey, Jr., J. G. White, and W. Krivit. Cholestyramine therapy in patients with a paucity of intrahepatic bile ducts. *J. Pediatr. 71,* 723-736 (1967).
62. N. B. Javitt, K. P. Morrissey, E. Siegel, H. Goldberg, L. M. Gartner, M. Hollander, and E. Kok. Cholestatic syndromes in infancy: Diagnostic value of serum bile acid pattern and cholestyramine administration. *Pediatr. Res. 7,* 119-125 (1973).
63. S. Shefer, S. Hauser, and E. H. Mosbach. 7α-Hydroxylation of cholestanol by rat liver microsomes. *J. Lipid Res. 9,* 328-333 (1968).
64. R. J. West and J. K. Lloyd. Use of cholestyramine in treatment of children with familial hypercholesterolemia. *Arch. Dis. Child. 48,* 370-374 (1973).

65. C. J. Glueck, R. C. Tsang, R. W. Fallat, and M. Mellies. Therapy of familial hypercholesterolemia in childhood: Diet and cholestyramine resin for 24 to 36 months. *Pediatrics 59,* 433-441 (1977).
66. W. J. Cohn, J. J. Boylan, R. V. Blanke, M. W. Fariss, J. R. Howell, and P. S. Guzelian. Treatment of chlordecone (Kepone) toxicity with cholestyramine. *N. Engl. J. Med. 298,* 243-248 (1978).
67. J. D. Lloyd-Still. Cholestyramine therapy and intestinal obstruction in infants. *Pediatrics 59,* 626-627 (1977).
68. J. V. Hartline. Hyperchloremia, metabolic acidosis, and cholestyramine. *J. Pediatr. 89,* 155 (1976).
69. W. G. Thompson. Cholestyramine. *Can. Med. Assoc. J. 104,* 305-309 (1971).
70. D. G. Gallo, K. R. Bailey, and A. L. Sheffner. The interaction between cholestyramine and drugs. *Proc. Soc. Exp. Biol. Med. 120,* 60-68 (1965).
71. R. J. West and J. K. Lloyd. The effect of cholestyramine on intestinal absorption. *Gut 16,* 93-98 (1975).

PART III

Intestinal Absorption Disorders

13 Penetration of Epithelial Barriers by Macromolecules: The Intestinal Mucosa

SAUL TEICHBERG / Cornell University Medical College, New York, New York, and North Shore University Hospital, Manhasset, New York

I. Introduction

A number of cellular barriers impede the passage of macromolecules across epithelia. These barriers include: (1) the properties of the cell surface, particularly certain immunoglobulins (reviewed in Ref. 1; see also Chapter 7 of this volume) that appear to inhibit the adsorption of foreign proteins to the plasma membrane of the epithelial cells; (2) tight junctional seals [2-7] that are impermeable to all but the smallest molecules and are formed by the very close apposition of the plasma membranes of adjacent epithelial cells [7-9] ; and (3) an intracellular lysosomal degradative mechanism capable of digesting all classes of foreign macromolecules that enter the cell by endocytosis [10-15] . Furthermore, intact foreign macromolecules that manage to penetrate these barriers and cross the epithelium are also susceptible to engulfment by wandering tissue macrophages.

Despite these defenses against the transepithelial flow of intact macromolecules, there is normally a significant penetration of some intact protein and partially degraded protein fragments [16] across several epithelia in experimental animals, including neonatal and adult intestinal mucosa [4, 17-19], choroid plexus from cerebrospinal fluid to blood [2, 20] , seminal vesicle [21] , and yolk sac [22] epithelia. This transport is increased by damage to the barrier systems during disease (or experimentally induced intestinal stress) [1, 23-28] .

This chapter reviews the organization of the structural barriers that regulate the penetration of macromolecules across epithelia and discusses how these barriers may be modified or damaged. We will principally focus out attention on the mucosal epithelium of the small intestine. (In Chapter 7 a comprehensive review is made of the development of host defense mechanisms and the mucosal barrier to the uptake of intestinal antigens and microorganisms.)

II. Epithelial Absorptive Barriers

A. Adsorption

An initial step necessary for the penetration of intact macromolecules across epithelia involves adsorption onto the surface of the epithelial cell. This adsorption appears to be controlled by several factors, including cell secretions [29, 30], surface immunological characteristics [1, 31, 32], cell surface charge [33], net charge of the foreign protein [34, 35], and, in the case of the small intestine, the efficiency of normal intraluminal digestion [36].

In general, cells bear a net negative charge on their surface, because of the presence of sulfated mucopolysaccharides that extend out of the surface plasma membrane into the external environment. This surface coat is very well developed and readily visualizable by routine transmission electron microscopy as the "fuzzy" coat on the microvilli of the jejunal epithelium [37, 38]. In the small intestine this coat also consists of a number of digestive enzymes, particularly oligosaccharidases [39, 40]. A number of recent reports indicate that net positively charged macromolecules have an appreciably greater affinity than neutrally charged or negatively charged macromolecules for cell surfaces. For example, cationic ferritin binds more avidly to pituitary cell surfaces than anionic ferritin [34]. A similar, though not exactly parallel, relationship between net positive charge and increased binding capacity has been demonstrated for variously charged peroxidase or dextran tracers along the basement membrane of the glomerular capillary loop [35]. While no direct evidence on this electrostatic relationship has been presented in the case of intestinal epithelia, in view of the sulfated mucopolysaccharides present on the surface of the microvilli, we think it likely that similar processes are operative. It is of interest that the most frequently utilized macromolecular tracer used in experimental systems is horseradish peroxidase (HRP), a basic protein with a net positive charge; HRP is readily adsorbed to cell surfaces, including the intestinal mucosa.

The interactions of exogenous proteins with the surface of epithelial cells may also be modified by cellular secretions. For example, Walker, Wu, and Bloch [30] demonstrated an increased production of goblet cells secreting mucus—an increase induced by the presence of absorbable protein. It has been suggested that the mucus "washes off" adherent antigens.

The role of local intestinal antibodies in the absorption of foreign antigens is a subject of growing interest [1, 28, 31, 32]. In brief, immunoglobulins on the mucosal surface, principally secretory IgA, but IgG as well, are thought to bind to undigested foreign protein and prevent adsorption to the cell surface. The role of this inhibition of macromolecular absorption by intestinal antibodies is emphasized by the work of Walker et al. [32], who showed that oral prefeeding of rats with HRP inhibited its subsequent absorption [32] (see Chapter 7).

Furthermore, clinical studies show that patients with secretory IgA (SIgA) deficiency have immunological sensitivities that can be related to oral antigen absorption; such an association has, for example, been recently demonstrated for milk protein hypersensitivity following gastroenteritis [28] in patients with SIgA deficiency. The mode of action of secretory IgA in preventing antigen absorption is not thoroughly understood. It has been suggested that binding and immobilization of antigens by SIgA promotes their digestion by intraluminal proteases [1, 41].

In addition to immunoglobulins and other cell secretions, luminal physiological conditions may affect antigen absorption. Rodewald [42] has presented evidence that intestinal luminal pH plays a role in the regulation of neonatal immunoglobulin absorption in rats. In our own experience pH does not appear to play a role in peroxidase absorption by the adult rat intestine.

Exogenous proteins or other particles that are successfully adsorbed to the cell surface could cross the epithelium either by migrating in small vesicles from one surface to the other, in a manner analogous to the "bulk" transport seen in endothelial cells [43-45], or by passing between the epithelial cells through the intercellular spaces. There are, however, substantial obstacles against macromolecular penetration via either of these routes.

B. Tight Junctional Barriers

Epithelia, such as the intestinal mucosa, renal tubular epithelium, or choroid plexus, contain a well-developed junctional complex [7-9] between adjacent cells. These specializations of the plasma membranes of adjacent cells are usually located toward the apical luminal surface of the epithelium and consist of three regions: a tight junction (zonula occludens), belt desmosome (zonula adhaerens), and button desmosomes (macula adhaerens). Another junctional structure located randomly over epithelia is the gap junction (reviewed in Ref. 46), which mediates the exchange of small molecules between the cells.

For purposes of the present discussion the most important structure is the tight junction. In these complexes located at the most apical region of the epithelium, plasma membranes of adjacent cells are practically fused (Figs. 1-4)—forming a barrier usually impenetrable to macromolecules moving from either direction. Freeze-fracture electron microscopy has demonstrated that this zone is composed of a series of interconnected, crisscrossed bands made of intramembranous particles [7-9] and surrounding the epithelium like a belt [37]. Under routine transmission electron microscopy one can occasionally obtain an image of a completely obliterated intercellular space, or a series of loci where plasma membranes touch (Fig. 1). If tracer macromolecules such

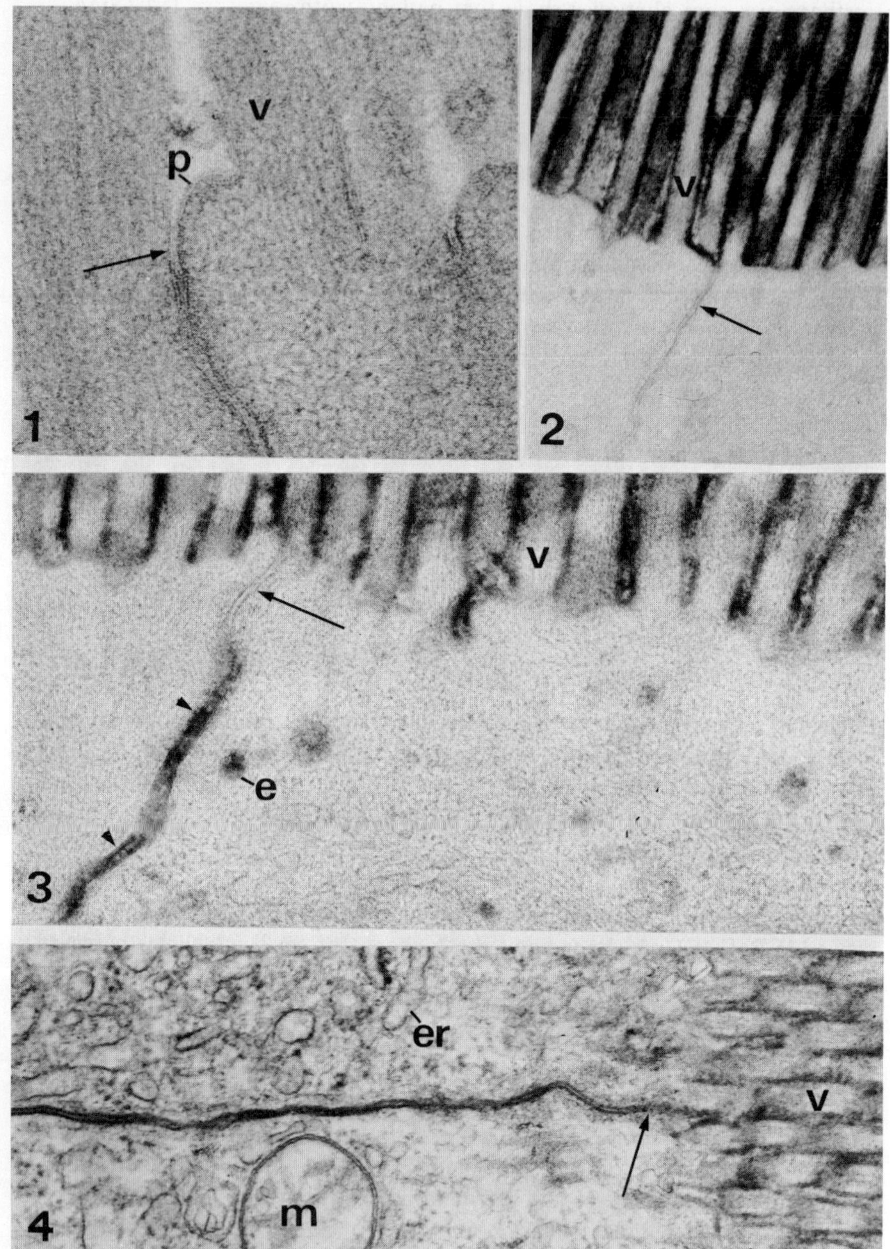
1
v
p
2
v
3
v
e
4
er
v
m

as horseradish peroxidase or colloidal lanthanum hydroxide suspension are added to the cell surface or injected into the circulation, tracer penetration normally ceases at the tight junction (Fig. 2). This barrier function is seen in a variety of epithelia including intestinal mucosa [4, 17, 26], renal tubular epithelium [4, 5, 47], and the choroid plexus epithelium of the blood-brain barrier [3, 48]. In addition to their barrier function, it is thought that tight junctions also prevent the lateral movement of intramembranous proteins and lipids [49-53] within the plane of the membrane [8, 9].

On the other hand, the tight junctional zone does permit the flow of water and ions through the intercellular spaces. Certain "leaky" epithelia, including the small intestinal epithelium have low resistance tight junctions that are readily permeable to the flux of small ions [54].

Figure 1 Electron micrograph of apical region of two rat absorptive jejunal epithelial cells, indicating tight junctional zone (arrow) where adjacent plasma membranes (p) are almost fused, forming barrier to penetration of intact macromolecules. Microvilli are at v. X 102,000.

Figure 2 From rat jejunal preparation exposed to macromolecular tracer, horseradish peroxidase (mol 40,000), while being perfused with "control" isotonic (280 mosM) NaCl-glucose solution. Reaction product localizing tracer is seen along microvilli (v). However, tracer is not demonstrable in intercellular space between adjacent epithelial cells (arrow). Under these control perfusion conditions, there is only a minimum of tracer absorption, and none is seen in the tight junctional zone. X 25,000.

Figure 3 Portion of two absorptive epithelial cells from jejunal preparation of a rat fed 60% lactose diet for 1 week. Jejunum was then perfused in vivo with same horseradish peroxidase control solution as in Figure 2. In addition to reaction product for peroxidase along microvilli (v), tracer is also found in endocytotic vesicles (e) and in intercellular spaces between absorptive epithelial cells (arrowheads). Note that since there is no demonstrable peroxidase in tight junctional zone (arrow). Tracer found in deeper regions of intercellular spaces may have been transported via endocytotic vesicles or may have leaked through tight junctional zones that are not in the plane of section of this micrograph. X 55,500.

Figure 4 Jejunal absorptive epithelial cells from preparation perfused with NaCl-glucose solution containing 5 mM deoxycholate, a secondary 7α-dehydroxylated, deconjugated bile salt, and horseradish peroxidase. Reaction product for peroxidase is seen on microvillar brush border (v), and tracer also appears to pass through tight junctional zone (arrow) into deeper regions of intercellular space between epithelial cells. Endoplasmic reticulum at er; mitochondrion at m. X 40,000.

The other junctional specializations, desmosomes and gap junctions, present no barrier to macromolecular penetration. The belt desmosomes (zonula adhaerens) are specializations between adjacent cells with a 200-Å intercellular space. In this zone, numerous filaments focus on a plasma membrane region, and some dense material is deposited in the intercellular space. This structure may play a

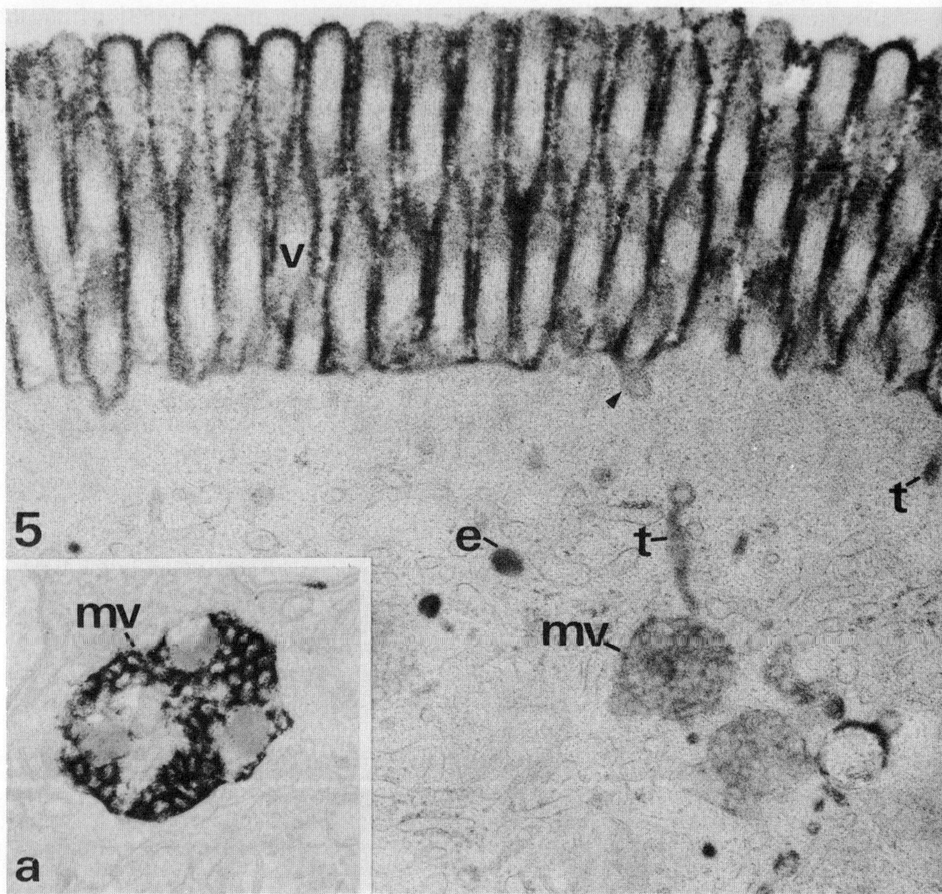

Figure 5 From jejunal preparation of rat fed 60% maltose diet, which appears to produce increased rate of pinocytotic activity. Preparation was then perfused with horseradish peroxidase-containing physiologic solution. Tracer is seen along microvillar brush border (v), in forming endocytotic vesicles (arrowhead), in mature endocytotic vesicles (e), tubules (t), and multivesicular bodies (mv). These multivesicular bodies incorporate much of the endocytosed horseradish peroxidase. The lysosomal, degradative nature of these bodies is illustrated in insert: from preparation incubated for localization of acid phosphatase, a characteristic lysosomal marker enzyme. Note strong acid phosphatase reaction in epithelial cell multivesicular body (mv). Figure, × 26,000; insert, × 41,000.

role in microvillar motility by acting as an anchorage zone for the 60-Å, thin, actin-like filaments that extend from the core of microvilli across the terminal web and into the desmosomal region. This structure may also be an important attachment site for adjacent cells. The button desmosomes (macula adhaerens) are also attachment sites between adjacent epithelial cells. Their discrete button-like structure obviates any barrier functions, since molecules of macromolecular dimensions are free to percolate around them.

C. Lysomal Barrier

Alternatively, macromolecules that are prevented from leaking across epithelial junctions may migrate across the cell in micropinocytotic vesicles. This vesicle transport plays a major role in the flow of serum proteins across capillary endothelia [43-45]. In most cell types, however, foreign proteins entering the cell by endocytosis are subject to degradation in lysosomes (reviewed in Ref. 10). Endocytosis consists of the budding into the cell of a small fragment of the surface membrane in the form of a vesicle roughly 1000-2000 Å in diameter. The endocytotic vesicles contain in their lumina foreign molecules that may have been attached to the cell surface or were in the immediately surrounding extracellular medium. Endocytotic structures may also be tubular in structure, and some of these tubules may fold back on themselves, forming doughnut-like structures [55], called cup-shaped bodies, that are thought to be precursor multivesicular bodies. In small-intestinal epithelium, endocytotic vesicles and tubules arise in the pits at the base of microvilli and enter the terminal web region (Figs. 3, 5). These vesicles may fuse to form the larger apical vacuolar structures, typical of renal tubular epithelium [5, 13]. As endocytotic vesicles form, "coats" of fibrillar material are often, though not always, seen attached to the vesicle membrane on its cytoplasmic side [10, 56, 57]. The role of these coats is not clear; they are transient structures and may conceivably exert some pulling action on the vesicles, in association with as yet undefined cellular contractile systems [6, 22].

The predominant fate of these endocytotic structures appears to be degradation in lysosomes (reviewed in Ref. 10). For a variety of cell types, including jejunal epithelia, neuronal perikarya, macrophages and other white blood cells, renal tubular epithelia, choroid plexus epithelia, and many other cell types, it has been demonstrated that endocytotic structures fuse with multivesicular bodies and other lysosomal structures (reviewed in Refs. 10, 13, 58). A multivesicular body (MVB) is a large, membrane-delimited vacuolar body containing small internal vesicles (Fig. 5). Fusion of an endocytotic vesicle with an MVB results in the dumping of the contents of the vesicle into the lumen of the MVB and incorporation of the endocytotic vesicle membrane into the surrounding membrane of the MVB. Some of the internal vesicles of the MVB are formed when a portion of the outer MVB membrane buds inward into the lumen of this structure. It is known that MVBs fuse with small primary lysosomes containing acid hydrolases that break down all classes of macromolecules (lipases, proteases, nucleases, carbohydrases) [10, 59, 60]. These primary lysosomes bud from Golgi apparatus-associated membrane systems [10], as described by Novikoff [61, 62]. The fusion of primary lysosomes with MVBs converts the latter into active lysosomal structure (Fig. 5), resulting in the release of small molecules for recycling as nutrients. This process of incorporation, sequestration, and degradation of intact proteins in lysosomes is very dramatically seen in renal tubular epithelium and is the core mechanism of protein reabsorption [5, 13].

Although lysosomal degradation provides a significant barrier to the penetration of macromolecules across cells, there may be important exceptions whereby materials escape these degradative processes. In endothelia, for example, materials move across the cell via small micropinocytotic vesicles that rarely if ever interact with lysomes [43-45]. This is probably due to the particular physical constraints of this system; there are few lysosomes in the thin rims of cytoplasm of the typical endothelial cells. The content of the micropinocytotic vesicle is released into the intercellular space by exocytosis (reverse pinocytosis). Another example of endocytotic structures escaping digestion concerns the double-stranded viral RNA of reovirus which is not susceptible to lysosomal nucleases. Thus, the virus taken up by endocytosis into lysosomes uses the lysosomal proteases for uncoating of the particle, and then the viral RNA begins to replicate within the lysosome, eventually spreading to the cytoplasm by some unknown mechanisms [63]. Certain other organisms, such as *Toxoplasma*, when phagocytized into macrophages [64], are able to live in these phagocytic vacuoles which lose their ability to fuse with lysosomal particles. A major immunologic puzzle related to these phenomena concerns immunologic memory mediated by macrophages. Initial endocytosis of antigen by a macrophage is known to increase tremendously the subsequent response of lymphocytes to the reappearance of antigen. A possible mechanism underlying this process is that some endocytotic vesicles in macrophages escape fusion with lysosomes and are re-released onto the macrophage surface where they can interact with lymphocytes [65].

Another important exception to the degradation of endocytosed macromolecules concerns the flow of maternal antibody and absorption of other intact proteins in the neonatal intestine and the leakage of intact protein from the circulation into the intestinal lumen. Such leakage may become very marked and lead to hypoproteinemia during certain diseases. These intestinal epithelial processes will be discussed in detail below.

III. Normal Transepithelial Penetration of Intact Macromolecules

Although the tight junctions, lysosomal degradative functions, and secreted immunoglobulins may impede the translocation of macromolecules across epithelia, they do not always entirely abolish this process. The chief route for the normal penetration of intact macromolecules across epithelia is probably endocytosis coupled to exocytosis. Thus, extracellular tracers such as HRP that are endocytosed at the base of microvilli of the small intestine appear to move in small vesicles to the lateral cell margins beyond the tight junctional zone (Fig. 3). At this site it is thought that the tracer-containing membrane-delimited vesicles fuse with the lateral plasma membrane of the cell, allowing the release of vesicular content into the intercellular space between epithelial cells [2, 4, 17-19, 21, 22]. It appears that some of the endocytotic vesicles avoid fusion with multivesicular bodies or other lysosomal structures; however, the relative proportions of vesicles that meet each of these fates is unclear. We do not understand what controls the fusions between the relevant cellular compartments (see discussion in Ref. 10). Perhaps these are in part random quantitative processes depending on the frequency of collisions between endocytotic vesicles and MVBs, other lysosomes, or lateral plasma membrane. That more than such a random phenomenon is involved is indicated by the fact that some membrane-delimited organelles never fuse, despite their proximity, while others readily do. Perhaps fusions are related to the presence of a "coat"; or perhaps certain membrane rearrangements or molecular exchanges occur during the formation of endocytotic vesicles—that lead to an alteration in their ability to fuse with the membranes of MVBs.

A similar endocytotic shuttle system is thought to transport IgA from the lamina propria across the intestinal epithelium to the microvillar surface, where it is presumably released by exocytosis [66]. In this case, the complexing of IgA with secretory component at the basal face of the epithelial cell is a significant step in the process. It is not clear whether or not secretory component prevents incorporation of the IgA into lysosomal structures. In the choroid plexus, transepithelial penetration of HRP from the cerebrospinal fluid into the circulation also occurs by means of endocytotic vesicles which escape the lysosomal system (Ref. 2; for a contrary view, see Ref. 3). On the other hand, blood-to-cerebrospinal-fluid flow of HRP appears entirely blocked by the choroid plexus epithelium utilizing both the tight junctions and lysosomal degradation [3]. In the case of renal tubular epithelium there is no evidence that protein reabsorbed at the luminal surface by endocytosis ever crosses the epithelium; the lysosomes in this epithelium are very large and active, and reports of protein leakage may be due to perfusion-pressure artifacts [47].

In summary, the best available evidence lends support to the view that the normal transport of intact macromolecules across epithelia of the small intestine and other systems occurs via the movement of endocytotic vesicles that escape the lysosomal system of the cell and go around the tight junctional barrier. We think it is highly unlikely that macromolecules which enter phagocytic structures that are incorporated into multivesicular bodies, are able to be released from these into the intercellular space. Firstly, only those particles or macromolecules with very special properties (e.g., double-stranded RNA of reovirus) [10, 63] appear able to elude digestion, once enveloped within lysosomal structures. Secondly, there are no compelling morphologic studies demonstrating this process, whereas fusion of endocytotic vesicles with the lateral cell margin has been demonstrated [2]. Where phagocytic or heterophagic lysosomal processes have been studied in detail, macromolecules incorporated into lysosomes are invariably degraded, and only small metabolites are released.

Even if larger macromolecules were released from lysosomes into the cytosol, it seems unlikely that such rather large molecules could cross the plasma membrane unless they were to have certain special properties. Plasma membrane permeability is known to decrease with increasing molecular size, and molecules of macromolecular dimension cannot normally be transported across the plasma membrane. Yet, one should not come to hard and fast conclusions. It is known, for example, that certain proteins can be inserted into membranes from their cytoplasmic face; that is, these "endoproteins" probably migrate in the cytosol and stick into the bimolecular leaflet of the plasma membrane on its cytoplasmic face (see Ref. 49 for review). Furthermore, some evidence has been presented indicating that the catalase of peroxisomes enters into the cisternal lumen of these membrane-delimited cytoplasmic structures via a cytosolic route.

A further mystery concerns the eventual fate of lysosomes, about which almost nothing is known. Only in hereditary lysosomal storage diseases do these structures accumulate in large numbers in cells and thereby disrupt cellular metabolism. Cells appear to have some means, as yet unknown, to dispose of lysosomes. Until these processes are more fully understood, we cannot rule out the possibility of more subtle events mediating the flow of intact molecules. Despite the caveats discussed here, the best positive evidence that can be mustered favors the view that a vesicle shuttle mechanism transfers macromolecules across epithelia under normal physiological conditions. A schematic outline of the possible movements of the pertinent intracellular compartments is seen in Figure 6.

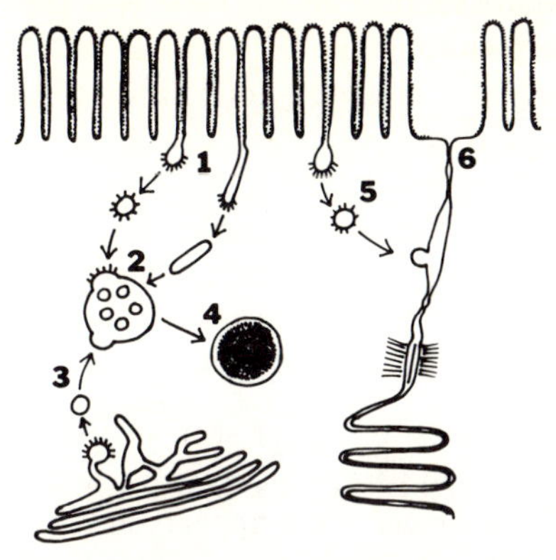

Figure 6 Schematic diagram illustrating some probable routes taken by exogenous macromolecules coming into contact with intestinal epithelial cell. At 1, endocytotic vesicles and tubules at base of microvilli are seen forming by budding into epithelial cell cytoplasm. Typically, these endocytotic structures are believed to fuse with multivesicular bodies seen at 2. Golgi apparatus derived vesicles (3) containing lysosomal acid hydrolases can then fuse with multivesicular bodies, converting these structures into functional lysosomes that eventually appear as dense bodies (4) containing residual undigested or partially digested material. Some endocytotic material apparently escapes fusion with multivesicular bodies, and, instead, fuses with plasma membrane at lateral cell margin (5), releasing its contents by exocytosis into intercellular space beyond apical tight junctional region (6). Any macromolecules absorbed by this route are able to diffuse in intercellular spaces to lamina propria. Tight junctional barrier (6) normally prevents gross leakage of macromolecules from lumen to blood or vice versa. This barrier can break down under some conditions of intestinal stress.

IV. Pathophysiologic Alterations in Intestinal Macromolecular Transport

Under certain conditions of pathophysiologic stress the normal barriers to the transepithelial migration of macromolecules may be functionally or structurally altered, leading to an increased leakage of intact proteins across epithelia. These conditions have been examined in the small intestine for lumen-to-blood as well as blood-to-lumen flow. Surgical trauma to the intestine [25], chronic protein-calorie malnutrition [23], luminal hyperosmolality [26], alcohol feedings [67], and deconjugated bile salts [68] have all been reported to alter the tight junctional barrier to macromolecular absorption (Table 1). The evidence for this process derives from cytochemical and quantitative analysis of the lumen-to-blood transport of a macromolecular tracer, horseradish peroxidase. Reaction product for this tracer has been demonstrated in the tight junctional zone, in deeper regions of the intercellular spaces, and in capillaries of jejunal epithelia during some of the above intestinal stresses (Fig. 4). Even in these pathophysiologic preparations the tracer is most frequently found only on the brush border and in deeper regions of the intercellular spaces [26]. Depending

Table 1 Experimental Pathophysiologic Conditions Associated with Increased Intestinal Macromolecular Absorption

Surgical trauma	Bile salt deconjugation
Malnutrition	Alcohol
Hyperosmolality	Lactose diarrhea

on conditions, there is a greater or lesser frequency of tracer seen in the tight junctional zone. For example, with luminal hyperosmolality [26] and deconjugated bile salts such as deoxycholate, the tracer often appears in the tight junctional zone, while with conjugated bile salts (at high concentrations) this is only a very occasional event. The latter observations have been interpreted as indicating that small breaks in the integrity of the tight junctional barrier [25, 26] may lead to significant leakage of tracer into deeper regions of the intercellular spaces. Clearly, these processes may be quite complex; for example, in hypertonically perfused jejunal preparations we also noted increased rates of endocytosis into the epithelium. Therefore, an acceleration of the normal rate of endocytotic vesicle transport, as described in Section III.C may also contribute to the tracer translocation.

We have been studying the effects of intraluminal bile salts and their 7α-dehydroxylated and deconjugated derivatives that may arise in the small intestine as a result of the metabolism of colonic bacteria that proliferate in the upper gastrointestinal tract during chronic diarrhea [69, 70]. Our studies indicate that elevated levels (5 mM) of all cholate salts, conjugated or deconjugated, increase the intestinal absorption of HRP from lumen to blood [68]. The increased jejunal absorption of HRP, seen with the primary conjugated salt taurocholate (Tch) at a 5 mM perfusion concentration, is quantitatively small, but is significant in comparison to bile salt-free controls. When the concentration of Tch is lowered to 0.5 mM, the HRP absorption is indistinguishable from that in controls. This penetration of HRP is most marked with the deconjugated salts, and greatest with the secondary dehydroxylated salt, deoxycholate. At lower luminal bile salt concentrations, 0.5 mM, only the deconjugated salts increase the absorption of HRP over levels seen in controls. With the deconjugated salts, especially at higher concentrations, HRP is demonstrable in the tight junctional zone between epithelial cells. Perhaps the detergent properties of the deconjugated bile salts, particularly deoxycholate, extract important membrane molecules, damaging the tight junctional barrier. Or, the deconjugated salts may sequester cell surface components such as secretory IgA–increasing rates of tracer

Recent studies in our laboratory on marasmatic protein-calorie malnutrition in young rats show that this condition leads to an increased sensitivity of the jejunal mucosa to the damaging effects of deoxycholate salts [71] ; thus, for example, HRP absorption from lumen to blood–induced by deoxycholate at low 0.5-mM levels–is even greater when the deoxycholate induction is superimposed on protein-calorie malnourishment in rats. It may be noteworthy that the 3-week malnourished young rats, who gain no weight, show a compensating increase in villus height, and have remarkably intact jejunal mucosal absorptive epithelial cells under the electron microscope, with a well-developed microvillar brush border. Clinically, malnourished children possess a severely damaged intestinal mucosa which is generally associated with intestinal infection. The notion that infection induces the damage to the intestinal mucosa of malnourished children is further supported by our findings of an increased sensitivity of the jejunum of malnourished rats to deoxycholate-induced macromolecular absorption.

We have also investigated the effects of jejunal luminal hyperosmolality on macromolecular absorption. Luminal hypertonicity arising as the result of nutrient malabsorption is a major cause of diarrhea and is well illustrated by the problem of lactose intolerance [72, 73]. Our initial studies focused on a purely nonabsorbable hyperosmotic agent, mannitol [26]. Perfusion of rat jejunum with hypertonic mannitol clearly increased cytochemically demonstrable jejunal HRP absorption in rats.

More recently, we have been evaluating the more clinically relevant case of lactose intolerance (see also Chapter 23 in this volume). The rats we use are lactase deficient, and lactose feedings, at a high (60%) concentration, induce diarrhea. Our evidence shows that rats fed 60% lactose for 1-7 days have an increased rate of HRP absorption (Fig. 3). This is also seen after 21 days of lower dose (5-20%) lactose feedings that do not induce diarrhea.

Clinical studies have now shown that milk protein allergy can be associated with lactose intolerance and a secretory IgA deficiency [28]. Several other intestinal disorders have been associated with an apparent increased antigen absorption. For example, Gruskay and Cooke [24] demonstrated increased egg albumin absorption following acute gastroenteritis. A good body of evidence favors the view that celiac disease is mediated by a local intestinal sensitivity to absorbed gluten [74]. Children with soy protein sensitivity, apparently induced during the course of enteritis, have been described [75, 76].

Clearly, the conditions and mechanisms that can increase the absorption of potential antigens from the intestine and the consequences to the host of this process are of major clinical importance and require further intensive study.

Acknowledgment

This work was supported in part by U.S. Public Health Service Grant 508 RR09128-07A1.

References

1. W. A. Walker and K. J. Isselbacher. Intestinal antibodies. *N. Engl. J. Med. 297,* 767-773 (1977).
2. B. Van Deurs, M. Miller, and O. Amtorp. Uptake of horseradish peroxidase from CSF into the choroid plexus of the rat, with special reference to transepithelial transport. *Cell Tissue Res. 187,* 215-234 (1978).
3. M. W. Brightman. Ultrastructural characteristics of adult choroid plexus: Relation to the blood-cerebrospinal fluid barrier to proteins. In *The Choroid Plexus in Health and Disease* (M. G. Netsky and S. Shuangshati, Eds.). Univ. Press of Virginia, Charlottesville, 1975, pp. 86-112.
4. W. A. Walker, R. Cornell, M. Davenport, and K. J. Isselbacher. Macromolecular absorption: Mechanism of horseradish peroxidase uptake and transport in adult and neonatal rat intestine. *J. Cell Biol. 54,* 195-205 (1972).
5. R. C. Graham and M. J. Karnovsky. The early stages of absorption of injected horseradish peroxidase in the proximal tubules of mouse kidney: Ultrastructural cytochemistry by a new technique. *J. Histochem. Cytochem. 14,* 291-302 (1966).
6. H. S. Bennet. The cell surface: Components and confirgurations. In *Handbook of Molecular Cytology* (A. Lima-de-Faria, Ed. Elsevier North Holland, Amsterdam, 1969, pp. 1261-1293.
7. M. G. Farquhar and G. E. Palade. Junctional complexes in various epithelia. *J. Cell Biol. 17,* 375-412 (1963).
8. L. A. Staehelin. Structure and function of intercellular junctions. *Int. Rev. Cytol. 39,* 191-283 (1974).
9. L. A. Staehelin and B. E. Hall. Junctions between living cells. *Sci. Am. 238*(5), 141-152 (1978).
10. E. Holtzman. *Lysosomes: A Survey.* Springer-Verlag, Vienna, 1976.
11. C. deDuve. The lysosome in retrospect. In *Lysosomes in Biology and Pathology* (J. T. Dingle and H. B. Fell, Eds.), Vol. 1. Elsevier North-Holland, Amsterdam, 1969, pp. 3-40.
12. B. Van Deurs. Endocytosis in high endothelial venules. Evidence for transport of exogenous material to lysosomes by uncoated "endothelial" vesicles. *Microvasc. Res. 16*:280-293 (1978).
13. A. B. Maunsbach. Functions of lysosomes in kidney cells. In *Lysosomes in Biology and Pathology* (J. T. Dingle and H. B. Fell, Eds.). Elsevier North-Holland, Amsterdam, 1969, pp. 115-154.

14. R. Wattiaux. Biochemistry and function of lysosomes. In *Handbook of Molecular Cytology* (A. Lima-de-Faria, Ed.). Elsevier North-Holland, Amsterdam, 1969, pp. 1159-1178.
15. D. S. Friend. Cytochemical staining of multivesicular bodies. *J. Cell. Biol. 41,* 267-279 (1969).
16. W. A. Hemmings and E. W. Williams. Transport of large breakdown products of dietary protein through the gut wall. *Gut 19,* 715-723 (1978).
17. R. Cornell, W. A. Walker, and K. J. Isselbacher. Small intestinal absorption of horseradish peroxidase. A cytochemical study. *Lab. Invest. 25,* 42-48 (1971).
18. R. Rodewald. Intestinal transport of antibodies in the newborn rat. *J. Cell Biol. 58,* 189-211 (1973).
19. D. Orlic and R. Lev. Fetal rat intestinal absorption of horseradish peroxidase from swallowed amniotic fluid. *J. Cell Biol. 56,* 106-119 (1973).
20. K. Mollgard, D. H. Malipowska, and N. R. Saunders. Lack of correlation between tight junction morphology and permeability properties in developing choroid plexus. *Nature 264,* 293-294 (1976).
21. L. R. Mata. Dynamics of HRPase absorption in the epithelial cells of the hamster seminal vesicles. *J. Microsc. Biol. Cell. 25,* 127-132 (1976).
22. L. A. Moxon, A. E. Wild, and B. S. Slade. Localization of protein in coated micropinocytotic vesicles during transport across rabbit yolk sac endoderm. *Cell Tissue Res. 171,* 175-193 (1976).
23. B. S. Worthington, E. S. Boatman, and G. E. Kenny. Intestinal absorption of intact proteins in normal and protein-deficient rats. *Am. J. Clin. Nutr. 27,* 276-286 (1974).
24. F. L. Gruskay and R. E. Cooke. The gastrointestinal absorption of unaltered protein in normal infants and in infants recovering from diarrhea. *Pediatrics 16,* 763-770 (1955).
25. R. S. Rhodes and M. J. Karnovsky. Loss of macromolecular barrier function associated with surgical trauma to the intestine. *Lab. Invest. 25,* 220-229 (1971).
26. M. Cooper, S. Teichberg, and F. Lifshitz. Alterations in rat jejunal permeability to a macromolecular tracer. *Lab. Invest. 38,* 447-454 (1978).
27. E. J. Eastham and W. A. Walker. Effect of cow's milk on the gastrointestinal tract: A persistent dilemma for the pediatrician. *Pediatrics 60,* 477-481 (1977).
28. M. Harrison, A. Kilby, J. A. Walker-Smith, N. E. Frace, and C. B. S. Wood. Cow's milk protein intolerance: A possible association with gastroenteritis, lactose intolerance and IgA deficiency. *Br. Med. J. 1,* 1501-1504 (1976).
29. D. R. Strombeck and D. Harrold. Binding of cholera toxin to mucins and inhibition by gastric mucin. *Infect. Immun. 10,* 1266-1272 (1974).
30. W. A. Walker, M. Wu, and K. J. Bloch. Stimulation by immune complexes of mucus release from goblet cells of the rat small intestine. *Science 197,* 370-372 (1977).
31. W. A. Walker. Host defense mechanisms in the gastrointestinal tract. *Pediatrics 57,* 901-916 (1976).
32. W. A. Walker, K. J. Isselbacher, and K. J. Bloch. Intestinal uptake of

macromolecules: Effect of oral immunization. *Science 177,* 608-610 (1972).

33. F. Grinnell, M. Q. Tobleman, and C. Hackenbrock. The distribution and mobility of anionic sites on the surfaces of baby hamster kidney cells. *J. Cell Biol. 66,* 470-479 (1975).
34. M. G. Farquhar. Recovery of surface membrane in anterior pituitary cells. *J. Cell Biol. 77,* R35-R42 (1978).
35. B. M. Brenner, T. H. Hostretter, and D. H. Humes. Molecular basis of proteinuria of glomerular origin. *N. Engl. J. Med. 298,* 826-833 (1978).
36. S. C. Kraft, R. M. Rothberg, and C. M. Knauer. Gastric output and circulating antibovine serum albumin in adults. *Clin. Exp. Immunol. 2,* 321-330 (1967).
37. J. S. Trier. Morphology of the epithelium of the small intestine. In *Handbook of Physiology,* Sect. 6, The Alimentary Canal, Vol. 3. The American Physiological Society, Washington, D.C., 1968, pp. 1125-1175.
38. S. Ito. The enteric surface coat on the cat intestinal microvilli. *J. Cell Biol. 27,* 475-491 (1965).
39. D. Miller and R. K. Crane. The digestive function of the epithelium of the small intestine. II. Localization of disaccharide hydrolysis in the isolated brush border portion of intestinal epithelial cells. *Biochim. Biophys. Acta 52,* 293-298 (1961).
40. D. H. Alpers and B. Seetharan. Pathophysiology of diseases involving intestinal brush-border proteins. *N. Engl. J. Med. 296,* 1047-1050 (1977).
41. A. L. Wu and W. A. Walker. Immunologic control mechanism against cholera toxin: Interference with toxin binding to intestinal receptors. *Infect. Immun. 14,* 1034-1042 (1976).
42. R. Rodewald. pH Dependent binding of immunoglobins to intestinal cells of the neonatal rat. *J. Cell. Biol. 71,* 666-669 (1976).
43. M. C. Williams and S. L. Wissig. The permeability of muscle capillaries to horseradish peroxidase. *J. Cell Biol. 66,* 531-555 (1975).
44. N. Simionescu, M. Simionescu, and G. E. Palade. Permeability of intestinal capillaries; pathway followed by dextrans and glycogen. *J. Cell Biol. 53,* 365-392 (1972).
45. F. Clementi and G. E. Palade. Intestinal capillaries. I. Permeability to peroxidase and ferritin. *J. Cell Biol. 41,* 33-58 (1969).
46. N. B. Gilula. Gap junctions and cell communication. In *International Cell Biology, 1976-77* (B. R. Brinkley and K. R. Porter, Eds.). Rockefeller Univ. Press, New York, 1977, pp. 61-69.
47. A. B. Maunsbach, E. L. Christensen, P. D. Ottosen, and L. Larsson. Uptake, transport and digestion of proteins in kidney cells. In *Proceedings of the Fourth International Congress of Histochemistry and Cytochemistry* (T. Takeuchi, K. Ogawa, and S. Fujita, Eds.). Nakanishi Printing Co., Kyoto, 1972, p. 65.
48. D. A. Davis and T. H. Milhorat. The blood-brain barrier of the rat choroid plexus. *Anat. Rec. 181,* 779-790 (1975).
49. J. E. Rothman and J. Lenard. Membrane asymmetry. *Science 195,* 743-753 (1977).

50. M. Bretscher. Membrane structure: Some general principles. *Science 181*, 622-629 (1973).
51. D. Branton and D. W. Deamer. *Membrane Structure*. Springer-Verlag, Vienna, 1972.
52. J. Schlesinger, D. Axelrod, D. E. Koppel, W. W. Webb, and E. L. Elson. Lateral transport of a lipid probe and labeled proteins on a cell membrane. *Science 195*, 307-308 (1977).
53. M. S. Bretscher and M. D. Raff. Mammalian plasma membranes. *Nature 258*, 43-49 (1975).
54. C. J. Edmonds. Salts and water in biomembranes. In *Intestinal Absorption*, Vol. 4B (D. H. Smyth, Ed.). Plenum Press, London, 1974, pp. 711-740.
55. E. Holtzman and R. Dominitz. Cytochemical studies of lysosomes, Golgi apparatus and endoplasmic reticulum in secretion and protein uptake of adrenal medulla cells of one rat. *J. Histochem. Cytochem. 16*, 320-326 (1968).
56. T. F. Roth and K. R. Porter. Yolk protein uptake in the oocyte of the mosquito, *Aedes aegypti*. *J. Cell Biol. 20*, 313-322 (1964).
57. E. Holtzman, A. B. Novikoff, and H. Villaverde. Lysosomes and GERL in normal and chromatolytic neurons of the rat ganglion nodosum. *J. Cell Biol. 33*, 419-436 (1967).
58. Z. Cohn and M. D. Fedorko. The formation and fate of lysosomes in *Lysosomes in Biology and Pathology*, (J. T. Dingle and H. B. Fell, Eds.). Elsevier North-Holland, Amsterdam, 1969, pp. 43-114.
59. H. G. Hers and F. van Hoff, (Eds.). *Lysosomes and Storage Diseases*. Academic Press, New York, 1973.
60. A. J. Barret. Lysosomal enzymes. In *Lysosomes: A Laboratory Handbook* (J. T. Dingle, Ed.). Elsevier North-Holland, Amsterdam, 1972, pp. 46-135.
61. A. B. Novikoff. Enzyme localization and ultrastructure in neurons. In *The Neuron* (H. Hyden, Ed.). Elsevier North-Holland, Amsterdam, 1967, pp. 255-318.
62. A. B. Novikoff. Lysosomes: A personal account. In *Lysosomes and Storage Disease* (H. G. Hers and F. Van Hoff, Eds.). Academic Press, New York, 1973, pp. 1-41.
63. S. Silverstein, C. Astell, D. Levin, M. Schonberg, and G. Acs. The role of lysosomes in the uncoating and activation of the reovirus genome. *Adv. Biosc. 11*, 1-26 (1973).
64. T. C. Jones and J. G. Hirsch. The interaction between *Toxoplasma gondii* and lysosomes. *J. Exp. Med. 136*, 1173-1194 (1972).
65. E. Kolsch. Patterns of handling and presenting antigen by macrophages. In *Mononuclear Phagocytes* (R. Van Furth, Ed.). Davis Co., Philadelphia, 1970, pp. 548-561.
66. M. E. Lamm. Cellular aspects of immunogloblin A. *Adv. Immunol. 22*, 223-290 (1976).

67. B. S. Worthington, L. Meserole, and J. A. Syrotuck. Effect of daily ethanol ingestion on intestinal permeability to macromolecules. *Digest. Dis. 23,* 23-32 (1978).
68. U. Fagundes-Neto, S. Teichberg, M. A. Bayne, B. Morton, and F. Lifshitz. Bile salt enhanced jejunal macromolecular absorption. *Fed. Proc. 37,* 699 (1978).
69. D. N. Challacombe, J. M. Richardson, and S. Edkius. Anaerobic bacteria and deconjugated bile salts in the upper small intestine of infants with gastrointestinal disorders. *Acta Paediatr. Scand. 63,* 581-587 (1974).
70. B. S. Drasar, M. J. Hill, and M. Shiner. The deconjugation of bile salts by human intestinal bacteria. *Lancet 1,* 1237-1238 (1966).
71. S. Teichberg, U. Fagundes-Neto, M. A. Bayne and F. Lifshitz. Increased susceptibility of malnourished rats to the effects of deoxycholate on jejunal macromolecular absorption. *Fed. Proc. 38*:764 (1979).
72. F. Lifshitz, P. Coello-Ramirez, G. Gutierrez-Topete, and M. C. Cornado-Coronet. Carbohydrate intolerance in infants with diarrhea. *J. Pediatr. 79,* 760-767 (1971).
73. F. Lifshitz, P. Coello-Ramirez, and M. L. Contrearas-Gutierrez. The response of infants to carbohydrate oral loads after recovery from diarrhea. *J. Pediatr. 79,* 612-617 (1971).
74. A. Ashkenazi, Z. T. Handzel, D. Idar, M. Ofarim, and S. Levin. An immunologic assay for diagnosis of coeliac disease. *Lancet 1,* 627-629 (1978).
75. K. Goel, F. Lifshitz, E. Kahn, and S. Teichberg. Monasaccharide intolerance and soy protein hypersensitivity in an infant with diarrhea. *J. Pediatr. 93,* 617-619 (1978).
76. M. E. Ament and G. E. Rubin. Soy protein another cause of the flat intestinal lesion. *Gastroenterology 62,* 227-234 (1972).

14 Digestion and Absorption in the Newborn and Low-Birth-Weight Infant

JOHN B. WATKINS / University of Pennsylvania School of Medicine, and Children's Hospital of Philadelphia, Pennsylvania

I. Introduction

Interest in neonatal gastrointestinal function has been recently stimulated by the remarkable clinical successes achieved in the care of the small premature infant. With improved survival has come the recognition that major transitions must also occur in gastrointestinal function as an infant adapts to an extrauterine environment. Trace elements such as iron, zinc, and calcium, which normally accumulate during the last trimester of pregnancy, must be efficiently absorbed. Many interrelated metabolic changes occur, including the switch from carbohydrate, the major fuel source in utero, to a dependency on dietary lipid to provide a major portion of the nutrient calories [1]. From these and other factors has grown an awareness that nutritional formulations specifically designed for the premature infant may be needed, and, further, that more knowledge is required concerning the development of the structural and functional aspects of the gastrointestinal tract in the preterm infant. This chapter will center upon the mechanisms of lipid absorption in the neonate, with emphasis on those aspects which represent new developments in understanding of the process of fat digestion and absorption, or which may provide insight into significant alternatives for improving nutrient lipid absorption in the immature infant.

II. Lipid Absorption in Infancy

Dietary lipid is the nutrient of the highest caloric density, and although it represents only 3-3.5% of the standard infant formula by weight, it contains nearly 40-50% of the total calories. In the adult, fat absorption is a relatively efficient process whereby 95% of intake is absorbed, or less than 5 g per day is excreted in the feces. By contrast, the newborn infant absorbs lipid inefficiently, so that the preterm infant of 32-34 weeks of gestation may normally absorb as little as 65-75% of intake, resulting in losses of 9-20 kcal/kg body weight, which are rarely recovered by increasing intake. Improved absorption occurs gradually, however; adult levels of absorptive efficiency are not routinely achieved in most infants until 4-6 months of age. Interestingly, there are marked variations in rates of fat absorption, depending upon the source of the nutrient lipid (e.g., breast milk versus butterfat or vegetable fat) and upon differences in the functional maturity of the gastrointestinal tract at birth [2].

The overall process of fat digestion and absorption can be described as a series or sequence of events which occur in three distinct phases: an intraluminal phase, a mucosal phase, and a transport or delivery phase. The events which occur within the intraluminal phase are dominated by the fact that dietary lipids (principally triglycerides) are largely nonpolar and thus water-insoluble. They contain, chiefly, saturated and unsaturated long-chain fatty acids (chain lengths greater than 14 carbon atoms) esterified to glycerol. The process of fat digestion is initiated by hydrolysis of the triglycerides to form fatty acids and monoglycerides, lipids which are more polar (i.e., water-soluble) and capable of being solubilized within the aqueous environment of the intestine.

A. Pharyngeal Lipase

Recent evidence indicates that lipolysis is initiated by lipases synthesized and secreted from the glands (of Ebner) located at the base of the tongue [3]. The characteristics which differentiate pharyngeal lipase from pancreatic lipase are listed in Table 1. Of note is the fact that pharyngeal lipase functions in the absence of bile salts; its pH optimum is near or at the pH of the stomach during meals, and the hydrolytic reaction may go to completion, producing fatty acids and glycerol in the presence of a fatty acid acceptor. This enzyme is recognized to play a major role in fat digestion in several animal species. It has been demonstrated to be present at birth in the human, even in premature infants and in children with esophageal atresia [4]. The data obtained from animals with a surgically created esophageal fistula [5] and, inferentially, from infants fed transpylorically [6] would suggest that lipolysis in the stomach serves to provide amphophiles necessary for the stabilization of the triglyceride emulsion particles, a requisite for efficient lipolysis in the duodenum. In addition, gastric lipolysis provides free fatty acids in the duodenum—which would stimulate cholecystokinin release, control gastric emptying, and promote contraction of the gallbladder, thereby increasing intraluminal bile acid

Table 1 Comparison of Pharyngeal and Pancreatic Lipase in Man

Absorption factors	Pharyngeal (gastric)	Pancreatic
Apparent mol wt	40,000-50,000	46,000
Inactivation by acid	Little	Marked
Resistance to trypsin	Little	Moderate
pH Optimum	4.5-5.4	7.5
Cofactor	?	(+) Colipase
Bile salts	Inhibit	Stabilize
Chain length specificity	$4>6>8\gg 18$	$4>6>8>18$
Positional specificity	$1>2$	$1\gg 2$
Esterification of FA acceptor[a]	Moderate	Marked
Hydrolysis of milk TG[b]	Moderate	Absent unless bile acids present
Primary role	Facilitate emulsification	Quantitative TG hydrolysis

[a]Fatty acid (FA).
[b]Triglyceride (TG).
Source: Data from Refs. 3, 29, and 30.

concentrations. Recent data from infant feeding studies further support the concept that gastric lipolysis may play a major role in fat digestion for the premature [7]. Specifically, much further work will be needed to characterize the lipases present in human milk, which also appear to have activity under the intragastric conditions found in the newborn infant [8]. These data could do much to provide information useful for optimizing lipid absorption in the preterm infant, as well as to provide an explanation for the improved lipid absorption observed with fresh or frozen breast milk, but not pasteurized breast milk.

B. Intraluminal Phase of Fat Digestion

In the adult and probably in the infant fed commercial formulas, the greater part of triglyceride hydrolysis takes place within the intestinal lumen. This process is efficient, but occurs only under a narrow range of physiologic conditions. The reaction is governed by the fact that pancreatic lipase is a water-soluble enzyme which acts only on the surface of the triglyceride emulsion particle at the oil-water interface. Proper orientation of the enzyme at the surface requires the presence of calcium, bile salts, and a cofactor, termed "colipase," which serves as an acceptor to the enzyme [9]. Enzyme activity is also affected by the chain length and the solubility (of the fatty acid) within the aqueous environment of the duodenum—a fact which accounts for the rapid hydrolysis and solubilization of medium-chain triglycerides [10]. In general, pancreatic lipase is specific for the 1- and 3-ester linkages of the triglyceride molecule, so that the hydrolysis of 1 mol triglyceride results in the production of 2 mol fatty acid and 1 mol monoglyceride. These lipids are in themselves potentially absorbable; however, it can be predicted that without the addition of bile acid, the lipolytic reaction would be incomplete and the lipid suboptimally absorbed [11].

III. Bile Salts in Fat Digestion

In the newborn infant and particularly in the preterm infant, during the first weeks of life both intraluminal bile acid concentrations and pancreatic lipase levels are diminished [12]. Pancreatic enzyme secretion does appear to respond to exogenous cholecystokinin administration [13]; however the presence of unhydrolyzed glycerides found in the feces of the full-term infant [14] and in the duodenal aspirates obtained from premature infants [15] during meals indicates that lipid hydrolysis is usually incomplete. This deficiency of the intraluminal phase of fat digestion is clearly related to the inability of the infant to maintain adequate intraluminal bile acid concentrations. In fact, a correlation in the infant occurs among intraluminal bile acid concentration, postnatal age, and the coefficient of fat absorption [15]. This is due to the fact that bile acids are a unique group of compounds which have physicochemical characteristics similar to all detergents in that they are amphipaths; i.e., they possess hydrophobic and hydrophilic regions. Conjugated bile acids are very soluble in water, and at low concentrations they exist as unassociated molecules (monomers); however, at high concentrations the individual molecules aggregate to form polymolecular complexes termed micelles. Bile acid micelles are spherical or cylindrical in shape, with the hydrophobic regions oriented inward toward the center of the micelle and the hydrophilic regions oriented to the outside of the micelle, facing the aqueous environment (Fig. 1). The concentration at which monomeric bile acids aggregate to form micelles is termed the "critical micellar concentration." This concentration varies for individual acids and is influenced by, among other things, the intraluminal pH, the chemical nature of the molecule solubilized within the micelle, the electrolyte concentration, and the temperature of the environment [16]. Under the physiologic conditions encountered in the jejunum, the critical micellar concentration for the conjugated bile acids is in the range of 1-2 mM.

A bile acid micelle has the capacity of solubilizing with its hydrophobic core less polar or water-insoluble lipids, including fatty acids and monoglycerides, the products of lipolysis, as well as other lipids such as cholesterol, phospholipids, and the fat-soluble vitamins A, D, and E. When these lipids are

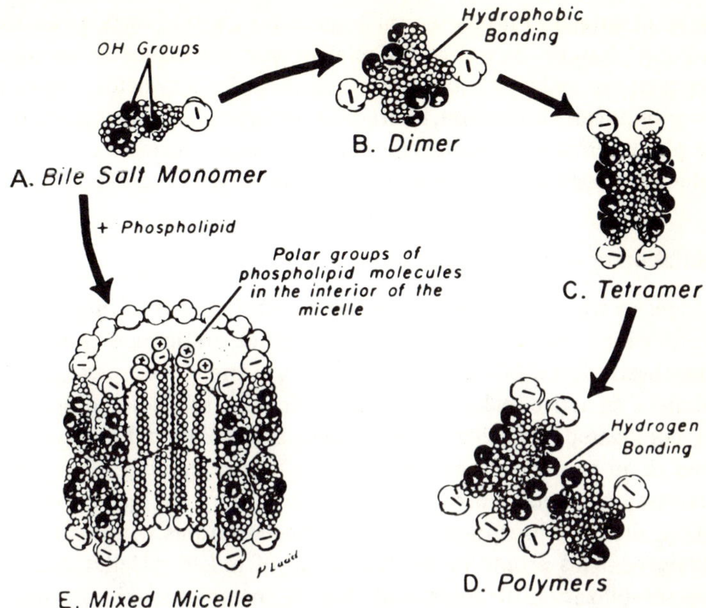

Figure 1 Formation of pure and mixed micelles in bile. Parts A-D represent process of micelle formation from bile salt monomers (A) to bile salt aggregates or micelles (B, C) at concentrations above critical micellar concentration. Self-association of pure bile micelles as in D, or of mixed micelles (E), may occur at high bile salt concentrations. Mixed micelle E is composed of outer shell consisting of bile acid molecules which then solubilize, within an inner core, phospholipids, cholesterol, and other lipids including the products of lipolysis. (Reproduced from Ref. 31, with the permission of the publisher.)

solubilized within the micelle, micellar size increases, and this aggregation of different lipids is termed a mixed micelle. It is by this process of micellar solubilization that water-insoluble lipids gain access to the aqueous environment of the intestine; therefore it represents a major physiologic role for bile acids within the luminal phase.

The fat-laden bile acid micelles neither bind to the microvillus membrane of the intestinal mucosal cell nor are they absorbed intact, but rather micelle formation serves to reduce the diffusion barrier posed by the unstirred water layer adjacent to the mucosal cell membrane. The kinetics of this process recently have been elegantly characterized and defined in terms of the micelle-water partition coefficient for each lipid [17]. These data explain the mechanisms and the tremendous physiologic importance of micellar solubilization to the mucosal uptake of nonpolar lipids, such as saturated fatty acids, sterols, and fat-soluble vitamins, as well as the relative lack of enhanced absorption in the presence of bile salts for short- and medium-chain fatty acids. Thus, with the absence of micelle formation, short- and medium-chain fatty acid absorption may take place normally; however, there is a moderate decrease in long-chain unsaturated fatty acid absorption and essentially no cholesterol absorption.

IV. Regulation of Bile Acid Metabolism

The mechanisms which are responsible for the maintenance of intraluminal bile salt concentrations above the critical micellar concentration are twofold: (1) hepatic synthesis of new bile salt from cholesterol and (2) the presence, in the distal ileum, of an active reabsorption mechanism for bile salt conjugates. In the adult, conjugated bile acids at the normal intraluminal pH are not passively reabsorbed to an appreciable degree in the proximal jejunum; hence most bile acids pass unabsorbed into the ileum, where they are reabsorbed [18]. By means of distal reabsorption, bile acid concentrations within the jejunum are maintained. This promotes the formation of mixed micelles, permits continued solubilization of lipids, and thereby maximizes lipid absorption. In the adult the reabsorptive capacity of the ileum for bile acid is immense, and it normally conserves 95-98% of each cycle of the bile acid pool. This forms an enterohepatic circulation in which 5-15% (i.e., 300-500 mg) of the bile salt secreted each day is lost in the feces. The total amount of bile acid contained within the enterohepatic circulation is called the bile salt pool—which remains nearly constant in size because of a sensitive enzymatic feedback mechanism through cholesterol 7α-hydroxylase.

It is evident then, that, although part of the inefficiency of neonatal fat absorption may be the result of an immaturity of pancreatic and/or intestinal function, bile acids clearly play a central role. What then is the functional maturity of the mechanisms for bile acid synthesis and turnover at birth? Much of the available information is schematically represented in Figure 2. This would indicate that bile acid synthesis and secretion begin in the fetus early in gestation. In the human, data obtained early in gestation are incomplete, but bile acids are found in the gallbladder bile of human fetuses as early as 14-16 weeks of gestation. Chenodeoxycholic acid is the predominant bile acid early in gestation, with cholic acid appearing in the bile obtained from fetuses later in gestation. Bile acids in the fetus and infants are conjugated primarily with taurine—in contrast to the adult where glycine conjugates predominate [19]. Bile acid sulfates have been recovered from the meconium of normal infants, and sulfated bile acids are routinely observed in the urine of cholestatic infants.

The developmental processes of bile acid synthesis and secretion have been best characterized in animal studies. The majority of evidence would indicate

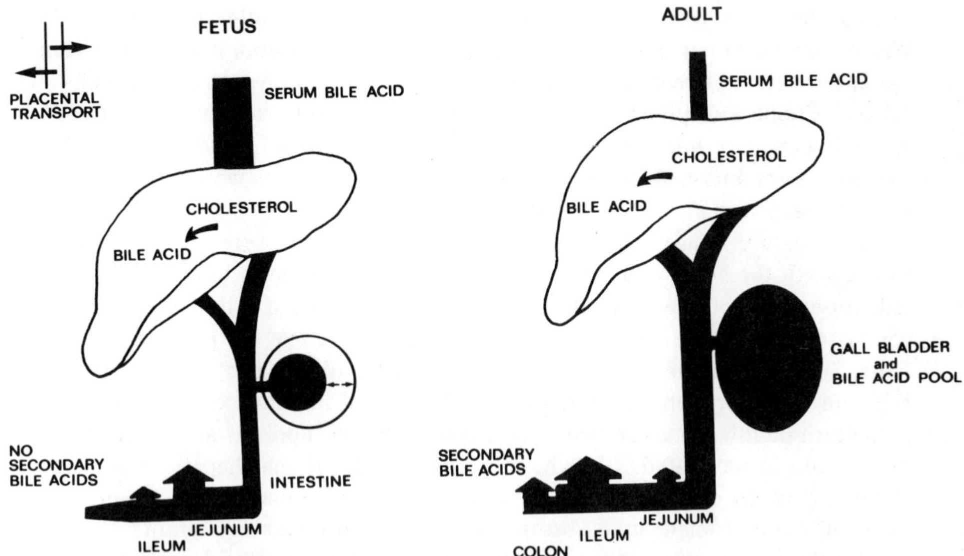

Figure 2 Comparison of bile acid metabolism in fetus and adult. In this schematic representation, relative magnitude of each process is indicated by width of dark line. Bile acids are synthesized from cholesterol in both fetus and adult, yet bile acid pool is contracted in the fetus, and gallbladder concentrations are reduced. Conjugated bile acids are secreted into the intestine; however, significant jejunal reabsorption of bile acid occurs in the fetus, in contrast to the adult, and no secondary bile acids are produced. Serum bile acid concentrations are high in the fetus, and bidirectional placental transport has been demonstrated. (Reproduced from Ref. 19, with the permission of the publisher.)

that bile acid synthesis and conjugation are existent in the near-term fetal animal, but that bile acid secretion may lag. Individual species show considerable variation in the ability to excrete a bile acid load or to respond to bile drainage with an increase in bile acid secretion or synthesis. Thus, the fetus and neonate may experience a functional cholestasis with bile acid synthesis in the presence of inadequate secretion. This may be demonstrated histologically in the fetal and neonatal liver by the presence of "bile plugs" within the canaliculi [20], suggesting that there may be variation in the development maturation of the mechanisms for the secretion of bile acids.

In the human infant, evidence obtained using stable, isotopically labeled bile acids (nonradioactive) indicates that a similar degree of hepatic immaturity may also exist. Through the use of these methods, it has been possible to measure bile acid pool size and synthesis rates in normal full-term infants [21]. When normalized per unit of body surface, the bile acid pool contained within the enterohepatic circulation was reduced to approximately one-half adult values. Cholic acid predominated over chenodeoxycholic acid by a 3:1 ratio, and the secondary bile acids (e.g., deoxycholic acid) found in adult bile and in the meconium and gallbladder of fetal and newborn infants were absent, confirming the maternal origin of these secondary bile acids.

In premature infants, 32-36 weeks of gestation, values were further reduced to one-sixth the adult values and one-third those in full-term infants. The reductions in pool size correlated closely with the reduced intraluminal [22] concentrations of bile acid; these averaged less than 2 mM for premature infants, 5 mM for full-term infants, and 8 mM for adults. Thus, intraluminal bile acid concentrations are often below the critical micellar concentrations in premature infants, a factor that may clearly limit the lipolysis and dispersion of nonpolar dietary lipids. Furthermore, it is probable that hepatic immaturity in the regulation of bile acid synthesis and/or secretion plays a significant factor in the inefficient lipid absorption observed in premature infants.

The close correlation observed between intraluminal bile acid concentrations and bile acid pool size suggests that bile acid secretion may be at a maximum, and raises the possibility that the intestinal mechanisms required to maintain the bile salt pool may be limited or incomplete. This aspect has been investigated in the dog, in vivo by perfusion studies and in vitro through the use of everted intestinal rings [23]. Both methods would indicate that the ileal transport mechanisms for active reabsorption of bile acid are immature, and that they improve with increasing postnatal age. Similar data are available for human intestine with limited in vitro techniques [24]. Interestingly, the jejunum of the neonate appears also to be remarkably permeable to conjugated bile acids, in contrast to the jejunum of the adult—a factor which may result in short-circuiting of the enterohepatic circulation and a further reduction in the intraluminal bile acid concentration. It appears most likely that the low intraluminal bile acid concentrations observed in the premature infant are due to immaturity of both the hepatic and intestinal factors which regulate bile acid synthesis and serve to conserve intraluminal bile acid concentrations.

V. Final Considerations

Important questions, then, remain: What are the factors which lead to the maturation of hepatic and intestinal function? Does the type of dietary lipid ingested alter hepatic bile acid synthesis? Is the availability of dietary taurine or cholesterol a crucial factor in regulating bile acid conjugation patterns—or synthesis rates? Finally, are there possible mechanisms whereby the maturation of these factors may be influenced, as has been accomplished with the induction of pulmonary surfactant synthesis and release in the fetal lung [25]?

To date, only preliminary data are available to answer these questions. In a study similar to those mentioned previously, three premature infants whose mothers had received dexamethasone and one whose mother had received phenobarbital–for differing lengths of time, including the last week of pregnancy–were studied. Intraduodenal bile acid concentrations and bile acid pool sizes were three times larger than in similarly aged infants, close to those observed in the full-term infants. The fractional turnover rate of the bile acid pool was also reduced relative to that for the infants from untreated mothers–suggesting that both hepatic and ileal functions may be more mature [22]. These findings were noted only retrospectively and thus far have been unsupported by further clinical trials. Preliminary evidence reported from animal studies would tend to support the concept that exposure to adrenocortical steroids stimulates both ileal function and hepatic bile acid synthesis [25]. Further studies are needed, however, before conclusions can be drawn as to possible therapeutic benefits and risks of this approach, and information is needed concerning the development of these and other associated hepatic and intestinal functions. Finally, a last but important aspect of lipid absorption concerns the mucosal phase. As mentioned previously, the passive diffusion of lipids to the mucosa is limited by the diffusion barrier presented by the unstirred layer [17] and is markedly facilitated by micellar solubilization.

The majority of data suggest that lipids are absorbed as monomers at the intestinal mucosal cell membrane by a passive or nonenergy-requiring process. Within the intestinal mucosal cell, however, long-chain fatty acids are activated to their CoA derivatives, and bound intracellularly to a recently described fatty acid binding protein similar to ligandin [26]. The fatty acid CoA is then reesterified by two pathways, a monoglyceride pathway and an L-glycerophosphate pathway, of which the former is quantitatively the most important. The newly synthesized triglycerides, together with phospholipids and cholesterol esters, are then combined with free cholesterol and lipoproteins to form either chylomicrons or very low density lipoproteins. Chylomicrons have been demonstrated in the serum of newborn infants after 2-3 days of age, but there are as yet no data concerning the developmental aspects of this process [27]. In addition, there are no data in humans concerning the process of triglyceride synthesis, fatty acid acylation, or the distribution of the fatty acid binding protein. Preliminary data in the rat suggest that, with increasing fat loads to the distal intestine, the concentration of this protein may increase, as does the activity of the triglyceride synthetic enzymes [28].

In summary, the study of the mechanisms of dietary lipid absorption in the preterm infant involves aspects of developmental pharmacology, as well as requiring a knowledge of the physicochemical processes required for the solubilization of lipids and an understanding of the processes of membrane transport. At a practical level, changes in formula design and advances in developmental biology are by now clearly interrelated. Each presents new opportunities to expand knowledge of basic cellular processes and the nutrition of the developing infant.

Acknowledgment

Supported in part by U.S. Public Health Service Research Grant HD-08489 from the National Institute of Child Health and Development.

References

1. E. W. Page. Human fetal nutrition and growth. *Am. J. Obstet. Gynecol. 104,* 378-387 (1969).
2. J. B. Watkins. Mechanisms of fat absorption and the development of gastrointestinal function. *Pediatr. Clin. North Am. 22,* 721-730 (1975).
3. M. Hamosh, H. L. Klaeveman, R. O. Wolfe, and R. O. Scow. Pharyngeal lipase and digestion of dietary triglyceride in man. *J. Clin. Invest. 55,* 908-910 (1975).
4. C. Salzman-Mann, M. Hamosh, K. N. Sivasubramaninan, G. B. Avery, T. Plucinski, J. B. Watkins, and P. Hamosh. Lipolytic activity in esophageal and gastric aspirates from infants with esophageal atresia. *Fed. Proc. 37,* 854 (1978).
5. C. C. Roy, D. Lefebre, and L. Chartrand. The role of gastric lipolysis in fat absorption and bile acid metabolism in the rat. *Clin. Res. 25,* 689A (1977).
6. R. N. Roy, R. P. Pollinitz, J. R. Hamilton, and G. W. Chance. Impaired assimilation of nasojejunal feeds in healthy low-birth-weight newborn infants. *J. Pediatr. 90,* 431-434 (1977).
7. B. Alemi, M. Hamosh, J. W. Scanlon. Fat digestion in premature infants. III. Relationship between lipolytic activity in gastric aspirates and fat absorption in the tiny premature. *J. Pediatr.* In press.
8. O. Hernell. Human milk lipase. III. Physiological implications of the bile salt-stimulated lipase. *Eur. J. Clin. Invest. 5,* 267-272 (1975).
9. B. Borgstrom and C. Erlanson. Pancreatic juice co-lipase: Physiological importance. *Biochim. Biophys. Acta 242,* 509-513 (1971).
10. G. Benzonana and P. Desnuelle. Etude cinctique de l'action de la lipase pancreatique sur des triglycerides en emulsion: Essai d'une enzymologic en milieu heterogene. *Biochim. Biophys. Acta 105,* 121-136 (1965).
11. H. Westergaard and J. M. Dietschy. Normal mechanisms of fat absorption and derangements induced by various gastrointestinal diseases. *Med. Clin. North Am. 50,* 1413-1427 (1974).

12. A. Norman, B. Strandvik, and O. Ojamae. Bile acids and pancreatic enzymes during absorption in the newborn. *Acta Paediatr. Scand. 61,* 571-576 (1972).
13. O. Nernell and T. Olivecrona. Human milk lipases. II. Bile salt-stimulated lipase. *Biochim. Biophys. Acta 369,* 234-244 (1974).
14. J. B. Watkins, C. M. Bliss, R. M. Donaldson, and R. Lester. Characterization of newborn fecal lipid. *Pediatrics 58,* 511-115 (1974).
15. E. Singer, G. M. Murphy, S. Edkins, and E. M. Andersen. Role of bile salts in fat malabsorption of premature infants. *Arch. Dis. Child, 49,* 174-180 (1974).
16. M. C. Carey and D. M. Small. The characteristics of mixed micellar solutions with particular reference to bile. *Am. J. Med. 49,* 590-608 (1970).
17. F. A. Wilson and J. M. Dietschy. Characterization of bile acid absorption across the unstirred water layer and brush border of the rat jejunum. *J. Clin. Invest. 51,* 3015-3025 (1972).
18. R. H. Dowling, E. Mack, and D. M. Small. Effect of controlled interruption of the enterohepatic circulation of bile salts by biliary diversion and by ileal resection on bile salt secretion, synthesis and pool size in the rhesus monkey. *J. Clin. Invest. 49,* 232-242 (1970).
19. J. B. Watkins and J. A. Perman. Bile acid metabolism in infants and children. *Clin. Gastroenterol. 6,* 201-218 (1977).
20. C. DeWolf-Peeters, R. Devos, and V. Desmet. Histochemical evidence of a cholestatic period in neonatal rats. *Pediatr. Res. 5,* 704 (1971).
21. J. B. Watkins, D. Ingall, P. Szczepanik, P. D. Klein, and R. Lester. Bile salt metabolism in the newborn. Measurement of pool size and synthesis by stable isotope technic. *N. Engl. J. Med. 288,* 431 (1973).
22. J. B. Watkins, P. Szczepanik, J. B. Gould, P. D. Klein, and R. Lester. Bile salt metabolism in the human premature infant. Preliminary observations of pool size and synthesis rate following prenatal administration of dexamethasone and phenobarbital. *Gastroenterology 69,* 706 (1975).
23. R. Lester, R. A. Smallwood, J. M. Little, A. S. Brown, G. J. Piasecki, and B. T. Jackson. Fetal bile salt metabolism. The intestinal absorption of bile salt. *J. Clin. Invest. 59,* 1009-1016 (1977).
24. R. C. De Belle, V. Vaupshaf, B. B. Vaitulo, L. R. Haber, E. Shaffer, G. G. Mackie, H. Owen, J. M. Little, and R. Lester. Intestinal absorption of bile salts: Immature development in the newborn. *J. Pediatr. 94:*472-476 (1979).
25. J. E. Richey, J. M. Little, D. H. Van Thiel, and R. Lester. Steroid-induced bile acid synthesis and secretion in the fetal rat. Abstract. *Gastroenterology 72,* 119 (1977).
26. R. K. Ockner and J. A. Manning. Fatty acid binding protein in small intestine. Identification, isolation and evidence for its role in cellular fatty acid transport. *J. Clin. Invest. 54,* 326-338 (1974).
27. V. Melichar, M. Novak, P. Hahn, O. Koldovsky, and L. Zeman. Changes in the blood levels of lipid metabolites and glucose following a fatty meal in infants. *Acta Paediatr. 51,* 481-489 (1962).

28. T. G. Holtzapple, G. Smith, and O. Koldovsky. Uptake, activation and esterification of fatty acids in the small intestine of the suckling rat. *Pediatr. Res. 9,* 786-791 (1975).
29. M. Cohen, G. R. H. Morgan, and A. F. Hofmann. Lipolytic activity of human gastric and duodenal juice against medium and long chain triglycerides. *Gastroenterology 60,* 1-15 (1971).
30. M. Hamosh and W. A. Burns. Lipolytic activity of human lingual glands (Ebner). *Lab. Invest. 37,* 603-608 (1977).
31. J. M. Dietschy. Mechanisms for the intestinal absorption of bile acids. *J. Lipid Res. 9,* 297 (1968).

15 Genetic Factors in the Absorption of Protein Breakdown Products

RAUL A. WAPNIR / Cornell University Medical College, New York, New York, and North Shore University Hospital, Manhasset, New York

I. Introduction

The concept that the intestinal absorption of amino acids is affected by genetic or metabolic determinants followed the discovery of various kinds of aminoacidurias. These events were made possible by the development of partition and ion-exchange chromatographic techniques in the late 1940s and 1950s.

Amino acids, as well as other small molecules such as monosaccharides, electrolytes, water, and gases, are involved in the bulk of exchanges between the body and the environment. Molecules below 200 daltons are capable of easily crossing the semipermeable plasma membrane and tight junctions of epithelial cells in organs where nutrients and excreta enter and leave the body, namely, the gastrointestinal tract and the kidney [1, 2].

Teleologically, free *diffusion* along a chemical gradient is insufficient to assure the provision of small molecules required as energy sources and as building blocks of tissue proteins. The plasma membrane of cells contains protein molecules, carriers or translocases, which participate in the transfer and exchange of amino acids or monosaccharides for other functionally equivalent molecules (*facilitated diffusion*); or which, at the expense of chemical energy, incorporate those small molecules into the cells, against an electrochemical gradient (*active transport*) [3]. Such mechanisms are essential for most forms of life as we know them today. Their obliteration is incompatible with survival.

II. Absorption of Amino Acids

The amino acid carriers in cells of eukaryotes are selective for amino acids with the L-configuration. Bacteria handle both L- and D-enantiomers. Small peptides can enter the enterocyte but are not transported by the same carriers as single amino acids.

The active intestinal transport of amino acids has been studied by in vitro and in vivo techniques [4-7]. In the majority of cases the chemical balance of the electrical charges in the molecule is a key factor that directs the behavior of carriers toward their amino acid substrates. Using a broad criterion, amino acids of physiologic significance may be divided as follows [8]:

1. Monoamino monocarboxylic acids (neutral amino acids: e.g., alanine, serine, glycine, threonine, valine, leucine, isoleucine, methionine, phenylalanine, tyrosine, tryptophan, histidine, cysteine, glutamine, asparagine)
2. Imino acids (proline, hydroxyproline, glycine)
3. Diamino monocarboxylic acids (basic amino acids: e.g., lysine, ornithine, arginine, cystine)
4. Monoamino dicarboxylic acids (acidic amino acids: e.g., aspartic acid, glutamic acid)
5. β-Amino acids (β-alanine, taurine, β-amino isobutyric acid)

The above functional classification acknowledges the fact that glycine shares a compatibility with the first two groups of carriers, and that cystine, although its electrical charges are balanced, behaves as if it were a basic amino acid. Aspartic and glutamic acids are considered not to be transported by active mechanisms. These and other peculiarities are the result of many observations indicating that the gene or genes which regulate the transport of a specific amino acid will often alter the translocation of other amino acids assigned to the same group.

However, this postulate knows of many exceptions, some of which will be discussed below. Often, there have been diseases reported in the literature in which a single amino acid, e.g., tryptophan, was defectively transported, while other neutral amino acids were not affected. To explain these findings, the concept of a single carrier, capable of transporting any and all the amino acids in a specific group of the classification described earlier, has to be abandoned. Hence, it must be considered that either (1) the common carrier has multiple active sites, which could be sterically altered by a change in the carbon skeleton of the amino acid, or (2) separate, individual amino acid carriers are present, each specific for an individual amino acid and not inhibited, or only partially so, by either genetically determined or exogenously originated inhibitors or competitors.

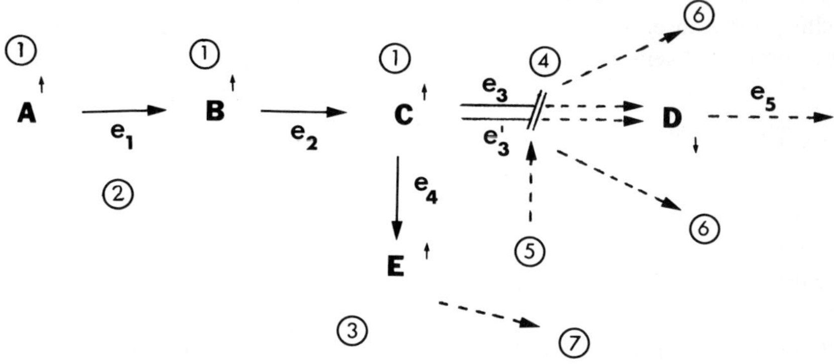

Figure 1 Schematic representation of inborn error of metabolism and its phenotypic effects. (1) Accumulation of metabolites proximal to site of enzymatic defect at e_3 step (A, B, C). Deficiency of metabolites distal to block (D). (2) Enzymatic steps (e_1 to e_5, etc.). (3) Increased production of normally insignificant metabolites by alternative pathways (E). (4) More than one allele (e_3, e_3') may be affected in enzymatic block. (5) External factors may affect expression of genotype. (6) Metabolic block may be expressed in more than one tissue. (7) Abnormal metabolites may interfere with other key enzymatic steps unrelated to original affected pathway.

An inherited defect of amino acid transport can be comparable to an inborn error of metabolism in a specific enzymatic step. In the latter case, alterations in the proportions of metabolites proximal and distal to the affected locus can occur. Thus, one amino acid or a group of amino acids may be malabsorbed, with consequent accumulation or deficit of these substances proximal to or distal from the absorptive step. Also, an enzymatic defect can manifest itself in one or several tissues, i.e., liver, kidney, or small-intestinal mucosa (Fig. 1). This phenotypic expression may vary with conditions peculiar to the tissue, e.g., elevation of plasma amino acid concentrations, hyperaminoaciduria, or bacterial attack of an unabsorbed amino acid in the gut.

III. Absorption of Peptides

It is now well accepted that the absorption of protein breakdown products does not take place exclusively at the amino acid level. The recent awareness of the important role that the translocation of di- or tripeptides may have in this physiologic process stems mainly from the work of Matthews [9]. The concept of intracellular hydrolysis of small peptides has filled a gap in the understanding of how metabolic defects of amino acid transport are substantially compensated for—by an intact capacity for uptake and liberation of amino acids poorly absorbed as single units. Yet, very little is known about the specificity and genetic determinants of intestinal transport of oligopeptides.

IV. The γ-Glutamyl Cycle

In addition to the concepts of group and specific amino acid membrane carriers for amino acids, a separate mechanism for the transport of amino acids and dipeptides across membranes has been proposed. A specific enzyme, γ-glutamyltranspeptidase, located in the cell membrane, is capable of catalyzing the reaction between glutathione (γ-glutamylcysteinylglycine) and an amino acid or dipeptide outside the cell, and translocating the substrate to the interior of the cell with formation of an intermediate peptide (γ-glutamylamino acid). A second enzyme, γ-glutamyl cyclotransferase, catalyzes the liberation of the amino acid and 5-oxoproline. Three more enzymatic steps are required for the regeneration of glutathione [10, 11].

The enzyme γ-glutamyltranspeptidase has been located and purified from preparations of rat small-intestinal villi. Certain dipeptides are especially effective as acceptors of glutamate. The fact that a gradient of activity exists from the crypts to the villi, and that it may parallel the location of (Na^+-K^+)-ATPase, contributes to support of the view that γ-glutamyltranspeptidase plays a significant role in the absorption of small peptides and amino acids from the small intestine [12]. Two isozymes have been separated from human intestine, which, in contradistinction to fractions obtained from other tissues (bone, liver, pancreas, kidney, placenta, and serum) cannot be activated by L-methionine or a detergent [13].

V. Specific Metabolic Disorders Associated with Abnormalities of Intestinal Transport

A. Cystinuria

Urinary cystine calculi were first described in 1810 by Wollaston. Cystinuria was included among the initial cluster of diseases designated as "inborn errors of metabolism" by Garrod, in 1908. Some forty years later, it was found that other dibasic amino acids also were present in excess in the urine of cystinurics [14]. Since cystine, lysine, arginine, and ornithine share a structure consisting of two amino groups separated by four to six carbon atoms, it was postulated that all these substances shared a common transport mechanism [15, 16]. Soon afterwards, it was demonstrated that an uptake and absorption defect identical to that existing in the kidney for dibasic amino acids was present in the small-intestinal mucosa of cystinurics [15, 17-19]. Such a transport defect seemed to be limited to tissues exchanging metabolites with the environment, since neither human leukocytes [20] nor cultured fibroblasts [21] displayed the translocation lesion present in kidney and small-intestinal mucosa.

More stringent metabolic and genetic studies paved the way for the division of cystinuria into three different entities [22]. In type I, patients have no active transport of cystine, lysine, or arginine in the gut, and their plasma cystine does not increase after a load of the amino acid. In type II there is active transport of cystine in the small-intestinal mucosa, but there is no active transport of lysine. In type III, intestinal transport of cystine and dibasic amino acids is reduced, but still present. The excretion of all these amino acids by the carriers of these conditions is different in each case. The demonstration of double heterozygosity has given added support to the above described classification [23].

A point of interest which demonstrated that the intestinal absorption of peptides was independent from that of free amino acids was the finding that lysine-containing peptides were absorbed normally by cystinuric patients who had an impaired absorption capacity for the free amino acid [24].

B. Hyperdibasic Aminoaciduria

The phenotype of hyperbasic aminoaciduria, the clinical condition originally described as a renal disturbance resembling cystinuria (i.e., an increased excretion of dibasic amino acids, with the exception of cystine) probably covers more than one genotype. Clusters of patients in Finland [25, 26] have been characterized by intolerance to protein, vomiting, diarrhea, failure to thrive, hepatomegaly, and cirrhosis. In spite of these symptoms, there were no studies that could verify the lesion at the intestinal level. A sibship in Japan apparently had a similar clinical presentation [27] as did 13 persons in a French-Canadian pedigree [28] who also had increased renal clearances of lysine, arginine, and ornithine. In the two latter instances, an intestinal transport defect for lysine was confirmed. In both of these populations, the trait was transmitted as a dominant. The findings in these patients confirm the existence of more than one mutant autosomal allele regulating the transport of cystine, on one side, and the dibasic amino acids, proper, on the other. The description of a patient with cystinuria, but without dibasic hyperaminoaciduria [29], has provided additional support to that condition.

C. Hartnup's Disease

The rare condition known as Hartnup's disease entails a defect in renal resorption and intestinal absorption of neutral amino acids. Tryptophan and indole derivatives originating from bacterial action on the unabsorbed amino acid in the gut is the most striking biochemical abnormality [30, 31]. A secondary deficiency of nicotinamide, due to an inappropriate endogenous production of the vitamin, produces some of the typical manifestations of pellagra, although it has been argued that the origin of the nicotinamide deficiency could be due to the inhibitory action of indolic compounds on the tryptophankynurenine enzymatic pathway leading to nicotinamide.

The finding that patients with Hartnup's disease, who were unable to absorb free neutral amino acids, did absorb dipeptides such as glycyltryptophan or phenylalanylphenylalanine explains the survival potential of these individuals, who otherwise would be deprived of essential amino acids [32]. Such evidence also emphasizes the importance of peptide absorption on the overall assimilation of protein breakdown products [9].

D. Tryptophan Malabsorption

The patients in a sibship first described in 1964 [33] were characterized as having urine that on exposure to air stained diapers dark blue—hence, the name of "blue diaper syndrome." This abnormality was traced to the excretion of indican. The origin of this product is related to the malabsorption of tryptophan and its partial degradation to indole, sulfated by the liver and excreted in the urine. Thus, it resembles the defect in Hartnup's disease. Nevertheless, the lesion seems to be restricted to tryptophan and seems not to include other amino acids. Furthermore, it is probably limited to the small-intestinal mucosa, since no gross tryptophanuria has been reported. It is not known whether the lack of tryptophanuria is related to hypotryptophanemia or to technical difficulties frequently experienced in the assay of tryptophan. If this disease is limited to the intestine, it obviously suggests a dissociation between transport mechanisms in the small intestine and the kidney.

E. Phenylketonuria

Without reaching the excessive levels of the excretion of indoles in Hartnup's disease or in tryptophan malabsorption, untreated phenylketonuric patients have been shown to excrete abnormally high amounts of indican and other indole derivatives [34, 35]. The possibility that the high blood levels of phenylalanine could be responsible for malabsorption of other amino acids was further explored by the administration of radioactive arginine and leucine. The levels of blood radioactivity from these compounds were markedly lower in phenylketonurics than in controls [36] or in patients treated with a low-phenylalanine diet. Tryptophan load tests showed that untreated phenylketonurics had a flat tolerance curve, as compared to controls, but patients on a low phenylalanine diet responded in a fashion indistinguishable from that of healthy children [37]. This presumed competition was further demonstrated by direct intestinal perfusion studies that indicated a generalized reduction in the absorption rates of amino acids [38]. Moreover, similar techniques showed that not only tryptophan, but phenylalanine itself was absorbed at a rate lower than that for controls in untreated patients with high blood phenylalanine levels. When the same individual was put on a low phenylalanine diet, and her blood phenylalanine levels were reduced from above 30 mg/dl to below 15 mg/dl, her amino acid absorption rates were not different from those of unaffected controls [39]. These studies suggest that rates of transport for specific amino acids across the small-intestinal mucosa may be determined, to a certain extent, by the circulating levels of the amino acids involved and those closely related in structure or sharing a common transport mechanism.

F. Methionine Malabsorption

The first patient described with methionine malabsorption had a urine strikingly unusual in odor, which eventually was traced to α-hydroxybutyric acid; the odor resembled that associated with drying ovens for hops–hence, its original name of oasthouse urine disease [40]. Chromatographic analysis indicated an excess of neutral amino acids, particularly methionine. Studies in another patient established that α-hydroxybutyric acid was the product of the bacterial fermentation of methionine remaining unabsorbed in the gut, a situation similar to that of the indicanuria in syndromes of tryptophan malabsorption [41]. Recently it has been shown that transient, milder forms of hypermethioninemia follow when an infant is unable to handle the load of sulfur-containing amino acids provided in some commercial formulas [42].

G. Iminoglycinuria

The first patient described with the syndrome of iminoglycinuria by Joseph et al. [43] presented with severe neurologic symptoms and a characteristic aminoaciduria. A series of nine patients in three Canadian kindreds was later reported [44]. The identity of these conditions served to support the concept of a common tubular resorption mechanism for glycine, proline, and hydroxyproline, in spite of the chemical differences between glycine and the two imino acids.

With the description of additional patients [45, 46], it was postulated that an intestinal transport defect might exist in some individuals with iminoaciduria, as suggested by a reduced increment of plasma proline following an oral challenge and by excessive fecal concentrations of glycine and imino acids.

H. Lowe's Syndrome

In 1952, Lowe et al. [47] described a new clinical entity characterized by organic aciduria, decreased renal ammonia production, and severe mental and neurologic handicaps, summarized by the descriptive nomenclature of oculocerebrorenal syndrome [48]. The aminoaciduria present was also of a generalized type and was accompanied by a loss of glucose, phosphate, potassium, and water. It was later reported that a defect in intestinal amino acid transport might coexist with the renal defect, which is the most striking feature of the disease [49].

VI. Nutrition and Genetics

There is a continuous interplay between the intake of protein as food, the absorption of oligopeptides and amino acids, the blood levels of amino acids, and the synthesis and breakdown of endogenous proteins (Fig. 2).

Dietary needs for humans have been extensively studied, although minimal and optimal requirements are under constant revision and updating [50, 51]. The quality and amino acid composition of the protein are undoubtedly vital to adequate nutrition. The classic division into "essential" and "nonessential" amino acids implies that an adequate supply of the amino acids that can be synthesized in the body will be available for protein synthesis. However, it is conceivable that suboptimal production of nonessential amino acids decreases the pool required for protein synthesis at maximum rates [52]. This may have consequences on the subject and, in pregnant females, on their fetuses

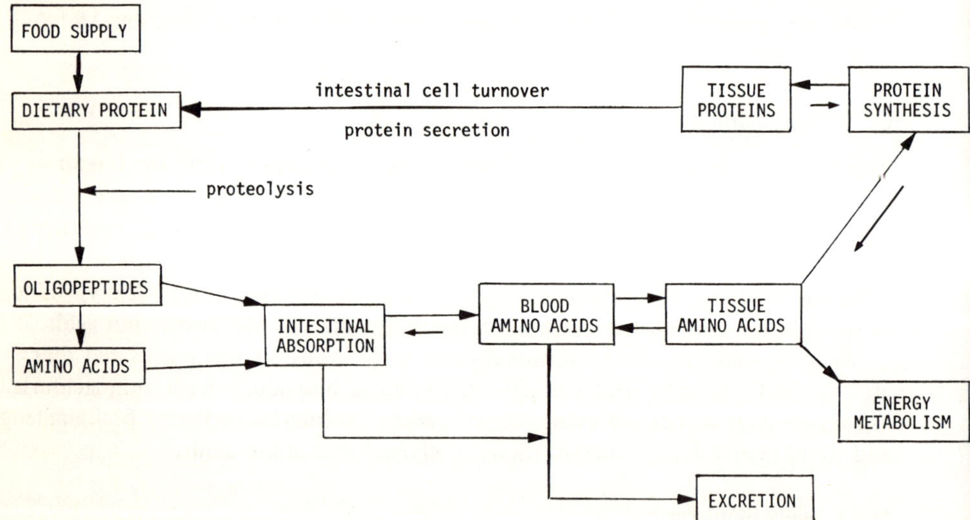

Figure 2 Interrelationships among dietary supply, absorption, and regulation of protein and its breakdown products.

during gestation. This is the basis for Bessman's "justification" theory [53], in which a combination of minimal metabolic disadvantages, due to heterozygosity for an amino acid metabolic defect and a relatively inadequate protein (or specific amino acid) intake, may combine and result in the birth of an infant who has suffered in utero from subclinical malnutrition.

It has been known for a number of years that a history of malnutrition may entail a deficiency of certain amino acids in the circulation [54]. How oscillations of blood levels of specific amino acids affect absorption rates of the same or structurally related amino acids has to be studied in experimental animals [55, 56]. In the rat, hypotyrosinemia induced as a consequence of malnutrition resulted in an increased intestinal absorption of tyrosine. Conversely, hyperphenylalaninemia or hypertyrosinemia, induced by massive feedings of the respective amino acids, depressed the absorption of the corresponding amino acids. These findings paralleled the situation in phenylketonuria described earlier [39].

There are several inborn errors of amino acid metabolism in humans, not necessarily associated with a defect in the intestinal transport of a specific substance, which have been treated by limiting, more or less severely, the intake of one or several amino acids or total protein, as the means to keep the amino acid proximal to the metabolic block from increasing to abnormal levels. In Table 1, adapted from Jonxis [57], are listed conditions requiring the limitation of certain amino acids or protein in an accepted standard therapeutic approach. As the figures indicate, certain situations may give rise to a true deprivation syndrome, as in the case of phenylketonuria and some urea-cycle disorders where the permissible intake is borderline or below normal dietary allowances.

The dietary control approach to other diseases, not listed in Table 1, has been less successful. In some cases, the risks and effort are not justified by the results. Such has been true of the attempts to ameliorate cystinuria [58, 59], or cystinosis [60] with low-methionine diets.

Recently, Scriver [61] introduced the concept of *euphenic nutrition*: that is, the manipulation of the environment in order to provide the optimal supply of nutrients for each individual. On a less dramatic level, humans and animals have instinctively chosen right, in most instances, and ingested the macro- and micronutrients required for growth, reproduction, and survival. Now it is possible to offset the handicap of deleterious genes with specially prepared diets and pre- and postnatal treatment of mutant individuals [62]. These are the "consumers with special needs" that can now be satisfied in most developed societies—possibly opening new avenues for exacting the greatest biological potential in all members of the community.

Table 1 Dietary Allowances of Key Amino Acids in the Treatment of Inborn Errors of Metabolism

Condition	Allowed Intake		Restricted amino acid or precursor	Normal allowance (per kg body wt per day)	
	Infant	Child (12 yr)		Infant (3-6 mo)	Child (10-12 yr)
Phenylketonuria	30-40 mg	10-20 mg	Phenylalanine	132 mg	22 mg
Tyrosinosis	-	25-30 mg	Phenylalanine and tyrosine		
Maple syrup urine disease	50 mg	20 mg	Isoleucine	80 mg	28 mg
	60 mg	40 mg	Leucine	128 mg	42 mg
	40 mg	30 mg	Valine	105 mg	33 mg
Methylmalonic aciduria	1.2 g (+ 100 μg B_{12})	-	Protein	2.0 g	0.6 g
Urea-cycle disorders	1.5 g	0.5 g	Protein	2.0 g	0.6 g
Hyperlysinemia and hyperdibasicamino-acidemia	100 mg	-	Lysine	97 mg	44 mg
Homocystinuria	-	10 mg (+ up to 400 mg B_6)	Methionine		
Cystathioninuria	-	200 mg B_6	Methionine and cystine	45 mg	22 mg
Methionine malabsorption	-	10 mg	Methionine		
Tryptophan malabsorption	-	?	Tryptophan	19 mg	4 mg

Source: Adapted from Jonxis [57].

Acknowledgment

This work was supported by U.S. Public Health Service Grant 1 508 RR 09128-01A1.

References

1. J. F. Danielli. The bilayer hypothesis of membrane structure. *Hosp. Pract. 8*(1), 63-71 (1973).
2. H. W. Davenport. *Physiology of the Digestive Tract,* 4th Ed. Year Book Med. Pub., Chicago, 1977, pp. 198-231.
3. S. O. Thier and D. H. Alpers. Disorders of intestinal transport of amino acids. *Am. J. Dis. Child. 117,* 13-23 (1969).
4. G. Wiseman. Absorption of amino acids using an in vitro technique. *J. Physiol. (Lond.) 120,* 63-72 (1953).
5. R. K. Crane. Na^+-Dependent transport in the intestine and other animal tissues. *Fed. Proc. 24,* 1000-1005 (1965).
6. E. Heinz. Transport through biological membranes. *Annu. Rev. Physiol. 29,* 21-58 (1967).
7. H. N. Christensen. Implications of the cellular transport step for amino acid metabolism. *Nutr. Rev. 35,* 129-133 (1977).
8. M. D. Milne. Disorders of amino acid transport. *Br. Med. J. 1,* 327-336 (1964).
9. 2222
   22222
10. M. Orlowski and A. Meister. The γ-glutamyl cycle: A possible transport system for amino acids. *Proc. Natl. Acad. Sci. USA 67,* 1248-1255 (1970).
11. A. Meister. On the enzymology of amino acid transport. *Science 180,* 33-39 (1973).
12. T. Q. Garvey, III, P. E. Hyman, and K. J. Isselbacher. γ-Glutamyl transpeptidase of rat intestine: Localization and possible role in amino acid transport. *Gastroenterology 71,* 778-785 (1976).
13. D. D. Jones, G. Williams, and B. Prochazka. Multiple molecular forms of γ-glutamyl transpeptidase during human pregnancy. *Enzyme 17,* 139-145 (1974).
14. M. L. Efron. *Aminoaciduria. N. Engl. J. Med. 272,* 1058-1067; 1107-1113 (1965).
15. M. D. Milne, A. M. Asatoor, K. D. G. Edwards, and L. W. Loughridge. The intestinal absorption defect in cystinuria. *Gut 2,* 323-337 (1961).
16. L. E. Rosenberg, S. J. Downing, and S. Segal. Competitive inhibition of dibasic amino acid transport in rat kidney. *J. Biol. Chem. 237,* 2265-2270 (1962).
17. C. F. McCarthy, J. L. Borland, H. L. Lynch, E. E. Owen, and M. P. Tyor. Defective uptake of basic amino acids and L-cystine by intestinal mucosa of patients with cystinuria. *J. Clin. Invest. 43,* 1518-1524 (1964).
18. S. O. Thier, M. Fox, S. Segal, and I. E. Rosenberg. Cystinuria: In vitro demonstration of an intestinal transport defect. *Science 143,* 482-484 (1964).
19. S. O. Thier, S. Segal, M. Fox, A. Blair, and L. E. Rosenberg. Cystinuria:

Defective intestinal transport of dibasic amino acids and cystine. *J. Clin. Invest. 44,* 442-448 (1965).

20. L. E. Rosenberg and S. J. Downing. Transport of neutral and dibasic amino acids by human leukocytes: Absence of defect in cystinuria. *J. Clin. Invest. 44,* 1382-1393 (1965).
21. V. Groth and L. E. Rosenberg. Transport of dibasic amino acids, cystine and tryptophan by cultured human fibroblasts: Absence of a defect in cystinuria and Hartnup disease. *J. Clin. Invest. 51,* 2130-2142 (1972).
22. L. E. Rosenberg, S. J. Downing, J. L. Durant, and S. Segal. Cystinuria: Biochemical evidence for three genetically distinct diseases. *J. Clin. Invest. 45,* 365-371 (1966).
23. C. L. Morin, M. W. Thompson, S. H. Jackson, and A. Sass-Kortsak. Biochemical and genetic studies in cystinuria: Observations on double heterozygotes of genotype I/II. *J. Clin. Invest. 50,* 1961-1976 (1971).
24. M. D. Hellier, D. Perrett, and C. D. Holdsworth. Dipeptide absorption in cystinuria. *Br. Med. J. 4,* 782-783 (1970).
25. J. Peerhentupa and J. K. Visakorpi. Protein intolerance with deficient transport of basic amino acids: Another inborn error of metabolism. *Lancet 2,* 813-816 (1965).
26. M. Kekkomaki, J. K. Visakorpi, J. Peerhentupa, and L. Saxen. Familial protein intolerance with deficient transport of basic amino acids. An analysis of ten patients. *Acta Paediatr. Scand. 56,* 617-630 (1967).
27. K. Oyanagi, R. Miura, and T. Yamanouchi. Congenital lysinuria: A new inherited transport disorder of dibasic amino acids. *J. Pediatr. 77,* 259-266 (1970).
28. D. T. Whelan and C. R. Scriver. Hyperdibasicaminoaciduria: An inherited disorder of amino acid transport. *Pediatr. Res. 2,* 525-534 (1968).
29. J. Brodehl, K. Gellissen, and S. Kowalewsko. Isolated cystinuria (without lysine-ornithine-argininuria) in a family with hypocalcemic tetany. In *Proceedings, Third International Congress of Nephrology.* Washington, D.C., 1976.
30. C. R. Scriver. Hartnup disease: A genetic modification of intestinal and renal transport of certain neutral alpha-amino acids. *N. Engl. J. Med. 273,* 530-532 (1965).
31. V. E. Shih, E. M. Bixby, D. H. Alpers, C. S. Bartsocas, and S. O. Thier. Studies of intestinal transport defect in Hartnup disease. *Gastroenterology 61,* 445-453 (1971).
32. A. M. Asatoor, B. Cheng, K. D. G. Edwards, A. F. Langt, D. M. Matthews, M. D. Milne, F. Navab, and A. J. Richards. Intestinal absorption of two dipeptides in Hartnup's disease. *Gut 11,* 380-387 (1970).
33. K. Drummond, A. Michael, A. Ulstron, and R. Good. *Blue diaper* syndrome: Familial hypercalcemia with nephrocalcinosis and indicanuria. *Am. J. Med. 37,* 928-948 (1964).
34. M. D. Armstrong and K. S. Robinson. On the excretion of indole derivatives in phenylketonuria. *Arch. Biochem. Biophys. 52,* 287-288 (1954).

35. S. P. Bessman and K. Tada. Indicanuria in phenylketonuria. *Metabolism 9,* 377-385 (1960).
36. F. Linneweh, X. X. Ehrlich, E. H. Graul, and H. Hundeshagen. Uber den-Amino-sauren transport bei phenylketonurischer Oligophrenia. *Klin. Wochenschr. 41,* 253-255 (1963).
37. M. T. Yarbro and J. A. Anderson. L-Tryptophan metabolism in phenylketonuria. *J. Pediatr. 68,* 895-904 (1966).
38. J. P. Farriaux, J. P. Delhaye, and G. Fontaine. Etude de l'absorption intestinale des acides amines chez le sujet phenylcetonurique par la methode de perfusion intestinale continue. *Path. Biol. 20,* 543-550 (1970).
39. R. A. Wapnir and F. Lifshitz. Intestinal transport of aromatic amino acids, glucose and electrolytes in a patient with phenylketonuria. *Clin. Chim. Acta 54,* 349-356 (1974).
40. A. J. Smith and L. B. Strang. An inborn error of metabolism with the urinary excretion of α-hydroxybutyric acid and phenylpyruvic acid. *Arch. Dis. Child. 33,* 109-113 (1958).
41. C. Hooft, J. Timmermans, J. Snoeck, I. Antener, W. Oyaert, and C. Van den Hende. Methionine malabsorption syndrome. *Ann. Paediatr. 205,* 73-84 (1965).
42. R. G. Meny, R. L. Gutberlet, P. T. Ozand, C. Morric, and C. H. Kim. Hypermethioninemia in an infant. *Am. J. Dis. Child. 132,* 261-262 (1978).
43. R. Joseph, M. Ribierre, J. C. Job, and M. Girault. Maladie familiale associante des convulsions à début très précoce, une hyperalbuminorachie et une hyperaminoacidurie. *Arch. Franc. Pediatr. 15,* 374-378 (1958).
44. C. R. Scriver. Renal tubular transport of proline, hydroxyproline and glycine. III. Genetic basis for more than one mode of transport in human kidney. *J. Clin. Invest. 47,* 823-835 (1968).
45. T. Morkawa, K. Tada, T. Ando, T. Yoshida, Y. Yokohama, and T. Arakawa. Prolinuria: Defect in intestinal absorption of imino acids and glycine. *Tohoku J. Exp. Med. 90,* 105-116 (1966).
46. S. I. Goodman, C. A. McIntyre, and D. O'Brien. Impaired intestinal transport of proline in a patient with familial iminoaciduria. *J. Pediatr. 71,* 246-249 (1967).
47. C. Lowe, M. Terrey, and E. A. MacLachlan. Organic aciduria. decreased renal ammonia production, hydrophthalmos and mental retardation. A clinical entity. *Am. J. Dis. Child. 83,* 164-184 (1952).
48. W. Richards, G. N. Donnell, W. A. Wilson, and D. S. Stowens. Oculo-cerebro-renal syndrome of Lowe. *Am. J. Dis. Child. 100,* 707-709 (1960).
49. C. S. Bartsocas, H. L. Levy, J. D. Crawford, and S. O. Thier. A defect in intestinal amino acid transport in Lowe's syndrome. *Am. J. Dis. Child. 117,* 93-95 (1969).
50. World Health Organization. *Energy and Protein Requirements.* Technical Report Series No. 522, 1973.

51. National Research Council, Food and Nutrition Board. *Recommended Dietary Allowances,* 8th Ed. National Academy of Sciences, Washington, D.C., 1974, p. 44.
52. S. P. Bessman, M. K. Williamson, and R. Koch. Diet, genetics, and mental retardation interaction between phenylketonuric heterozygous mother and fetus to produce nonspecific diminution of IQ: Evidence in support of the justification hypothesis. *Proc. Natl. Acad. Sci. USA 75,* 1562-1566 (1978).
53. S. P. Bessman. Genetic failure of fetal amino acid justification: A common basis for many forms of metabolic, nutritional, and "nonspecific" mental retardation. *J. Pediatr. 81,* 834-842 (1972).
54. R. G. Whitehead and T. R. Milburn. Amino acid metabolism in kwashiorkor II. Metabolism of phenylalanine and tyrosine. *Clin. Sci. 26,* 279-289 (1964).
55. R. A. Wapnir, R. L. Hawkins, and F. Lifshitz. Hyperaminoacidemia effects on intestinal transport of related amino acids. *Am. J. Physiol. 223,* 788-793 (1972).
56. R. A. Wapnir and F. Lifshitz. Absorption of amino acids in malnourished rats. *J. Nutr. 104,* 843-849 (1974).
57. J. H. P. Jonxis. The nutritional significance of inborn errors of amino acid metabolism. *Nutr. Metab. 21,* 33-48 (1977).
58. H. H. Zinneman and J. E. Jones. Dietary methionine and its influence on cystine excretion in cystinuric patients. *Metabolism 15,* 915-921 (1966).
59. F. O. Kolb, J. M. Earll, and H. A. Harper. "Disappearance" of cystinuria in a patient treated with prolonged low methionine diet. *Metabolism 16,* 378-381 (1967).
60. H. Bickel, D. Lutz, and H. Schmidt. The treatment of cystinosis with diet or drugs. In *Cystinosis* (J. D. Schulman, Ed.). U.S. Department of Health, Education, and Welfare Publication NIH 79-249, 1977, p. 199.
61. C. R. Scriver. Diet and genes: Euphenic nutrition. *N. Engl. J. Med. 297,* 202-203 (1977).
62. C. R. Scriver. Realized and potential neutralization of mutant genes in man by nutritional selection. *Fed. Proc. 35,* 2286-2290 (1976).

16
Carbohydrate Malabsorption

FIMA LIFSHITZ / Cornell University Medical College, New York, New York, and North Shore University Hospital, Manhasset, New York

I. Introduction

Many of the problems related to carbohydrate malabsorption that are currently being investigated have been apparent for some time. As early as 1901, Jacobi noted that some children showed "specific idiosyncrasies" to the carbohydrate of milk [1]. The first report on milk (sugar) malabsorption was recorded by Finkelstein and Meyer in 1911 [2]. In 1921 Howland described alterations in the absorption of other dietary disaccharides, such as sucrose, that occurred in children with diarrhea [3]. He suggested that the difficulties in digestion and absorption of carbohydrates were related to "the ferments of the intestine." There were thought to produce a prolongation and worsening of diarrhea.

At the beginning of this century important advances were also made in the biochemical field of carbohydrate malabsorption. In 1907 L. B. Mendel demonstrated that calf intestinal lactase activity was much greater in younger than in older animals [4]. This confirmed earlier studies, in 1906, by Plimmer [5]. These reports stimulated work pertinent to an understanding of lactose malabsorption and lactase deficiency. However, it took almost 50 years until observations similar to those in animals were documented in humans [6].

II. Carbohydrate Absorption

The subject of carbohydrate digestion and absorption has recently been extensively reviewed in detail [7-9]. Most ingested carbohydrates are absorbed in the small intestine; thus, little or no sugar normally reaches the terminal ileum or colon. Dietary carbohydrates are digested and absorbed by a series of specific mechanisms. Salivary α-amylase begins the digestion of polysaccharides (starch, glycogen, dextrins) into oligosaccharides and some disaccharides. Pancreatic α-amylase completes the digestion of these larger oligosaccharides to disaccharides. Dietary disaccharides, like lactose or sucrose, arrive intact in the small intestine. In the jejunum specific hydrolases, oligosaccharidases, split the disaccharides into their component monosaccharides.

The disaccharidases should, in fact, be regarded as oligosaccharidases, since they are capable of hydrolyzing sugars with three or more hexose units into the constituent monosaccharides. The oligosaccharides are large glycoproteins with a half-life of a few hours and a pH optimum of 6.0. There are two types of oligosaccharidases in the human jejunum, as shown in Table 1. The single hexose sugars resulting from hydrolysis are transported by specific mechanisms into the intestinal epithelial cells. Since the rate of hydrolysis of disaccharides is more rapid than the rate of absorption of monosaccharides, some hexoses may diffuse back into the lumen and subsequently be absorbed at a more distant small-intestinal segment. Beta-galactosidase activity is the rate-limiting enzyme in this process. It is slower and releases monosaccharides in quantities which are not sufficient to saturate the transport mechanism. The unstirred layer of intestinal contents overlying the surface membrane [10] constitutes an important physiologic means of regulating oligosaccharide hydrolysis and absorption. It may also act as an osmotic barrier, limiting the excessive pressure that might result if uncontrolled production of monosaccharides occurred.

Intestinal oligosaccharidases are located principally in the brush border of the epithelial cells. Maximum enzyme activity is present in the distal portion of villi, and, in the human, it increases caudally from the proximal duodenum, with its peak in the jejunum or proximal ileum. Oligosaccharidase activities are low in the distal ileum and are absent in the stomach and colon. In newborn children total oligosaccharidase activity remains relatively low for the first few days of life until the microvilli are fully developed.

Glucose is the major monosaccharide in dietary carbohydrates; about 80% of ingested sugars are eventually broken down in the intestine to glucose. Monosaccharides require a specific transport mechanism to move into the intestinal cells. The glucose carrier is a protein in the microvillus membrane that binds Na^+ and utilizes energy from the hydrolysis of ATP by a (Na^+-K^+)-activated ATPase [7]. This carrier releases glucose into the epithelial cell, where its concentration may exceed that of the lumen more than 15-fold. Glucose then leaves the cell by diffusion into the capillaries of the portal system. Galactose shares this transport mechanism with glucose, but fructose appears to be transported by an independent process of facilitated diffusion which does not require Na^+.

Table 1 Human Intestinal Brush Border Oligosaccharidase

Type	Name	Carbohydrate substrate	Dietary source	Products
β-Galactosidase	Lactase	Lactose	Milk	Glucose and galactose
α-Glucosidases	Glucoamylase (maltase[a])	Maltose and oligosaccharides	Starch	Glucose
	Sucrase-dextrinase (sucrase-isomaltase[a])	Maltose, sucrose, and dextrins	Starch and sugar	Glucose and fructose
	Trehalase	Trehalose	Mushrooms	Glucose

[a]Common nomenclature.

Source: Adapted from Gray [8]. There are three β-galactosidases, but only one is responsible for lactose absorption.

III. Lactose and Lactase

A. Lactose

It has been suggested that the disaccharide lactose and the intestinal enzyme lactase appeared at about the same time in evolution [11] and that they may be more than 100 million years old. The fact that lactose is a constituent of milk was discovered over 300 years ago. It was only recently synthesized in the laboratory. It may be of interest that some plants make a β-galactoside similar to the lactose of human milk.

Lactose is synthesized in the mammary glands and requires two proteins: one, the enzyme *N*-acetylgalactose transferase; and the other, the protein α-lactalbumin. The α-lactalbumin is not an enzyme, but it affects the transferase so that the K_m for glucose is considerably lower, and the enzyme shifts from the synthesis of *N*-acetyllactosamine to the synthesis of lactose. Very high concentrations of glucose can have the same effect as α-lactalbumin on galactosyl transferase. In the rat mammary gland, the activity of galactose transferase increases throughout gestation, but α-lactalbumin does not become evident until 18-19 days of gestation. Then it increases abruptly in concentration, coincident with a marked increase in lactose production at the 19th to 20th day of gestation. In vitro studies indicate that insulin, prolactin, and hydrocortisone participate in the synthesis of both the galactosyl transferase and α-lactalbumin, while progesterone is inhibitory to the synthesis of α-lactalbumin and consequently lactose.

Lactose is found in the milk of all mammals, except seals, sea lions, and walruses [12]. In these species there is no lactose; in fact there are no carbohydrates in the milk of these animals. The concentration of carbohydrate in milk varies considerably from species to species and bears an indirect relationship to the concentration of fat and protein. In the human, lactose intake constitutes a most important source of calories, particularly in infancy. In Table 2, the role of lactose intake via milk in the calorie supplies of human nutrition is shown. During the first year of life, lactose accounts for 40-50% of the total caloric intake. Thereafter, there is a gradual decrease in calories supplied by lactose to a minimum of 2% in an adult who may take one glass of milk per day. Why lactose was selected in evolution as such an important calorie source is a very interesting and unanswered question. One aspect which may have participated in its selection is the fact that lactose yields twice the caloric value of glucose at only one-half the osmolarity. Another aspect may be the fact that lactose does not diffuse from the mammary gland into the circulation.

B. Lactase

Lactase is an enzyme localized in the epithelial cells of the villi. In the dividing crypt cells there is no immunochemical, and only negligible biochemical, evidence of the presence of the enzyme. It is the most superficial and the

Table 2 Lactose Intake and Its Relationship to Calorie Supplies in Human Nutrition

Age of child (yr)	RDA[a] (cal/day)	% Total calories consumed as lactose[b,c]	
		1 Cup milk/day	4 Cups milk/day
0-1	-[d]	-[d]	40-50
1-3 (both sexes)	1,300	3.7	14.8
4-6 (both sexes)	1,800	2.7	10.7
11-14 (male)	2,800	1.7	6.8
11-14 (female)	2,400	2.0	8.0
$\overline{X}$, 11-14 (both sexes)	2,600	1.8	7.4
15-18 (male)	3,000	1.6	6.4
15-18 (female)	2,100	2.3	9.1
$\overline{X}$, 15-18 (both sexes)	2,550	1.9	7.5

[a]From *Recommended Dietary Allowance 1974,* Food and Nutrition Board, National Research Council, National Academy of Sciences of the United States.
[b]One cup whole milk (3.5% fat) contains 12 g lactose. (From C. E. Cburch and H. N. Church. *Food Values of Portions Commonly Used.* Lippincott, Philadelphia, 1970.)
[c]Based on 12 g lactose per cup: cup milk × 4 kcal/g carbohydrate = 48 kcal lactose/cup milk; 4 cups milk × 48 kcal lactose/cup = 192 kcal lactose/4 cups milk.
[d]Breast milk provides 6-7% lactose, and thus it supplies up to 42% of total calories ingested. Cow's milk provides 4-4.2% of lactose, and cow's milk formulas for babies from 4.8 to 7.6%.
Source: This table was kindly supplied by Dr. Lani Stephenson, Division of Nutrition Sciences, Cornell University, Ithaca, New York.

least efficient of all the oligosaccharidases. There are three β-galactosidases: a specific lactase with a maximum activity at pH 6.0, located in the brush border; a β-galactosidase with the same pH optimum, but which is inactive against lactose, located in the cytoplasm; and a β-galactosidase with a pH optimum of 4.5, present in the lysosomes. The specific brush border lactase is an extremely sensitive and rate-limiting enzyme, which is competitively inhibited in vitro by glucose, as well as by substances such as colchicine [13]. It has been postulated that the nonspecific β-galactosidase in the brush border is a precursor for the specific lactase, but this proposal has not been substantiated. The specific lactase has been partially purified, and antibodies have been developed to the enzyme derived from rat and human intestine [8].

There is a characteristic ontogenetic pattern of lactase activity in most mammals, including humans. In fetal life there is a gradual increase in lactase activity, presumably due to synthesis of the enzyme. Lactase activity in most mammals is greatest in the perinatal period; there is approximately 10 times as much lactase at birth as in adult mammals including the human adult. The continued feeding of lactose after weaning has little effect on enzyme levels. This was shown by studies first done in 1906 by Plimmer [5] and reconfirmed over the ensuing 70 years.

There are some interesting variations in this ontogenetic pattern of lactase. In guinea pigs lactase activity reaches a peak in utero. This animal also matures in utero and need not suckle at the mother's breast, but can be fed with vegetables at birth. As noted above, there are lactase-deficient mammals such as sea lions and walruses in the Pacific Basin [12].

In humans, lactase activity follows the same pattern of development as in other animal species, with the exception of certain groups of persons who maintain high lactase levels throughout life. These people are generally the northern Europeans (Anglo-Saxons); the Finns, Hungarians, and those related to the Mongols; and three tribes in Africa: the Fulani, the Tusi, and the Nasi. Therefore the majority of adult humans, like other adult mammals, are naturally lactase deficient [14, 15]; lactose malabsorption occurs almost invariably in most of the world's population after 3-5 years [16-18]. The ability of humans to tolerate lactose after age five may result from a mutation, since this enzymatic activity normally decreases after weaning in mammals. No other animal has been found that can digest lactose after weaning. Persistence of the infantile level of lactase activity throughout adult life is thus the exception, and may represent an evolutionary adaptive process which provided a selective advantage when humans were first exposed to increased lactose intake. Milk drinking can only be dated back to about 8000-10,000 B.C. The ability to tolerate lactose was thereafter inherited as a dominant characteristic, which helped in the natural selection process of the lactose digesters in some specific groups, particularly Anglo-Saxons and some African tribes.

It has been calculated that the gene for adult lactase production has an assumed frequency of 0.60 in tolerant populations and 0.05 in intolerant ones. The selection intensity against homozygotes required to produce a change in the gene frequency from intolerant to tolerant would thus require a passage of about 400 generations, or approximately 10,000 years, in order to change an ethnic group from predominantly lactase deficient to lactase sufficient in adult life.

IV. Carbohydrate Malabsorption Syndromes

Carbohydrate digestion and absorption are highly specific. A variety of alterations in any one of the steps in the process may result in carbohydrate malabsorption. Abnormalities may affect the absorption of specific dietary carbohydrates, or combinations of disaccharides and monosaccharides. Except for maldigestion of starch caused by amylase deficiency in newborn infants, the majority of carbohydrate malabsorption syndromes are related to alterations in the functional integrity of the intestinal mucosa and its epithelial cells. There are three types of carbohydrate malabsorption syndromes: (1) ontogenetic, (2) primary, and (3) secondary.

A. Ontogenetic

The ontogenetic type of carbohydrate malabsorption [11, 19, 20] has been comprehensively studied by Kretchmer et al. The term describes the lactose malabsorption which occurs during the time that lactase activity is normally low. This is seen in both the immediate neonatal period and beyond 3-5 years of age in many ethnic groups. Newborn babies do not absorb lactose well until the first week of life [21], whereas in premature infants, a normal response to lactose loading is not observed until 2-3 weeks of life [22]. Lactose malabsorption in newborn children is not usually associated with diarrhea; however, in preterm infants, there is metabolic acidosis following lactose loading [22]. The improvement in the neonatal period is independent of lactose ingestion, and may be due to the maturity of the microvilli, which is achieved after birth.

The striking regional and ethnic, or racial, incidence of lactose malabsorption usually becomes apparent after 3-5 years of age [16-18]. Conversely, individuals who are destined to be able to tolerate lactose continue to digest and absorb this carbohydrate throughout life. Several other hypotheses attempt to account for changes in the capacity to absorb lactose. The inductive hypothesis correlates lactase deficiency with decreased consumption of milk after weaning [23]. The inhibitory hypothesis emphasizes the capacity of certain sugars and drugs to inhibit lactase activity and hence to decrease lactose tolerance with age [13]. The adaptive hypothesis relates the increased incidence of enteric disease to those groups with nonspecific small-bowel injury and reduced lactase activity. The recent observation that lactase is the target enzyme for enteric rotaviruses fits with this explanation [24]. In addition, adaptation of the individual to intestinal stress may vary. The dependence of intestinal oligosaccharidases on dietary carbohydrate substrate susceptibility has been found to be enhanced during diarrhea induced by hyperosmotic loads [25]. However, the most widely accepted ontogenetic hypothesis [11, 14, 15, 19, 20] relates the persistence of lactase activity into adulthood to an adaptive human evolutionary trait of certain ethnic or racial groups, as described above.

B. Primary

The primary or congenital specific carbohydrate malabsorption syndromes are rare. Primary deficiencies have been described for each of the intestinal surface oligosaccharidases, and for the capacity of the intestine to transport glucose (Table 3). These entities may manifest themselves very early in life or may have a late onset in adults. The patients have a virtual absence of hydrolytic activity for a single disaccharide, or an absence of the intestinal capacity to transport glucose and galactose. However, they have no other abnormality of intestinal function or structure. The precise biochemical defect responsible for the absence of enzymatic activity has not been characterized in any primary deficiency state. There may be a complete deletion of the enzyme protein, or there may be an abnormal, biologically inactive molecule.

Congenital lactose malabsorption is a rare disorder [26]. There are very few patients with direct biopsy evidence of low intestinal lactase activity. The mode of inheritance has not be clarified. In the literature there are more males than females described with lactase deficiency, and three pairs of siblings have also been reported. Sucrase-isomaltase deficiency is an inherited autosomal recessive disorder, which is more common than other disaccharidase deficiencies [27]. This entity may be due to an abnormal sucrase protein [28], which is quite prevalent among Greenland Eskimos, with an incidence of up to 10% [29]. Children with this disease seem to tolerate dextrins because of the low osmotic force of these high molecular weight sugars. Trehalase deficiency has also been reported in a patient who had diarrhea after ingestion of mushrooms [30]. However, there may be other patients with this alteration who have no symptoms, since the intake of trehalose is minimal in the Western diet. Isolated maltase deficiency probably does not exist because of the existence of several brush border enzymes with maltase activity.

Table 3 Primary Carbohydrate Malabsorption

Age of onset
Newborn
Adult
Type
Deficiency of intestinal surface oligosaccharidases
Lactase
Sucrase-dextrinase
Trehalase
Deficiency of intestinal transport capacity
Glucose-galactose

A primary inability to absorb the products of disaccharide hydrolysis may also occur. Glucose-galactose malabsorption is a hereditary autosomal recessive disorder of actively transported monosaccharides, with effects upon the intestine and kidney tubules. It may result from an abnormality in the membrane binding sites for these carbohydrates [31]. Kinetic analysis of the absorption of glucose has indicated that there is a reduced transport capacity (V_{max}) and a normal affinity for the carbohydrate (K_m). These patients develop diarrhea and glycosuria as soon as milk feedings are begun. On the other hand, fructose is absorbed at normal rates and can, therefore, be utilized to supply carbohydrates in the diet.

Of interest is the late onset of any of the above-mentioned primary carbohydrate malabsorption syndromes [32-34]. The usual view is that these are genetically controlled diseases, which are first manifested in adult life. However, they may result from secondary or ontogenetic causes.

C. Secondary

Secondary carbohydrate malabsorption may be associated with any of the diverse systemic and/or intestinal disorders listed in Table 4. This type of

Table 4 Secondary Carbohydrate Malabsorption

- Age of onset
  - Any age following intestinal damage
- Type
  - Deficiency of intestinal surface oligosaccharidases
    - Selective lactase
    - Generalized brush border oligosaccharidases
  - Deficiency of intestinal transport capacity
    - Active transport (glucose)
    - Altered permeability (fructose)
- Associated disorders
  - Diarrheal disease
  - Protein-energy malnutrition, specific deficiencies (e.g., iron)
  - Malabsorption syndrome (celiac, sprue, and blind-loop)
  - Giardia lamblia infestation
  - Cystic fibrosis
  - Chronic inflammatory disease of the bowel
  - Gastric and intestinal surgery
  - Immune deficiency syndromes and cow's-milk allergy
  - Drugs (birth-control, neomycin, colchicine)
  - Hypoxia

carbohydrate malabsorption is usually related to a depression of small-intestinal oligosaccharidase activity due to mucosal damage induced by the primary disease process [20, 36] (see also Chap. 23). The lesion may affect one or all of the mucosal oligosaccharidases, as well as other intestinal transport processes, and at times even intestinal permeability. Secondary lactose malabsorption alone is the most frequent clinical alteration [36]; however, it may be complicated by malabsorption of sucrose and other disaccharides. When the alteration is more severe, there may also be malabsorption of all monosaccharides, including fructose [36]. Several factors may account for the high frequency of transient lactose malabsorption. Lactase is the most superficial enzyme of the intestinal oliogosaccharidases. Its activity is rate limiting for absorption, and lactase concentrations are lower than those of other mucosal enzymes [8]. Lactase may be a target enzyme for the rotavirus which produces infantile gastroenteritis–frequently leading to specific lactase deficiency [24]. In addition to a decrease in intestinal oligosaccharidase activity, there may be other factors leading to carbohydrate malabsorption. For example, a primary disease process might increase motility or decrease the absorptive surface area and, therefore, reduce the time of exposure of a disaccharide to the intestinal enzymes. There may also be interference in the binding of a substrate to its enzyme because of epithelial cell inflammation, anatomical disturbance, or other alterations [25]. For example, the carbohydrate malabsorption which follows hypoxia is due to factors other than altered intestinal disaccharidases, as described in Chapter 23 of this volume.

V. Clinical Assessment of Carbohydrate Malabsorption

Sugar malabsorption of all types is clinically characterized by watery, sour-smelling, diarrheal stools that have an acid pH and contain carbohydrates and organic acids, especially lactic acid. Weight loss, failure to thrive, dehydration, and electrolyte loss may be present. These symptoms decline when the offending carbohydrate is eliminated from the diet. These consequences of carbohydrate malabsorption are referred to as carbohydrate intolerance and are reviewed in detail in Chapter 23 of this volume. Since milk is the primary source of lactose, it may lead to the erroneous conclusion that lactose intolerance is synonymous with milk intolerance (see Section VI). Different investigators place reliance on different criteria for diagnosis of the capacity of patients to tolerate carbohydrates. These criteria vary from simple clinical sugar tolerance tests to measurements of disaccharidase activity of the intestinal mucosa, metabolic balance studies with quantitation of organic acid and carbohydrate excretion, and determination of intestinal absorptive rates for specific carbohydrates by transintestinal intubation.

Indications of carbohydrate malabsorption can be derived from simple, semiquantitative measurements of the amounts of reducing substances, glucose, and the pH of stools [36-38]. The indices for carbohydrate intolerance in infants with diarrhea include concentrations of reducing substances above 0.25%, 1+ glucose, and pH less than 6.0. Although these techniques are now widely employed, a very important source of error is commonly introduced by testing for these parameters in nonfresh stool specimens. Within minutes after excretion there is exogenous bacterial fermentation, the pH of the stool and its glucose concentration rapidly drop, and its lactic acid concentration rapidly increases. Thus the stool has to be tested immediately after it is excreted. We utilize a simple electronic device to signal the time of bowel movements to ensure that tests will be made on fresh stools.

It is important that the progress of patients with diarrhea be followed by stool testing throughout the time that they have abnormal stools. Most fecal samples analyzed at random with these simple bedside methods have a pH of 6.0 or more, and contain concentrations of carbohydrates below those of clinical significance. To assess the capacity of infants and children to tolerate specific carbohydrates, two to three fresh liquid stools should be checked daily throughout the illness, with changes in specific dietary intake. Severe lactose intolerance is diagnosed if most of the stools on a milk formula contain carbohydrates and are of acid pH. Mild intolerance is considered to be present if fewer than 30% of the stools are positive for these parameters [36].

Response to an oral carbohydrate load is frequently used to test the capacity to tolerate specific disaccharides or monosaccharides [37]. The absence of a rise in blood sugar levels after carbohydrate ingestion is often regarded as the sole criterion to establish impaired hydrolysis. A flat curve corresponds to a rise of less than 20 mg% above basal; a reduced absorption is considered to occur when less than 40 mg% rise is observed; and a normal absorption is that which produces more than 40 mg% rise above basal. However, up to 30% of healthy subjects with normal intestinal lactase activities may have flat tolerance tests following lactose loads. Blood sugar levels vary after carbohydrate ingestion, depending on the site from which blood is obtained. The blood sugar response of infants to an oral carbohydrate load after recovery from diarrhea is variable and does not correlate with the stool pattern [37]. It is therefore preferable to correlate carbohydrate intolerance with diarrhea, acid stools, and excretion of carbohydrates on ingestion of the offending sugar. There are a number of recent modifications in the carbohydrate oral test, including the barium-lactose roentgenologic study [39], the analysis of labeled CO_2 in the breath after administration of [^{14}C]L-lactose [40], and the analysis of hydrogen gas in the breath after lactose feeding [41]. A rise in breath hydrogen level greater than 10 ppm above baseline value at 90 to 120 min following ingestion of a standard dose of lactose is considered abnormal.

Lactosuria may be present following lactose ingestion in infants with lactose intolerance. However, it is not a feature specific to lactose malabsorption since it may be seen in other conditions such as infection or hyperthyroidism, as well as in normal young infants.

The most accurate test for disaccharidase deficiencies is the determination of these intestinal enzymes by peroral biopsy of the small intestine. Measurements of specific activity (units of enzyme per gram of protein) are accurate, but are not indispensable for diagnosis of the capacity to tolerate carbohydrates [36, 37]. Low lactase activity or lactase deficiency is defined as less than 2 units of lactase activity per gram of wet weight of mucosa. However, this measurement is not as accurate as when units are expressed per gram of protein, particularly in disease states where there may be inflammation of the cell with a reduction of the enzymatic capacity per gram of wet weight of mucosa, but with no alterations in disaccharidase specific activity. A value of less than 20 units of lactase specific activity is usually considered diagnostic of lactase deficiency. The sucrase and maltase values are usually two and four times higher than the lactase levels. Disaccharidase ratios are pertinent to ascertain the diagnosis of disaccharidase deficiency, particularly when the concentration of these enzymes are measured by wet weight of mucosa. The response to a disaccharide oral load can be, at best, only an indirect measurement of the disaccharidase activity, since there are many factors which influence the blood sugar rise, in addition to the presence of the specific disaccharidsae in the intestinal mucosa.

VI. Carbohydrate Malabsorption and Food Intolerance

Alterations in the digestion and absorption of carbohydrates of any type may lead to carbohydrate intolerance. A review of secondary carbohydrate intolerance is provided in Chapter 23 of this volume. Here, a brief review of the concept of lactose malabsorption and its association with milk intolerance is undertaken, since there is much disagreement over the practical relevance of lactose malabsorption. It is important to understand this issue so that those individuals who may enjoy the nutritional benefits of milk are not needlessly denied this valuable nutritional source, and those for whom dietary alterations are necessary may be properly advised. There is little question that the prevalence of lactose malabsorption is high among most peoples throughout the world, as reviewed above. Nevertheless, the question still remains: what is the practical relevance of these findings in healthy populations? The nomenclature in itself has been a source of confusion. There are three terms to keep in mind: Lactose malabsorption, lactose intolerance and milk intolerance. Lactose malabsorption is reduced absorption of lactose as determined by a lactose tolerance test. Usually there is a diminished rise in blood sugar after an oral lactose load as described above. This may or may not be accompanied by intolerance [37]. Lactose intolerance is defined as the development of clinical symptoms, particularly diarrhea (with excretion of acid stools and carbohydrates in feces) and/or other gastrointestinal symptoms, following ingestion of lactose mixed with water in a standard dose (i.e., 50 g/m^a of body surface area or 2 g/kg body weight).

Milk intolerance can be defined as the development of significant symptoms, similar to those described for lactose intolerance, following the consumption of usual amounts of milk-containing products [14, 42]. Not all patients with milk intolerance have lactose intolerance, since there are other constituents of milk which can induce similar symptoms with or without lactose intolerance. The obvious problems in evaluating "intolerance" relates to what is meant by "significant" and "usual amounts." Furthermore, who should decide on the significance of symptoms–a second-party observer or the individual involved? Should the term significant be applied only when the symptoms are sufficient to cause the individual to alter the serving size of milk consumed? An even more pertinent question is what, if any, is the relevance of symptoms to clinical and nutritional status?

Simoons et al. [17] raise three important considerations about practical questions concerned with milk intolerance: (1) whether a significant number of children who are lactose malabsorbers also are milk intolerant; (2) the amount of milk or lactose required to bring about symptoms in children who are lactose malabsorbers; and (3) the significance of the symptoms in terms of severity and likely detrimental effects on the child.

Lactose malabsorption has been found to be a common cause of gastrointestinal complaints among adults when they ingested one glass of milk per day [43, 44]. On the other hand, lactose malabsorption was found to be a clinically insignificant problem by others [45, 46] when milk was limited to a one-glass level of intake. However, among milk-intolerant black adolescents, few said they would stop drinking milk because of symptoms [47]. The majority of lactose-intolerant adults also said they would not stop drinking milk when the total amount of lactose taken at one time was less than 15 g [42]. On the basis of these and many other studies [48-52], it is fair to conclude that the milk-drinking habits of healthy populations who are lactose malabsorbers are modified in determining the extremes of milk ingestion (i.e., four glasses or more–or no milk ingestion), but that lactose malabsorption has little effect on the intermediate patterns of milk consumption. The above findings can be explained as due to the differences in absorption of lactose from aqueous solutions (for tolerance tests), as compared to absorption from milk. It has been aptly demonstrated that the form and the amount of the lactose challenge greatly affect the number and severity of symptoms [53-59]. The maximal safe dose of cow's milk for all age groups of lactose malabsorbers has been found to correspond to about 15 g lactose or 300 ml milk. This dose of lactose was fairly well tolerated even when it was given mixed in water [42]. Therefore, the response to a lactose tolerance test does not seem to be a good predictor of symptomatic response to normal milk consumption in healthy individuals. The classification of persons who are lactose malabsorbers and/or lactase deficient may thus be important for definition purposes, but in terms of predicting milk tolerance it is not operational in the healthy state. While more data are necessary to provide for sound conclusions on the effects of lactose malabsorption on utilization of nutrients of milk, the present data suggest that this is not a clinically significant problem [60]. At times the clinical significance may be difficult to ascertain unless double-blind studies are undertaken. However, when diarrhea and/or other symptoms occur, lactose and/or milk intolerance may be a most important problem (see Chap. 23).

VII. Therapeutic Considerations

A precise diagnosis of the type of carbohydrate malabsorption, as well as of the capacity to tolerate specific carbohydrates, is essential for rational treatment. It should be directed toward correcting the carbohydrate intolerance and the diarrhea. All the clinical symptoms will improve when the specific carbohydrate is eliminated from the diet. The dietary treatment of carbohydrate malabsorption should be instituted as soon as the diagnosis is made. During the acute stage of the illness there might be associated oligosaccharidase deficiencies secondary to the diarrheal course. Therefore, elimination of all the carbohydrates that are not tolerated is indicated. However, after recovery, only the specifically incriminated disaccharides need be eliminated from the diet. In patients with α-glucosidase deficiencies there is usually an intolerance to sucrose and isomaltose. Maltose is usually well tolerated; however, there have been a few patients described who have maltase deficiency and who are therefore unable to tolerate maltose as well. On the other hand, in patients with lactase deficiency, although lactose will have to be eliminated from the diet, the other disaccharides might be included since they are usually absorbed normally. In the primary forms of the disease a prolonged adherence to the dietary regimen is necessary. The disaccharide should be sufficiently restricted from the diet to keep the patient symptom-free and growing at a normal rate. In all instances of primary oligosaccharidase deficiencies a gradually increased tolerance of the specific carbohydrate might be observed. The patients may eventually tolerate an ordinary diet, but with certain limitations throughout life in regard to their specific intolerance. Even patients with lactase deficiency can consume some milk without any problem. However, these patients require a very strict adherence to the lactose-free diets for a limited time during the acute stage.

Infants with congenital glucose-galactose malabsorption cannot be kept free from symptoms unless they are fed a diet containing fructose as the only carbohydrate. However, gradually they might be offered some solid or semi-solid food items with low starch content. Between 2 and 3 years of age these patients may tolerate ordinary children's food, but with certain limitations in regard to milk- and starch-containing foods (bread, potatoes, and cereals). They can usually consume one glass of milk, two or three sandwiches, and two small potatoes daily without major trouble. These diet restrictions then have to be followed for the rest of their lives. Whenever diarrhea is induced there must be a reduction of the various carbohydrates that are being fed. On the other hand, if no gastrointestinal symptoms occur, the patient may have an intake of these nutrients to provide for normal growth and development.

The question of policy regarding ontogenetic lactose malabsorption and its relationship to milk consumption is of practical importance. It has been considered inappropriate to discourage worldwide milk consumption or programs for improving milk supply solely because of the fear of milk intolerance and lactose malabsorption [60]. Most children with mild ontogenetic lactose malabsorption experience no adverse effects and derive nutritional benefit from drinking moderate amounts of milk [42]. However, the reverse may occur in a particular child [61]. The pediatrician must therefore weigh carefully the use of milk, dairy products, and sugars other than lactose in individuals who exhibit carbohydrate intolerance, and permit consumption in accordance with clinical courses.

Premature infants also have a relative lactase deficiency that results in a diminished capacity to digest and absorb lactose. They usually do not have diarrhea while on milk formula feedings. However, they may develop metabolic acidosis, with a drop in blood pH and serum CO_2, when fed lactose. These patients may be treated by lactose-free formulas during the first 3 weeks of life.

References

1. A. Jacobi. Milk-sugar in infant feeding. *Trans. Am. Pediatr. Soc. 13,* 150-160 (1901).
2. H. Finkelstein and L. F. Meyer. Zur Technik und Indikation der Ernahrung mit Eiweissmilch. *Münch. Med. Wochenschr. 58,* 340-345 (1911).
3. J. Howland. Prolonged intolerance of carbohydrates. *Trans. Am. Pediatr. Soc. 33,* 11-19 (1921).
4. L. B. Mendel and P. H. Mitchell. Chemical studies on growth. I. The inverting enzymes of the alimentary tract, especially in the embryo. *Am. J. Physiol. 20,* 81-95 (1907).

5. R. H. A. Plimmer. On the presence of lactase in the intestine of animals and on the adaptation of the intestine to lactose. *J. Physiol. (Lond.) 35,* 20-31 (1906-1907).
6. N. S. C. Heilskou. Studies on animal lactase. II. Distribution in some of the glands of the digestive tract. *Acta Physiol. Scand. 24,* 84-89 (1951).
7. R. K. Crane. Hypothesis for mechanism of intestinal active transport of sugars. *Fed. Proc. 21,* 891-895 (1962).
8. G. M. Gray. Carbohydrate digestion and absorption. Role of the small intestine. *N. Engl. J. Med. 292,* 1225-1230 (1975).
9. H. B. McMichael. Disorders of carbohydrate digestion and absorption. *Clin. Endocrinol. Metab. 5,* 627-650 (1976).
10. F. A. Wilson and J. M. Dietschy. The intestinal unstirred layer: Its surface area and effect on active transport kinetics. *Biochim. Biophys. Acta. 363,* 112-126 (1974).
11. N. Kretchmer. Memorial lecture: Lactose and lactase-A historical perspective. *Gastroenterology 61,* 805-814 (1971).
12. P. Sunshine and N. Kretchmer. Intestinal disaccharidases: Absence in two species of sea lions. *Science 144,* 850-851 (1964).
13. J. J. Herbst, R. Hurwitz, P. Sunshine, and N. Kretchmer. Effect of colchicine on intestinal disaccharidases: Correlation with biochemical aspects of cellular renewal. *J. Clin. Invest. 49,* 530-536 (1970).
14. F. J. Simoons. Primary adult lactose intolerance and the milking habit: A problem in biologic and cultural interrelations. II. A cultural historical hypothesis. *Am. J. Dig. Dis. 15,* 695-710 (1970).
15. F. J. Simoons. New light on ethnic differences in adult lactose intolerance. *Am. J. Dig. Dis. 18,* 595-611 (1973).
16. N. S. Rosensweig and T. M. Bayless. Racial difference in the incidence of lactase deficiency. *J. Clin. Invest. 45,* 1064 (1966).
17. F. J. Simoons, J. D. Johnson, and N. Kretchmer. Perspective on milk-drinking and malabsorption of lactose. *Pediatrics 59,* 98-110 (1977).
18. E. Lebenthal, I. Antonowicz, and H. Schwachman. Correlation of lactase activity, lactose tolerance and milk consumption in different age groups. *Am. J. Clin. Nutr. 28,* 595-600 (1975).
19. N. Kretchmer. Lactose and lactase. *Sci. Am. 227*(4), 70-78 (1972).
20. J. D. Johnson, N. Kretchmer, and F. J. Simoons. Lactose malabsorption: Its biology and history. *Adv. Pediatr. 21,* 191-237 (1974).
21. S. W. Boellner, A. G. Beard, and T. C. Panos. Impairment of intestinal hydrolysis of lactose in newborn infants. *Pediatrics 36,* 542-550 (1965).
22. F. Lifshitz, S. Diaz-Bensussen, V. Martinez-Garza, F. Abdo-Bassols, and E. Diaz del Castillo. The influence of disaccharides on the development of systemic acidosis in the premature infant. *Pediatr. Res. 5,* 213-225 (1971).
23. T. D. Bolin and A. E. Davis. Primary lactase deficiency. Genetic or acquired? *Am. J. Dig. Dis. 15,* 679-692 (1970).

24. I. H. Holmes, R. D. Schnagi, S. Rodger, B. J. Ruck, I. D. Gust, R. F. Bishop, and G. L. Barnes. Is lactase the receptor and uncoating enzyme for infantile enteritis (rota) viruses? *Lancet 1,* 1387-1388 (1976).
25. R. Pergolizzi, F. Lifshitz, S. Teichberg, and R. A. Wapnir. Interaction between dietary carbohydrates and intestinal disaccharidase in experimental diarrhea. *Am. J. Clin. Nutr. 30,* 482-489 (1977).
26. A. Holzel. Sugar malabsorption due to deficiencies of disaccharidase activities and of monosaccharide transport. *Arch. Dis. Child. 42,* 341-352 (1967).
27. M. E. Ament, D. R. Perea, and L. J. Esther. Sucrase-isomaltase deficiency—A frequently misdiagnosed disease. *J. Pediatr. 83,* 721-727 (1973).
28. H. Preizer, D. Menard, R. K. Crane, and J. J. Cerda. Deletion of enzyme protein from the brush border membrane in sucrase-isomaltase deficiency. *Biochim. Biophys. Acta 363,* 279-282 (1974).
29. A. McNair, E. G. Hyer, S. Jarnum, and L. Orrid. Sucrose malabsorption in Greenland. *Br. Med. J. 2,* 19-21 (1972).
30. R. Bergoz. Trehalose malabsorption causing intolerance to mushrooms. Report of a probable case. *Gastroenterology 60,* 909-912 (1963).
31. L. J. Elsas, R. E. Hillman, J. H. Patterson, and L. E. Rosenberg. Renal and intestinal hexose transport in familial glucose-galactose malabsorption. *J. Clin. Invest. 49,* 576-585 (1970).
32. G. Neale, M. Carlk, and B. Levin. Intestinal sucrase deficiency presenting as sucrose intolerance in adult life. *Br. Med. J. 2,* 1223-1225 (1965).
33. J. D. Welsh. Isolated lactase deficiency in humans: Report on 100 patients. *Medicine 49,* 257-277 (1970).
34. S. F. Phillips and D. B. McGill. Glucose-galactose malabsorption in an adult: Perfusion studies of sugar, electrolyte and water transport. *Am. J. Dig. Dis. 18,* 1017-1024 (1973).
35. P. Coello-Ramirez and F. Lifshitz. Enteric microflora and carbohydrate intolerance in infants with diarrhea. *Pediatrics 49(2),* 233-242, 1972.
36. F. Lifshitz, P. Coello-Ramirez, G. Gutierrez-Topete, and M. C. Cornado-Cornet. Carbohydrate intolerance in infants with diarrhea. *J. Pediatr. 79,* 760-767 (1971).
37. F. Lifshitz, P. Coello-Ramirez, and M. L. Contreras-Gutierrez. The response of intants to carbohydrate oral loads after recovery from diarrhea. *J. Pediatr. 79,* 612-617 (1971).
38. F. Lifshitz. Clinical studies in diarrheal disease and malnutrition associated with carbohydrate intolerance. In *Proceedings of the Ninth International Congress of Nutrition,* Vol. 1, Mexico, 1972 (A. Chavez, H. Bourges, and S. Basta, Eds.). S. Karger, Basel, 1975, pp. 173-181.
39. C. J. Rosenquist, J. W. Heaton, G. W. Friedland, G. M. Gray, and F. F. Zboralske. Assessment of a radiographic method for diagnosis of intestinal lactase deficiency: A perspective study. *Invest. Radiol. 6,* 40-43 (1971).

40. Y. Sasake, M. Ilo, H. Kameda, H. Ueda, T. Aoyagi, N. Christopher, T. Bayless, and H. Wagner. Measurement of ^{14}C-lactose absorption in the diagnosis of lactase deficiency. *J. Lab. Clin. Med. 76,* 824-835 (1970).
41. A. D. Newcomer, D. G. McGill, P. H. Thomas, and A. F. Hofmann. Prospective comparison of indirect methods for detecting lactase deficiency. *N. Engl. J. Med. 293,* 1232-1236 (1975).
42. L. S. Stephenson and M. C. Latham. Lactose intolerance and milk consumption: The relation of tolerance to symptoms. *Am. J. Clin. Nutr. 27,* 296-303 (1974).
43. T. M. Bayless, B. Rothfeld, C. Massa, L. Wise, D. Paige, and M. Bedine. Lactose and milk intolerance: Clinical implications. *N. Engl. J. Med. 292,* 1156-1159 (1975).
44. J. D. Welsh. Diet therapy in adult lactose malabsorption: Present practices. *Am. J. Clin. Nutr. 31,* 592-596 (1978).
45. M. Unger. *Comparative Tolerance of Adults of Differing Ethnic Backgrounds to Lactose-free and Lactose-containing Milk.* M. S. Thesis, Massachusetts Institute of Technology, 1978.
46. M. H. Rorick. *The Prevalence of Milk Intolerance Secondary to Lactose Malabsorption in Elderly Americans.* M.S. Thesis, Massachusetts Institute of Technology, 1978.
47. T. M. Bayless. Recognition of lactose intolerance. *Hosp. Pract. 11,* 97-102 (1976).
48. D. M. Paige, T. M. Bayless, and W. S. Dellinger, Jr. Relationship of milk consumption to blood glucose rise in lactose intolerance individuals. *Am. J. Clin. Nutr. 28,* 677-680 (1975).
49. D. M. Paige, T. M. Bayless, G. D. Ferry, and G. G. Graham. Lactose malabsorption and milk rejection in Negro children. *Johns Hopkins Med. J. 129,* 163-169 (1971).
50. L. S. Stephenson, M. C. Latham, and D. V. Jones. Milk consumption by black and by white pupils in two primary schools. *J. Am. Diet. Assoc. 71,* 258-262 (1977).
51. D. M. Paige, T. M. Bayless, and G. G. Graham. Milk programs: Helpful or harmful to Negro children? *Am. J. Public Health 62,* 1486-1488 (1972).
52. R. Lisker, L. Aguilar, and C. Zavala. Intestinal lactase deficiency and milk drinking capacity in the adult. *Am. J. Clin. Nutr. 31,* 1499-1503 (1978).
53. J. Leichter. Comparison of whole milk and skim milk with aqueous lactose solution in lactose intolerance testing. *Am. J. Clin. Nutr. 26,* 393-396 (1973).
54. D. M. Paige, E. Leonardo, A. Cordano, J. Nakashima, B. Adrianzent, and G. G. Graham. Response of lactose intolerance children to different lactose levels. *Am. J. Clin. Nutr. 25,* 467-469 (1972).
55. V. Reddy and J. Pershad. Lactase deficiency in Indians. *Am. J. Clin. Nutr. 25,* 114-119 (1972).

56. A. D. Newcomer, D. B. McGill, P. S. Thomas, and A. F. Hoffman. Tolerance to lactose among lactase deficient American Indians. *Gastroenterology 74,* 44-46 (1978).
57. T. M. Bayless and D. M. Paige. Lactose intolerance by lactose malabsorbing Indians. Editorial. *Gastroenterology 74,* 153 (1978).
58. G. Flatz, C. Saengudom, and T. Sanguanbhokhai. Lactose intolerance in Thailand. *Nature 221,* 758-759 (1969).
59. P. Vlachos, D. Liakakos, and E. Boviatis. Childhood lactose intolerance. *N. Engl. J. Med. 294,* 163-164 (1976).
60. Committee on Nutrition, American Academy of Pediatrics. Should milk drinking by children be discouraged? *Pediatrics 53,* 576-582 (1974).
61. J. P. Stanfield. The diarrhea-malnutrition circle. *J. Trop. Pediatr. 12,* 53-54 (1966).

17
Malnutrition and the Intestine

ULYSSES FAGUNDES-NETO / Cornell University Medical College, New York, New York, and North Shore University Hospital, Manhasset, New York

I. The Natural History of Severe Protein-Energy Malnutrition

Malnutrition has been recognized for centuries all over the world, but only since the early 1930s has special attention been given to this major problem in the nutritional field. Cicely Williams [1], in the Gold Coast of Africa (now Ghana), was the first physician to describe kwashiorkor, protein malnutrition, as a disorder due to some amino acid or protein deficiency in children. Kwashiorkor was then considered the most serious and widespread nutritional disorder known to medical and nutritional sciences, while marasmus was totally neglected. Officials from the World Health Organization (W.H.O.) and Food and Agriculture Organization (F.A.O.) of the United Nations [2], in 1953, reinforced the idea that kwashiorkor was the most important problem, and it soon became known as protein malnutrition [3]. The theory of the "protein gap" appeared, and all the efforts to improve this condition were directed to the production of essentially protein-rich food mixtures [4]. At the present time, it is accepted that kwashiorkor is the most common clinical picture of severe protein-energy malnutrition, occurring mostly in the rural zones, in children after the first year of life. On the other hand, marasmus is the most important type of severe protein-energy malnutrition, associated with diarrhea, that affects bottle-fed infants, especially in the large urban centers [5]. Since the early 1920s the dangers of bottle feeding-induced malnutrition and the need to advocate the proper utilization of nature's best protein source for infants, breast milk, has been recognized [6].

Present Affiliation:
Escola Paulista de Medicina, Sao Paulo, Brazil

Our contention is that, under the influence of rapid social change, we are assisting "the rise of marasmus." This situation is generally due to a massive migratory movement from rural zones and other small centers toward the large cities. This very important sociological situation is actually occurring today in most countries of Latin America, West Africa, and Asia. Native people who experience an abrupt change in their habits, whose own culture is subverted, and who are trying to adopt the uses and customs of the most advanced technological societies, suffer an almost invariable process of disintegration of their social organization. They lose their basic traditions, and at the same time they cannot attain the technological benefits of the industrialized societies. These people suffer the full impact of an abrupt transition into a new culture.

In general, these migratory masses are composed of low-income families with numerous problems, who are compelled to live in wretched conditions in a contaminated environment. There is also precocious weaning and the use of diluted formulas in the early stages of life, because of the high price of food. In addition, there may be repeated bouts of infectious processes, mainly diarrhea [6], and a decreased food intake. These factors acting synergistically may lead to severe protein-energy malnutrition.

II. Malnutrition, Energy Gap, and Infection

The theory of the "protein gap" was based on the direct relationship "created" between kwashiorkor and protein deficiency; the obvious answer to combat this problem was considered to be the production of more and better protein. As a matter of fact, in 1961, the FAO made its position very clear, emphasizing that the "number-one" problem for FAO itself and for national agricultural departments, was the production of protein foods of good quality. Numerous local sources of protein were sought, and a "protein-rich food mixture" began to be formulated, not just as a treatment for kwashiorkor, but as the main driving force to prevent childhood malnutrition. The results of this policy, however, were a total failure. McLaren [7] called it "the great protein fiasco," and considered that the wrong measures were taken to identify and combat the problem.

The idea that the main point to be considered in the etiology of kwashiorkor was protein deficiency was based upon erroneous worldwide generalization—made from probably correct, but limited, observations in atypical situations, such as rural Africa. Lack of nutriment in general, with an "energy gap" rather than a protein gap, is a much more realistic approach to the subject, especially if we consider marasmus as a cause of severe protein-energy malnutrition at least equal in importance to kwashiorkor.

Indeed, Waterlow and Payne [8], in a very elegant paper, recently agreed that the protein gap is a myth, and that what really exists, even for vulnerable groups, is a food gap and an energy gap. Measurements of energy and protein intakes of children under 2 years of age in various countries where malnutrition is endemic showed that a greater deficit of energy than of protein is the real problem.

The importance of an unfavorable environment as an aggravating factor in malnutrition was recently stressed in a long-term study in a Guatemalan village [9]. The factors predisposing to malnutrition in this population were of a cultural as well as of a socioeconomic nature. These included low-yield agriculture, low income, inadequate knowledge of child feeding during weaning, deficient sanitation and personal hygiene.

The study of the Guatemalan village clearly shows that the origin of malnutrition in young children rests on two factors: lack of an adequate maternal technology for preparing foods for weanling children and the lack of knowledge of how to avoid some omnipresent microbial pathogens in the environment. Infectious disease, mainly diarrhea due to environmental contamination, especially during the weaning period, is the most important single cause that leads to malnutrition.

Infection and malnutrition, with a consequent elevation in the morbidity and mortality rates, are a monotonous constant seen in the countries of the Third World and presenting an "eternal" challenge to the governmental organs of public health.

III. A Model of Good Nutrition in a Primitive Society

There are very few studies concerning the nutritional status of so-called "primitive" people, living in their natural habitat. These few studies, however, almost always stress that malnutrition has no major role in these communities [10, 11]. On the other hand, there are a large number of observations concerning the nutritional status of the pediatric population in communities of low socioeconomic level in Third World countries—showing that malnutrition is a major problem. The prevalence of malnutrition can reach values as high as 55% in children under 5 years of age [12].

The study described below, performed in an Indian reservation in Brazil, showed that malnutrition is a minor problem when people, even those with a very rudimentary technology, live in an environment relatively free of fecal contamination—although malaria is endemic in this community—and rationally utilize the natural resources of food, including prolonged breast feeding.

The Xingo National Park in the Amazonas region, Brazil, is practically unique in that the inhabitants of this reservation, the Indians, are allowed to live in the most "authentic" conditions, protected against indiscriminate contact with another kind of civilization. It is one of the few areas in the country, and even in the world, where it is possible to find people of the so-called primitive culture, living in their natural habitat and maintaining their traditions and customs.

The National Park, due to its geophysical aspects and to the cultural characteristics of the Indian tribes inhabiting the region, can be divided into two main areas: one at the north, called Medio Xingu, and the other in the south, called Alto Xingu.

There are nine tribes living in their own villages distributed around the 10,000-km^2 area of the Alto Xingu region. The state of isolation from other societies and the occupation of the same area for a long period of time by those nine tribes–with a great facility of internal movements–have contributed to the development of close social and cultural relationships among themselves, but not with the outside world. These tribes, despite their organization into totally independent nations, are considered to belong to a common culture known as "Xinguana" culture, the present population of which is 811 people.

Since this is a very large, water-rich area, fishing is highly developed, and fish is the most important source of food of animal origin–although during the rainy season, the Indians pursue some hunting activities. The Indians also have agriculture. The main crop is "mandioca" (*Manihot utillissima*), a special kind of tapioca, followed by corn (*Zea mays*) and sweet potato (*Ipomoea batatas*). Some wild fruits are also consumed in significant amounts, especially "piqui," which is an oily fruit rich in vitamin A. The practice of breast feeding is universal, and human milk is practically the only kind of food that children receive during their first year of life. Although lactation extends until 2-3 years of age, at the end of the first year new foods are introduced into the diet–namely, fish and mandioca. Cow's milk is never utilized, since the Indians do not tend any grazing animals.

Since 1965, this population has been receiving medical care from the Institute of Preventive Medicine of the Escola Paulista of Medicine. Medical teams go to the Indian reservation year-round, basically to check the health conditions of the Indians, to provide medical attention as needed, and to apply any prophylactic measures possible to preserve a good state of health in the community. Except for malaria, which is endemic, and for a mild degree of parasitosis, there are no important health hazards in the population, since the Indians receive routine immunizations, including BCG, pertussis, tetanus, diphtheria, poliomyelitis, and measles vaccine.

The apparently good nutritional status of the children in this population was just a subjective impression, since no objective study or assessment of the nutritional status has been undertaken in this population since the creation of the Indian reservation by the Brazilian government in 1961.

In order to assess the magnitude of malnutrition and the possible causes, as well as to propose adequate measures to correct the abnormalities found, a project to evaluate the nutritional status of the pediatric population was designed. Because of the peculiarities of the conditions in the field, we chose to utilize two of three direct methods of nutritional assessment: (1) physical examination and (2) anthropometric evaluation.

The anthropometry was oriented to measure the variation among the different segments of the body as age-independent indices to be compared with reference patterns of both local and international growth charts–including weight, height, head circumference, and tricipital cutaneous fold, that are already tabulated as age-independent values.

The weight-height adequacy index [13] was utilized in the assessment of the nutritional status of the Indian children. The *Harvard Standard Curve* [14] was adopted as a reference, and the classification of the nutritional status was done following the Macias criteria [15] modified by Batista-Filho [16].

The field work was undertaken in the first two weeks of July during three consecutive years (1974, 1975, 1976). At the end of this period, 175 children were studied, 97 male and 78 female, all with an estimated age of 5 years or younger. Two types of studies were done: cross-sectional and longitudinal. In the cross-sectional study we examined the children from each year of the three years of study. The longitudinal assessment was done by a yearly follow-up of all children examined during each session.

The groups of children included in this nutritional survey were classified according to the year and the type of studies undertaken. In the cross-sectional study 175 children were evaluated; 79 in 1974, 45 in 1975, and 51 in 1976. In the longitudinal study, 108 children were followed up, 46 for two consecutive years, 9 for two alternate years, and 53 for three consecutive years.

During the 3-year period of study, 336 clinical examinations were performed, and we could not detect any sign of third-degree malnutrition. On only three occasions were clinical manifestations of malnutrition classified as group I of Jelliffe [13] observed: two cases of angular stomatitis and one of seborrheic dermatitis. Splenomegaly was the most frequent clinical abnormality found. In 185 (55%) of the 336 clinical examinations performed, the spleen was palpable. The following distribution for the splenic size calculated as Hackett index [17] was found: splenic index 1 in 52 children, 2 in 81, 3 in 45, and 4 in 7. There was no case of splenic index 5 detected.

The anthropometric evaluation in the cross-sectional study showed that the prevalence of malnutrition was low and remained essentially the same in each year of the survey (Table 1). The intensity of malnutrition was almost always mild in degree, and severe malnutrition was never detected. The longitudinal study provided evidence that 47 of 53 children remained well nourished for three consecutive years. One child that was detected with

Table 1 Nutritional Status of Brazilian Indian Children

			Malnourished					
	Well-nourished		D_1[a]		D_2[a]		Total	
Year	No.	%	No.	%	No.	%	No.	%
1974	76	96.2	2	2.5	1	1.3	79	100.0
1975	43	95.5	2	4.5	0	0	45	100.0
1976	49	96.1	2	3.9	0	0	51	100.0
Total[b]	168	(96.0)	6	(3.4)	1	(0.6)	175	(100.0)

[a]Degree of malnourishment indicated by subscripts 1, 2.
[b]Values in parentheses based on 3-yr cumulative data.
Note: Assessment based on eight-height adequacy distributed according to nutritional status and year of study.

first-degree malnutrition during the first year of the survey recovered nutritional status during the second year and remained well nourished in the third year of the study. Three children were classified malnourished in the second year but recovered their nutritional status the next year. Two children that were classified as well nourished during the two previous years appeared malnourished during the third year. The intensity of malnutrition in all the cases was always classified as first degree (Table 2).

The weight-height adequacy index is useful only to detect the current state of malnutrition; it does not identify past history of malnutrition. In fact, the prevalence of malnutrition shown by using this index is almost always smaller than when the weight-age criteria are utilized. The longitudinal study, however, allowed us to establish the growth rhythm of the children. It was possible, then, to apply the Seoane and Latham criteria [18], not only in order to study the prevalence of current malnutrition, but also in order to look for malnutrition in the past and for chronic evolutive malnutrition.

The prevalence of malnutrition in the different forms cited above was: current malnutrition 4.66%, past malnutrition 7.54%, and chronic evolving malnutrition 2.9%—the total value being 15.12%.

In conclusion, the data obtained in this survey have led us to state that the prevalence of malnutrition in these Indian children is dramatically lower than that reported in studies of similar communities where the native population experiences an indiscriminate contact with the so-called "civilized" societies. Furthermore, the prevalence of malnutrition is strikingly lower than that seen in children belonging to low-income families that have migrated from rural areas to the periphery of the large urban centers [12]. The prevalence of

Table 2 Evolution of Nutritional Status of Brazilian Indian Children

Years of study			Number of children with each pattern
1974	1975	1976	
WN[a]	WN	WN	47
M_1	WN	WN	1
M_1	M_1	WN	0
M_1	WN	M_1	0
M_1	M_1	M_1	0
WN	M_1	WN	3
WN	M_1	M_1	0
WN	WN	M_1	2
Total			53

[a]WN = well-nourished.
[b]M_1 = malnutrition, first degree.
Note: Assessment based on weight-height adequacy index.

malnutrition in the Alto Xingu region is minimal, and of a lower degree than that reported in the city of São Paulo [16], the largest and richest city of the country.

Brazil has an area of 8,511,965 km^2 and a population of approximately 110 million people. After World War II the nation entered a phase of accelerated industrialization which resulted in the growth of very large cities in the southern part of the country and, consequently, in an exodus of rural populations to urban centers [19]. The fraction of the population living in cities increased from 36% in 1950 to 45% in 1960 and 56% in 1970 [20].

São Paulo is the largest city in the country, with a population of 12 million people (estimated for the metropolitan area known as greater São Paulo). It is the most important industrial center of the nation and constitutes a constant attraction for migratory movements that come mainly from the poorest rural areas of the country, the North and Northeast. As a natural consequence, the population in São Paulo is growing at a rate of 4.2% per year. The per capita income in São Paulo is 2900 U.S. dollars per year, double that of the rest of the country; but the infant mortality rate is showing a permanent rise that now has reached the level of 100 per 1000, up from 70 per 1000 fifteen years ago.

The prevalence of malnutrition in children under five, as cited previously, is 31.4% [16], and the majority of the cases of hospital admissions for severe protein-energy malnutrition is due to marasmus [21].

IV. Malnutrition and Malabsorption

The abnormalities reported in the digestive-absorptive function in malnutrition may be a direct consequence of malnutrition and may also be a reflection of life in a contaminated environment. The wide range of abnormalities of the digestive system which occurs in severe malnutrition has been, until recently, ascribed to a low protein intake leading to a severe deficiency of essential amino acids, with the consequent atrophy of the organ systems that have a fast cell turnover [22]. However, it is now well established that additional factors, apart from deficient protein consumption, play a major role in the pathophysiology of the malabsorption which is seen in children with protein-energy malnutrition [23].

The alterations in the physiology of the digestive-absorptive processes represent a summation of effects. The unfavorable contaminated environment is considered to be the triggering agent of the intestinal infection and, in combination with malnutrition per se, may be a perpetuating cause for a continuous alteration. This interaction may lead to several morphological and functional derangements of the gastrointestinal tract of the host. Atrophy of the gastric mucosa and hypochlorhydria have been reported in children with severe protein-energy malnutrition [24]. The intestinal wall may become thin and hypotonic, and there is also decreased intestinal motility [25].

Pancreatic structure and function appear to be markedly affected in malnutrition as observed by Barbezat and Hansen [26]. Pancreatic output after secretin and pancreozymin stimulation is markedly decreased. Lipase, trypsin, chymotrypsin, and amylase activities are all reduced in the malnourished child, but these alterations seem to be transitory, and the normal functions are resumed very soon, as nutritional recovery begins [27].

There is general agreement that most of the morphologic changes during malnutrition are nonspecific, although alterations in the enteric mucosa like those observed in untreated celiac disease have been described in as many as 10-60% of children with kwashiorkor [28]. On the other hand, marasmic patients do not have significant changes in small-intestinal morphology [29], but have a slow mitotic index in the crypt cells, suggesting a low rate of cellular proliferation in the crypts.

An increase in protein excretion by the intestinal tract has been reported, as well as steatorrhea, the latter being due to partial pancreatic dysfunction [30] and to low bile salt concentration in the intestinal lumen [31]. Tests which measure the intraduodenal capacity to form fat micelles have shown a marked impairment of this function in children with protein-energy malnutrition. Malnourished children have an increased incidence and severity of lactose intolerance with diarrhea [32]. These patients have been shown to have a deficiency of the intestinal disaccharidases [33], and the deleterious effect of lactose in diarrheal disease among malnourished children has long been recognized [34]. Impaired digestion of other dietary disaccharides, as well as deficient absorption of monosaccharides, may also be an important feature of deranged intestinal function [35].

Ileal function is also defective in severe protein-energy malnutrition as demonstrated by an impairment of vitamin B_{12} absorption and a great loss of bile salts in the stools [36].

A striking feature of protein-energy malnutrition is bacterial overgrowth in the small intestine [37]. Gastric hypochlorhydria, intestinal hypotonia and hypomotility [25], and immunologic deficiencies [38] are factors that, together with environmental conditions, will favor a chronic overgrowth of colonic flora in the small intestine. A disruption in the most important intestinal microfloral regulatory mechanisms may favor a fecal flora overgrowth within the upper intestinal lumen in concentrations exceeding 10^4 colonies/ml, with serious consequences to the host [39].

The common feature in this syndrome is massive bacterial proliferation in the proximal small bowel, secondary to stasis. The overgrowth of bacteria competes against host food utilization. Dietary proteins as well as folic acid are metabolized by bacteria [40]. The bacteria, mainly the anaerobes such as *Bacteroides* and *Veillonella,* are also capable of causing deconjugation of primary bile salts and their 7α-dehydroxylation in the intestinal lumen. Deconjugated and/or dehydroxylated bile salts cannot produce the necessary micellar solution and fat malabsorption [41]. On the other hand, the presence of these bile salts in elevated concentrations in the jejunal lumen has been shown to induce glucose malabsorption, sodium and water secretions, and also morphologic abnormalities in the intestinal mucosa [42].

V. Functional and Morphologic Abnormalities of the Small Intestine in Malnourished Patients

We studied 22 patients of both sexes, admitted to the pediatric ward of Hospital São Paulo, Escola Paulista de Medicina, in the city of São Paulo, Brazil [43]. Intestinal function was investigated as described below. Ages varied from 3 to 36 months, with an average age of 10.7 months. All the children were bottle-fed, belonged to families with low incomes, had chronic diarrhea, and also had had at least one previous hospital admission for an episode of acute diarrhea. All had third-degree malnutrition according to Gomez [44] and were classified as marasmic according to McLaren et al. [45]. On admission, the children received parenteral hydration when clinical conditions made it necessary. Cow's-milk formula full strength was started as soon as fluid imbalance was repaired, furnishing a minimum caloric intake of 150 kcal/kg body weight per day.

In the presence of diarrhea, fecal samples were collected for determination of pH and testing for reducing substances, by means of pH paper strips and Clinitest tablets, respectively. Fecal pH values under 6 and/or the presence of reducing substances in stools indicated the need for replacement of the milk formula by soybean lactose-free formula (Sobee). Persistence of diarrhea was followed by replacement of the disaccharide-containing soybean formula with one containing only monosaccharide. When this type of sugar was also not tolerated, glucose was administered intravenously, and an oral sugar-free formula was fed.

The small-intestinal functional and morphologic evaluations were started when the patients were clinically stabilized, usually after 5-10 days of hospitalization. The small-intestinal function was evaluated by D-xylose absorption and carbohydrate tolerance tests. After a 4-hr fasting period, the patient received an oral load of D-xylose in doses of 15 g/m^2 in a 10% aqueous solution. Blood samples were obtained by venipuncture before, and 1 and 2 hr after, the oral load. The D-xylose blood levels were assayed by the Roe and Rice method [46].

Carbohydrate tolerance tests were performed on alternate days for each of the sugars studied: lactose, sucrose, and glucose. An oral load of a 10% aqueous solution containing 2 g/kg body weight for the disaccharides and 1 g/kg body weight for the monosaccharide. Blood glucose was measured from capillary puncture at 0, 30, 60, and 90 min [47]. The jejunal biopsy was performed with a pediatric Crosby-Kugler capsule [48]. The morphologic interpretation of the intestinal fragment was based on Schenk and Klipstein protocol [49].

The D-xylose absorption test in marasmic patients gave mean values of 24.8 ± 9.2 mg% at the first hour and 28.0 ± 8.2 mg% at the second hour, while in "normal" children the mean values were 42.4 ± 9.6 mg% and 37.6 + 8.9 mg%, respectively, at the first and second hours. Difference between the marasmic and the normal values were significant, in both the first and second hours ($P < 0.01$). The malabsorption of D-xylose indicated an alteration of the enteric mucosa. Another hypothesis, however, to explain this finding is that the pentose in the jejunum may be consumed by the bacterial flora, which can be abnormally overgrown at this level of the intestine in the undernourished patient [50].

It is worth pointing out that our results agree with those of Bowie et al. [51] and Viteri et al. [52] in undernourished patients with kwashiorkor, even though the doses were different. There was malabsorption of lactose in 73% of our patients, and sucrose malabsorption occurred in 23% of them. Only one patient had malabsorption of glucose. A deficiency of intestinal disaccharidases [51-53], especially of lactase, and malabsorption of sugars is a well-known complication of malnutrition in infancy. Lactose malabsorption, in some circumstances, is considered to be a limiting factor in the recuperation of the child [34, 54], and there is a decrease in mortality when it is abolished from the diet [55]. The presence of lactose in the diet leads to aggravation of diarrhea, increase in fecal volume, increased lactic acid excretion, and loss of sugar in feces.

The jejunal biopsy showed alterations in most of the patients; only one child had a normal intestinal mucosa. In approximately half the biopsy specimens studied, the morphologic alterations were nonspecific. In 12 of the 22 biopsy specimens analyzed, the intestinal mucosa clearly revealed a reduction in the number of villi in relation to the normal, leading us to designate this group "decreased villus population." These alterations were similar to those found by Barbieri [56] in marasmatic patients and by Burman [57], Schneider and Viteri [58], and Barbezat et al. [59] in kwashiorkor. We did not find villus atrophy like that of celiac disease as reported by Creamer et al. [60] or like that reported by Stanfield et al. [28] and Brunser et al. [29] in patients with kwashiorkor.

VI. Conclusions

The current evidence seems to be clear about the multiplicity of factors which may induce malnutrition. A prepondenant sociological problem is that of families with numerous problems and low income who are compelled to live in wretched conditions, with poor hygiene. This life-style contributes to the existence of high indices of environmental contamination. On the other hand, the constant decrease in frequency in the practice of breast feeding in favor of bottle feeding may contribute significantly to an increase in the incidence of infectious disease, mainly bacterial diarrhea. Repeated diarrheic bouts may thus lead to malnutrition.

The Indian community, although "technologically delayed," teaches us that the rational use of the elements that nature provides is sufficient to maintain a good state of nutrition in the general population. Breast feeding practiced for a prolonged period of time and the use of the natural resources of food are the basic points stressed by the Indian community experience. This should be learned by the organs of public health of the underdeveloped countries for correction of this worldwide problem.

Several studies done as long as five decades ago already emphatically stated the alarming hazards of bottle feeding [61, 62]. It was claimed then that breast feeding is better than—and preferable to—bottle feeding under practically all conditions, and that it should be continued for the most protracted period possible.

Unfortunately, however, in the underdeveloped countries, food industries are more powerful than those who make any of these numerous scientific claims. The final result is the increase in diarrhea associated with malnutrition that has always been the first cause of infant mortality.

References

1. *A Special Number Marking the Eightieth Year of Cicely D. Williams. Nutr. Rev. 31,* 331-383 (1973).
2. Joint FAO/WHO Expert Committee on Nutrition. Monograph Series. *World Health Organization Third Report,* No. 72, 1953, pp. 3-30.
3. J. F. Brock, J. D. L. Hansen, E. E. Howe, P. J. Pretorious, and J. G. A. Davel. Kwashiorkor and protein malnutrition. A dietary therapcutic trial. *Lancet 2,* 355-360 (1955).
4. M. Autret. *Meeting Protein Needs of Infants and Children.* Publication 843. National Academy of Sciences, National Research Council, Washington, D.C., 1961, p. 537.
5. F. Monckeberg. *Pre-School Child Malnutrition.* Publication 1282. National Academy of Sciences, National Research Council, Washington, D.C., 1961, p. 168.
6. R. M. Woodbury. *Causal Factors in Infant Mortality. A Statistical Study Based on Investigation in Eight Cities.* U. S. Department of Labor, Child Bureau Publication 142, 1925, p. 48.
7. D. S. McLaren. The great protein fiasco. *Lancet 2,* 93-96 (1974).
8. J. C. Waterlow and P. R. Payne. The protein gap. *Nature 258,* 113-117 (1975).
9. L. J. Mata, R. A. Kromal, J. J. Urrutia, and B. Garcia. Effect of infection on food intake and the nutritional state: Perspectives as viewed from the village. *Am. J. Clin. Nutr. 30,* 1215-1227 (1977).
10. D. B. Jelliffe, J. Woodburn, F. J. Bennett, and E. F. P. Jelliffe. The children of the Hadza hunters. *J. Trop. Pediatr. 60,* 907-913 (1962).
11. P. B. Eveleth, F. M. Salzano, and P. E. Lima. Child growth and adult physique in Brazilian Xingu Indians. *Am. J. Phys. Anthropol. 41,* 95-102 (1974).
12. J. C. S. Guitti. Condição nutricional de crianças de zero a seis anos de idade na periferia da cidade de Londrina— Influencia da condição socioeconomica. Medical Thesis, Centro de Cien. da Saúde da Univ. Est. de Londrina, Londrina, 1975.
13. D. B. Jelliffe. Evaluacion del estudo de nutrición de la comunidad. Organizacion Mundial de la Salud (O.M.S.), serie Monografias No. 53, 1968.
14. H. C. Stuart and S. A. Stevenson. Physical growth and development. In *Textbook of Pediatrics,* 7th Ed. (W. Nelson, Ed.). Saunders, Philadelphia, 1959, pp. 12-61.
15. J. A. Macias. Metodo para la evaluación del crecimiento de hombres y mujeres desde el nacimiento hasta los 20 años para uso a nivel nacional e internacional. *Arch. Latinoamer. Nutr. 22,* 531-546 (1972).

16. M. Batista-Filho. Prevalencia e estagios da desnutricão proteico-calórica em criancas da cidade de São Paulo. Medical Thesis, Fac. de Saúde Publ. Univ. SP, São Paulo, 1976.
17. WHO. *Terminology of Malaria and Malaria Eradication.* World Health Organization, Geneva, 1963.
18. N. Seoane and M. C. Latham. Nutritional anthropometry in the identification of malnutrition in childhood. *J. Trop. Pediatr. 17,* 98-104 (1971).
19. J. Goldenberg. Brazil: Energy options and current outlook. *Science 200,* 158-160 (1978).
20. Estatistica Brasileira de Energia. *Biannual Bulletin of the Brazilian National Committee of the World Energy Conference,* No. 19. Rio de Janeiro, 1974, p. 50.
21. O. Rosenburgo. Aleitamento no lo ano de vida de criancas internadas em hospital assistencial do municipio de São Paulo. *Rev. Saúde Publ. 7,* 381-388 (1973).
22. M. Behar, G. Arroyave, and C. Tejada. Desnutricion severa en la infancia. *Rev. Col. Med. (Guatemala) 7,* 221-278 (1956).
23. R. E. Viteri and R. E. Schneider. Gastrointestinal alterations in protein-calorie malnutrition. *Med. Clin. North Am. 58,* 1487-1505 (1974).
24. J. J. Herbst, P. Sunshine, and N. Kretchmer. Intestinal malabsorption in infancy and childhood. *Adv. Pediatr. 16,* 11-64 (1969).
25. W. P. T. James. Sugar absorption and intestinal motility in children when malnourished and after treatment. *Clin. Sci. 39,* 305-318 (1970).
26. G. O. Barbezat and J. D. L. Hansen. The exocrine pancreas and protein-calorie malnutrition. *Pediatrics 42,* 77-92 (1968).
27. R. E. Schneider and F. E. Viteri. Luminal events of lipid absorption in protein-calorie malnourished children; relationship with nutritional recovery aspirates. *Am. J. Clin. Nutr. 27,* 788-796 (1974).
28. J. P. Stanfield, M. S. R. Hutt, and R. Tunnicliffe. Intestinal biopsy in kwashiorkor. *Lancet 2,* 519-523 (1965).
29. O. Brunser, A. Reid, and R. G. F. Monckeberg. Jejunal mucosa in infant malnutrition. *Am. J. Clin. Nutr. 21,* 976-983 (1968).
30. J. E. D. Oliveira and E. Rolando. Fat absorption studies in malnourished children. *Am. J. Clin. Nutr. 15,* 287-292 (1964).
31. R. E. Schneider and F. E. Viteri. Luminal events of lipid absorption in protein-calorie malnourished children; relationship with nutritional recovery and diarrhea. I. Capacity of the duodenal content to achieve micellar solubilization of lipids. *Am. J. Clin. Nutr. 27,* 777-787 (1974).
32. M. D. Bowie, G. L. Brinkman, and J. D. L. Hansen. Acquired disaccharide intolerance in malnutrition. *J. Trop. Pediatr. 66,* 1083-1091 (1965).
33. W. P. T. James. Effects of protein-calorie malnutrition on intestinal absorption. *Ann. N.Y. Acad. Sci. 176,* 244-261 (1971).
34. F. Lifshitz. Clinical studies in diarrheal disease and malnutrition associated with carbohydrate intolerance. In *Proceedings of the Ninth International Congress in Nutrition, Mexico, 1972* (A. Chavez, H. Bourges, and S. Basta, Eds.). S. Karger, Basel, 1975, pp. 173-181.

35. W. P. T. James. Comparison of the methods used in assessment of carbohydrate absorption in malnourished children. *Arch. Dis. Child. 47,* 531-536 (1972).
36. J. Alvarado, W. Vargas, N. Dias, and F. E. Viteri. Vitamin B_{12} absorption in protein-calorie malnourished children and during recovery: Influence of protein and of diarrhea. *Am. J. Clin. Nutr. 26,* 595-599 (1973).
37. L. J. Mata, F. Jimenez, and M. Cordon. Gastrointestinal flora of children with protein-calorie malnutrition. *Am. J. Clin. Nutr. 25,* 1118-1126 (1972).
38. R. G. Bell, J. Turner, M. Gracey, J. Suharjona, and W. Sunoto. Serum and small intestine immunoglobulin levels in undernourished children. *Am. J. Clin. Nutr. 29,* 393-397 (1976).
39. R. M. Donaldson, Jr., C. McConnell, and N. Deffner. Bacteriological studies in clinical experimental blind loop syndrome. *Gastroenterology 52,* 1082 (1967).
40. R. M. Donaldson, Jr. Studies of the pathogenesis of steatorrhea in the blind loop syndrome. *J. Clin. Invest. 44,* 1815-1825 (1965).
41. M. E. Ament, S. S. Shinmoda, D. R. Saunders, and C. E. Rubin. Pathogenesis of steatorrhea in three cases of small intestinal stasis syndrome. *Gastroenterology 63,* 728-747 (1972).
42. M. Gracey, V. Burke, and A. Oshin. Bacteria, bile salts, and intestinal monosaccharide malabsorption. *Gut 12,* 683-692 (1971).
43. U. Fagundes-Neto, J. Wehba, F. S. R. Patricio, and N. Machado. Morphologic and functional study of the small intestine in marasmic patients. *Arq. Gastroenterol. 14,* 241-248 (1977).
44. Gomez, F. Desnutricion. *Bol. Med. Hosp. Infant. Mex. 3,* 543-551 (1946).
45. D. S. McLaren, P. L. Pellet, and W. W. C. Read. A simple scoring system for classifying the severe forms of protein-calorie malnutrition of early childhood. *Lancet 1,* 533-534 (1967).
46. J. H. Roe and E. W. Rice. Photometric method for determination of free pentoses in animal tissues. *J. Biol. Chem. 173,* 507-512 (1948).
47. A. G. Huggett and D. A. Nixon. Enzymatic determination of blood glucose. *Biochem. J. 66,* 12 (1957).
48. H. Toccalino and J. O. O'Donnell. Tecnica para la introduction de la sonda-capsula de Crosby en niños. *Rev. Hosp. de Niños de Buenos Aires 12,* 29-30 (1962).
49. E. A. Schenk and F. A. Klipstein. A protocol for the evaluation of small bowel biopsies. *Am. J. Clin. Nutr. 25,* 1108-1117 (1972).
50. M. Gracey, D. E. Stone, J. Suharjona, and W. Sunoto. Microbial contamination of the gut: Another feature of malnutrition. *Am. J. Clin. Nutr. 26,* 1170-1174 (1973).
51. M. D. Bowie, G. O. Barbezat, and J. D. L. Hansen. Carbohydrate absorption in malnourished children. *Am. J. Clin. Nutr. 20,* 89-97 (1967).
52. F. E. Viteri, J. M. Flores, J. Alvarados, and M. Behar. Intestinal malabsorption in malnourished children before and during recovery. Relation between severity of protein deficiency and malabsorption process. *Am. J. Dig. Dis. 18,* 201-211 (1973).

53. W. P. T. James. Jejunal disaccharide activities in children with marasmus and with kwashiorkor. *Arch. Dis. Child. 46,* 218-220 (1971).
54. J. G. Prinsloo, W. Wittman, and P. J. Pretorius. Effect of different sugars on diarrhea of acute kwashiorkor. *Arch. Dis. Child. 44,* 593-599 (1969).
55. A. E. Ifekwuingwe. Emergency treatment of large numbers of children with severe protein-calorie malnutrition. *Am. J. Clin. Nutr. 28,* 79-81 (1975).
56. D. Barbieri. *Mucosa jejunal na má nutricão proteica primaria grave da criança.* Tese de Doutoramento apresentada a Faculdade de Medicina da Universidade de São Paulo, 1971. Medical Thesis.
57. D. Burman. The jejunal mucosa in kwashiorkor. *Arch. Dis. Child. 40,* 526-531 (1965).
58. R. E. Schneider and F. E. Viteri. Morphological aspects of the duodeno jejunal mucosa in protein-calorie malnourished children and during recovery. *Am. J. Clin. Nutr. 25,* 1092-1102 (1972).
59. G. O. Barbezat, M. D. Bowie, R. O. C. Kaschula, and J. D. L. Hansen. Studies on the small intestinal mucosa of children with protein-calorie malnutrition. *S. Afr. Med. J. 41,* 1031-1035 (1967).
60. B. Creamer, W. Dutz, and C. Post. Small intestine lesion of chronic marasmus in Iran. *Lancet 1,* 18-20 (1970).
61. H. K. Faber and T. L. Sutton. A statistical comparison of breast-fed and bottle-fed babies during the first year. *Am. J. Dis. Child. 40,* 1163-1176 (1930).
62. M. M. Glazier. Comparing the breast-fed and the bottle-fed infant. *N. Engl. J. Med. 230,* 626-628 (1930).

PART IV

Diarrheal Disorders

18
Childhood Diarrhea: An Overview

FIMA LIFSHITZ / Cornell University Medical College, New York, New York, and North Shore University Hospital, Manhasset, New York

I. Introduction

The study of human excreta dates back to ancient times. Indeed, this may have been the first scientific endeavor of medical people. For many thousands of years we have known about the high morbidity and mortality of diarrheal disease. The Greek word *diarrhoia,* which means to flow through, already defined an abnormal condition which was known to frequently afflict animals as well as human beings throughout recorded history. Hippocrates defined diarrhea as an abnormal frequency and liquidity of fecal discharges. Today this definition still holds! Moreover, diarrheal disease continues to be a leading cause of infant morbidity and mortality in all parts of the world. In 1975 there were approximately 500 million episodes of diarrhea among children throughout the world [1]. In healthy individuals this disease is usually a somewhat troublesome illness, but self-limited. However, this illness killed between 5 and 18 million children in 1975 [1]. Moreover, it had a greater devastating effect, causing or contributing to malnutrition [2, 3]. In debilitated children, diarrhea is often the precipitating event that brings the child to the hospital—or the "coup de grace."

II. Etiology

Some of the causes of childhood diarrhea are listed in Table 1. The illness may be acute or chronic. The frequent morbidity of diarrheal disease may be due to the great susceptibility of the gastrointestinal tract to a variety of noxious agents. The intestinal cell turnover as well as the cell function and

Table 1 Causes of Diarrhea

General type	Typical causes
Infectious	Viruses, bacteria, protozoans, fungi
Metabolic	Gastrointestinal alkalosis, disaccharidase deficiencies, monosaccharide intolerance, celiac disease
Nutritional	Malnutrition, marasmus, kwashiorkor
Allergic	Milk, foodstuffs
Mechanical	Shunt, obstruction, short gut, blind loop
Hyperosmolar	Overfeedings, hyperosmolar formulas
Chemical	Heavy metals, boric acid, toxins
Neoplastic	Ganglioneuroma, lymphoma, Whipple's disease
Psychogenic	Stress
Idiopathic	Chronic inflammatory disease of the bowel

enzymatic content may be affected rapidly by factors such as infection, metabolic disease, toxic toxins, and chemicals. The frequency of gastrointestinal symptoms in any systemic disease in children, and particularly in malnutrition, is probably a reflection of these rapid alterations in the intestinal mucosa. Indeed, diarrhea is the most common problem which might be the primary—or the only—manifestation in many diseases of known and unknown cause.

III. Physiology

Diarrhea occurs whenever there is an increase in the volume of stools. Since the volume is primarily determined by the water content of feces, diarrhea might be considered to result from a decrease in the adequate net movement of water from the intestinal lumen to plasma. Theoretically, there may be three main factors responsible for decreased net movement of water in the intestine. "Factor 1"—less time for reabsorption (e.g., because of a short gastrointestinal tract)—is rare and generally is a problem only after major surgical resections. Much emphasis has been put on another possibility—rapid transit—as a cause of diarrhea. However, it has long been known that in many instances diarrhea is seen in patients with distended fluid-filled loops, an observation suggesting that adequate time does exist for reabsorption of water. Furthermore, it must be remembered that fluid remaining within the intestinal tract serves as a stimulus to peristaltic action, and hyperirritability may be the result, rather than the cause, of decreased transport of water. "Factor 2"–less reabsorption per unit time, as occurs with a decreased surface area–may be of importance in chronic diseases such as ulcerative colitis, with major scarring and loss of normal epithelium. However, factor 3–the most important factor–seems to be an altered transport per unit surface area, which results in either less reabsorption or more secretion of water and electrolytes.

Under normal circumstances the fluxes of water across the small intestine are very large [4, 5]. However, the conservation of water by the intestine is so efficient that only a small amount is excreted in the feces. Therefore, a slight change in transport per unit of surface area in either absorption or secretion of any solute can cause a very marked change in the net intestinal flow of water. Consequently, even relatively minor alterations of solute fluxes induced by gastrointestinal flora may significantly alter the delicate balance of water movement in the intestine. Microorganisms or their metabolic by-products or other noxious agents must therefore interfere with the net movement of water across intestinal cell membranes in order to induce water loss and diarrhea. This may be achieved either by increasing secretion or by inhibiting absorption of actively transported solutes, principally sodium and glucose, to which water transport is linked. It may also follow alterations in permeability of the cell membranes or the intestinal motor activity. Diarrhea will result when the excess in the volume of fluid delivered to the colon from the upper segments of the small intestine surpasses the reabsorptive ability of the large intestine.

IV. Classification

There is a tendency to classify the different types of diarrhea according to the primary alteration in water transport: i.e., secretory, osmolar, absorptive, and motor. Secretory diarrhea is considered to be present when diarrhea is severe and persists even after oral feedings have been discontinued. Characteristically, the stools contain large quantities of sodium (more than 80 mEq/kg, body weight, since this electrolyte is being secreted together with water by the patient. On the other hand, osmolar or absorptive types of diarrhea, which are more frequently found in infants with this illness, classically improve whenever oral feedings are not given. The stools of these patients have smaller quantities of sodium but may contain carbohydrates. However, in all patients with diarrhea there may be secretory, osmolar, absorptive, and motor alterations intermingled and associated with each other, and these may all be simultaneously ongoing in any one patient.

There are several factors responsible for the type of diarrhea observed clinically. The luminal osmolar gradients seem to be the most important factor in determining the type of diarrhea [6]. Indeed, whatever the initial event (usually an infection), the presence or absence of diarrhea, as well as the severity of the illness, may be dependent on the presence of active osmotic carbohydrates or other molecules within the intestinal lumen. It has long been known that fasting reduces fluid loss in diarrhea. This may be related to hormones and other factors. However, it seems to be mainly the result of the presence or absence of free carbohydrates within the lumen. The details of the cycle of events that results whenever there is carbohydrate malabsorption, as occurs in diarrheal disease, are described in Chapter 21 of this volume. However, any other condition associated with excess water-soluble molecules remaining in the bowel may be sufficient to cause retention of water or secretory disturbances in the small bowel, as described elsewhere in this volume.

V. Pathogenic Mechanisms

Diarrhea may result whenever a microorganism or any other noxious agent induces one of the following intestinal alterations: (1) pathogenicity by invasion, penetration, and/or disruption of the intestinal epithelium; (2) pathogenicity by secretory enhancement of fluid and electrolytes where the mucosal integrity is generally preserved; and (3) pathogenicity by substances injurious to the intestine; these are usually generated by the metabolic activity of bacteria on foodstuff and/or host secretions. In this volume special attention is given to several of the most frequent causes of diarrhea of infectious origin, namely viral, bacterial, and parasitic.

Any agent which is capable of inducing diarrheal disease will do so only when there is an imbalance with the immune mechanisms of the host in defense against enteric disease [7]. Even the most pathogenic bacteria will not produce disease if the patient is not exposed to an infective dose. In Chapter 21 of this volume the variability of infectious doses of several bacterial species is discussed. Bacteria capable of inducing disease by invasion and penetration of the enterocyte requires a small innoculum to produce disease, whereas bacteria producing disease by other mechanisms will only do so when present in large number.

General host factors, such as age and nutritional status of the patient, are also important in determining whether diarrhea results [8]. Previous treatment with antibiotics and/or other medications might also facilitate the development of enteric infections due to overgrowth of bacteria not susceptible to antibiotic treatment. In addition, the use of medications which influence intestinal motility may allow bacteria to infect the host, due to increased time of contact between the organism and the host [9].

In the past few years, great emphasis has been placed on "breast feeding" as a factor in defense against disease [10]. It is not possible to review here all the evidence suggesting that breast feeding decreases the incidence and severity of enteric infections. The benefits of breast milk are principally related to decreased contamination as well as general and local immune factors. Several studies done as long as five decades ago already showed the alarming hazards of bottle feedings [11, 12]. It was claimed that breast feeding is better and preferable to bottle feeding under nearly all conditions. This is particularly important in the underdeveloped world. However, the practice of breast feeding has become less frequent and commerciogenic feeding has become popular, replacing the natural food supply that these populations would use in the normal "primitive habitat," thus contributing to malnutrition.

The local gastrointestinal defense factors are probably of greatest significance; included are the gastric acidity and the diarrhea per se. One reduces the viability of the germs and the other decreases the time exposure of the intestine to the infecting organism or noxious agent. Other important factors include intestinal antibodies and bacterial flora.

It has been shown that, regardless of the cause of diarrhea, there is a frequent proliferation of nonspecific fecal and colonic bacteria in the upper segments of the small intestine of these patients [13]. These increased enteric microbial populations may be directly responsible for the diarrhea. However, in the majority of instances the microbial overgrowth appears to be a secondary alteration which may result from the disease process per se. It has been postulated that the initial infection which triggers diarrhea (probably a virus in the majority of instances) may induce a disordered small-bowel function with subsequent overgrowth of host colonic and fecal flora in the upper segments of the small intestine. Among the factors which may influence enteric bacterial dissemination and proliferation in the upper bowel segments in diarrhea are disturbed motility, the presence of free carbohydrates in the lumen [14], the presence of plasmids in bacteria [15], and/or the metabolic interactions among intestinal microorganisms [16, 17]. Whatever the reason, small-bowel colonization with enteric microflora may directly aggravate the intestinal function alterations [13, 14, 18, 19].

In contrast, proliferation of intestinal microflora in the upper segments of the bowel has been reported to occur in malnourished children even when they have no diarrhea [20]. However, quantitative and qualitative differences in small-bowel microflora may account for variation in the production of factors injurious to the small intestine and therefore the presence or absence of diarrhea [21].

When bacteria proliferates in the small intestine they may produce disease by altering foodstuffs and/or host secretions. Such bacterial metabolic activity generates a variety of substances: e.g., deconjugated bile salts [21] and/or hydroxy fatty acids [22], short-chain organic acids [23], or alcohol [24, 25]. These can be injurious to the intestine, with induction of alterations in the transport of solutes and water, resulting in diarrhea. Ultrastructural and functional abnormalities of the intestine have all been related to these bacterial metabolites. A wide spectrum of enteric microorganisms may alter intestinal function when present in excessive numbers in the small intestine [26]. Bacterial overgrowth can be the primary cause of acute illness, or it can be secondarily associated with monosaccharide intolerance, gastrointestinal surgery, blind-loop syndrome, achlorhydria, inflammatory bowel disease, and alterations of intestinal motility, as well as other conditions [13, 14, 18, 19, 27]. However, it may play its most important role in the secondary pathogenic alteration of diarrhea, often causing prolongation and aggravation of the disease.

VI. Clinical Assessment

The traditional evaluation of the patients should also include an assessment of the diarrhea in relation to the cause of the disease as well as to the patient's tolerance to carbohydrates. Examination of the stools should include analysis of fecal leukocytes, pH, and carbohydrate excretion, in addition to the customary cultures. This will allow a more accurate clinical assessment of the type of process which may be involved in the cause of the diarrhea, as well as provide tools for rational decisions regarding treatment of these patients. Diagnosis of bacterial diarrhea by clinical features is often difficult [28]. The analysis of fecal leukocytes provides a rapid diagnosis of the possible infective process which will later be confirmed by the classic cultural isolation of the microorganisms induced [29]. It provides immediate clues regarding bacterial viruses or nonbacterial causes. It may even shed light on the possible types of organisms and on whether antibiotic treatment may or may not be used [30]. A patient with diarrhea with marked leukocytosis and a high proportion of neutrophils in stools may require antibiotics for treatment before cultural isolation of the bacterium. It must be emphasized that this test should not be used alone to indicate the appropriateness of antibiotic therapy, since fecal leukocytes may be found in patients with certain types of bacterial infection, e.g., salmonellosis, where antibiotic therapy may be contraindicated [31]. However, the absence of fecal leukocytes may be a rapid and reliable way to identify patients with viral or nonspecific diarrhea, for whom antibiotic therapy is not indicated. In addition, the quantitative and qualitative cell analysis may be suggestive of other causes of diarrhea. For example, the presence of eosinophils in stools may give clues to a possible allergic manifestation.

The assessment of the capacity to tolerate carbohydrates should also be made by simple, semiquantitative methods that measure the presence of reducing substances, glucose, and the pH of the stools [32, 33]. These techniques are now widely employed; however, it is very important to remember to test for these parameters in fresh stool specimens throughout the time the stools are abnormal. Within minutes after excretion, there is exogenous bacterial fermentation, the stool pH and glucose concentrations rapidly drop, and lactic acid rapidly increases [33]. Thus, the stool has to be tested immediately after it is excreted. An alternative could be rectal examination, with the feces retrieved being tested immediately. The best clinical indices of carbohydrate intolerance in infants with diarrhea are: the presence of carbohydrates in the stools in concentraions above 0.25% reducing substances, 1+ glucose, and the presence of stools with a pH less than 6. These abnormalities may manifest at any time during the diarrheal illness [32].

VII. Therapeutic Considerations

Prevention is still the challenge to concern us in dealing with diarrhea, which is one of the most mortal diseases. Improvement in economic levels, nutrition, and sanitation are of paramount importance. Hand-washing, refrigeration, and proper cooking can be achieved by improvements in socioeconomic and environmental standards such as safe water supply and control of flies. For certain groups at high risk of developing specific enteric infections, it may soon be feasible to control diarrhea through the use of an oral vaccine. It is unlikely, however, that immunologic approaches will offer the solution in the widespread control of diarrheal disease among the general population, because of the myriad of bacterial, viral, and protozoal etiologies.

The natural history of diarrheal disease varies considerably within each specific etiologic group of diseases and between these groups, so that the effectiveness of antibiotics against these diseases can be demonstrated only by well-controlled, double-blind treatment studies. However, even the "proven" drugs have limited value because antibiotic-resistant organisms continue to emerge and will eventually nullify the effect of the drug therapy now available. Studies have shown that ampicillin is effective against *Shigella* [34], and neomycin or colistin (orally) against *Escherichia coli* [35]. On the other hand, antibiotics are not effective against *Salmonella* [31] or in treating nonspecific gastroenteritis. For a more exciting discussion of the principles for control and chemotherapy, the reader is referred to Chapter 22 of this volume.

Maintenance of fluid and electrolyte balance and dietary treatment remain the central vital factors in the successful treatment of diarrheal disorders. And, as approximately 80% of infants and children have no demonstrable bacterial pathogen, fluid and electrolyte therapy and a proper diet are often the only necessary forms of therapy.

Nonspecific antidiarrheal drugs (e.g., opium preparations, Lomotil) are not recommended for use in children. Drug efficacy studies are very limited and poorly controlled, and the studies that are available indicate that these drugs are either ineffective or may even prolong the illness [36]. Antispasmodic and nonspecific antidiarrheal agents are of little value. Other medicines, which are intended to modify the physical appearance of the stools, do not decrease water and electrolyte losses and may provide a false sense of security, since the stools appear improved [37].

The dietary treatment of secondary carbohydrate intolerance in diarrheal disease is strongly recommended. The general principles to be followed are described in Chapter 23 of this volue [7] and elsewhere [38].

References

1. J. T. Harries. The problem of bacterial diarrhea. In *Acute Diarrhoea in Childhood* (K. Elliott and J. Knight, Eds.). *CIBA Foundation Symposium 42* (new series). Elsevier-North Holland, Amsterdam. 1976, pp. 3-25.
2. D. S. Mclaren. The great protein fiasco. *Lancet 12,* 93-96 (1974).
3. J. C. Waterlow and P. R. Payne. The protein gap. Review article. *Nature 258,* 113-117 (1975).
4. P. F. Curran and S. G. Schultz. Transport across membranes: General principles. In *Handbook of Physiology,* Sect. 6, The Alimentary Canal, Vol. 3 (C. F. Code, Ed.). The American Physiological Society, Washington, D.C., 1968, pp. 1217-1243.
5. H. W. Davenport. *Physiology of the Digestive Tract,* 3d Ed.) Year Book Med. Pub., Chicago, 1971, pp. 171-182.
6. K. Launialia. The effect of unabsorbed sucrose and mannitol in the small intestinal flow rate and mean trancit time. *Scand. J. Gastroenterol. 39,* 665-671 (1968).
7. F. Lifshitz. The enteric flora in childhood disease—diarrhea. *Am. J. Nutr. 30,* 1811-1818 (1977).
8. J. E. Gordon. Diarrheal disease of early childhood—worldwide scope of the problem. Part 1. Factors determining host susceptibility and response to neonatal gastroenteritis. *Ann. N.Y. Acad. Sci. 176,* 9-15 (1971).
9. H. L. Dupont and R. B. Hornick. Adverse effect of lomotil therapy in shigellosis. *J. A.M.A. 226,* 1525-1528 (1973).
10. D. B. Jelliffe and E. F. P. Jelliffe. *Human Milk in the Modern World.* Oxford Univ. Press, Oxford, 1978.
11. H. K. Faber and T. L. Sutton. A statistical comparison of breast fed and bottle fed babies during the first year. *Am. J. Dis. Child. 40,* 1163-1176 (1930).
12. M. M. Glazier. Comparing the breast-fed and the bottle-fed infant. *New Engl. J. Med. 230,* 626-628 (1930).
13. P. Coello-Ramirez and F. Lifshitz. Enteric microflora and carbohydrate intolerance in infants with diarrhea. *Pediatrics 49,* 233-242 (1972).
14. V. Burke and C. M. Anderson. Sugar intolerance as a cause of protracted

diarrhea following surgery of the gastrointestinal tract in neonates. *Aust. Paediatr. J. 2,* 219-227 (1966).

15. T. Watanabe. Infectious drug resistance in enteric bacteria. *N. Engl. J. Med. 275,* 888-894 (1966).
16. R. Freter. Interactions between mechanisms controlling the intestinal microflora. *Am. J. Clin. Nutr. 27,* 1409-1416 (1974).
17. M. J. Wolin. Metabolic interactions among intestinal microorganisms. *Am. J. Clin. Nutr. 27,* 1320-1328 (1974).
18. P. Coello-Ramirez, G. Gutierrez-Topete, and F. Lifshitz. Pneumatosis intestinalis. *Am. J. Dis. Chil. 120,* 3-9 (1970).
19. F. Lifshitz, P. Coello-Ramirez, and G. Gutierrez-Topete. Monosaccharide intolerance and hypoglycemia in infants with diarrhea. I. Clinical course of 23 infants. *J. Pediatr. 77,* 595-603 (1970).
20. L. J. Mata, F. Jimenez, M. Cordon, R. Rosales, E. Prera, R. E. Schneider, and F. Viteri. Gastrointestinal flora of children with protein-calorie malnutrition. *Am. J. Clin. Nutr. 25,* 1118-1126 (1972).
21. T. Midtvedt. Microbial bile acid transportation. *Am. J. Clin. Nutr. 27,* 1341-1347 (1974).
22. H. J. Binder. Fecal fatty acids—Mediators of diarrhea? *Gastroenterology 65,* 847-850 (1973).
23. A. J. Chernov, W. F. Doe, and D. Compertz. Intrajejunal volatile fatty acids in the stagnant loop syndrome. *Gut 13,* 103-106 (1972).
24. F. A. Klipstein, L. V. Holdeman, J. J. Corcino, and W. E. C. Moore. Enterotoxigenic intestinal bacteria in tropical sprue. *Ann. Intern. Med. 79,* 632-641 (1973).
25. E. Baraona, R. C. Pirola, and C. S. Lieber. Small intestinal damage and changes in cell population produced by ethanol ingestion in the rat. *Gastroenterology 66,* 226-234 (1974).
26. M. Gracey, V. Burke, J. A. Thomasa, and D. C. Stone. Effect of microorganisms isolated from the upper gut of malnourished children or intestinal sugar absorption in vivo. *Am. J. Clin. Nutr. 28,* 841-845 (1975).
27. V. Burke and D. M. Danks. Monosaccharide malabsorption in young infants. *Lancet 1,* 1177-1180 (1966).
28. J. D. E. Knox, A. R. Laurence, G. MacNaughtan, and A. A. Robertson. Diagnosis of diarrhea in general practice, bacteriologic "self-help." *Lancet 2,* 1392-1394 (1967).
29. J. C. Harris, H. L. DuPont, and R. B. Hornick. Fecal leukocytes in diarrheal illness. *Ann. Int. Med. 76,* 697-703 (1972).
30. J. D. Nelson and K. C. Haltalin. Accuracy of diagnosis of bacterial diarrheal disease by clinical features. *J. Pediatr. 78,* 519-522 (1971).
31. B. Aserkoff and J. V. Bennett. Effect of antibiotic therapy in acute salmonellosis on the fecal excretion of salmonellae. *N. Engl. J. Med. 281,* 636-640 (1969).
32. F. Lifshitz, P. Coello-Ramirez, G. Gutierrez-Topete, and M. C. Cornado-Cornet. Carbohydrate intolerance in infants with diarrhea. *J. Pediatr. 79,* 760-767 (1971).

33. F. Lifshitz. Clinical studies in diarrheal disease and malnutrition associated with carbohydrate intolerance. *Proceedings of the Ninth International Congress in Nutrition 1972* (A. Chavez, H. Bourges, and S. Basta, Eds.). S. Karger, Basel, 1975, pp. 173-181.
34. K. C. Maltalm, J. K. Nelson, R. Ring II, M. Sladoje, and L. V. Minton. Double blind treatment study of shigellosis comparing ampicillin, sulfadiazine and placebo. *J. Pediatr. 70,* 970-981 (1967).
35. J. D. Nelson. Duration of neomycin therapy for enteropathogenic *Escherichia coli* diarrheal disease. *Pediatrics 48,* 248-258 (1971).
36. H. L. DuPont and R. B. Hornick. Adverse effect of Lomotil therapy in shigellosis. *JAMA 226*, 1525-1528 (1973).
37. M. Davidson. Chronic nonspecific diarrheal syndrome. In *Current Pediatric Therapy,* 6th Ed. (S. Gellis and B. M. Kagan, Eds.). Saunders, Philadelphia, 1973, pp. 192-193.
38. F. Lifshitz. Current therapy of the malabsorption syndrome and intestinal disaccharidase deficiencies. In *Current Pediatric Therapy,* 6th Ed. (S. Gellis and B. M. Kagan, Eds.). Saunders, Philadelphia, 1973, pp. 236-247.

19 Physiologic Bases of Secretory Disturbances in the Human Bowel

RAMON B. TORRES-PINEDO / University of Oklahoma Health Sciences Center, and Oklahoma Children's Memorial Hospital, Oklahoma City, Oklahoma

I. Introduction

A detailed discussion of electrolyte transport in mammalian intestine is beyond the scope of this brief review of secretory disturbances in the human bowel. An excellent review article on the subject has been recently published [1]. Notwithstanding, it needs to be stated that the rapid increase in understanding of the mechanisms involved in the secretory diarrheas has stemmed directly from recent developments in the field of mammalian epithelial transport. Particularly relevant to this discussion are the following observations:

1. The demonstration of the quantitative importance of the "shunt" pathway in the net movement of ions across the intestinal epithelium [2-4]
2. The localization of specific transport functions at the brush border and basolateral membranes of the epithelial absorptive cells [4-10]
3. The kinetic characterization of "coupled" transport at the level of the apical plasma membrane of these cells [10]
4. The elucidation of the prominent role of cyclic AMP (cAMP) on Na and Cl transport at the apical membrane [10]

Figure 1 is based on the model for transepithelial NaCl movement presented by Nellans et al. [10]. Ions (and probably also small nonelectrolytes) move across the intestinal epithelium through inter and transepithelial pathways. As shown in vitro [4, 11, 12] and in vivo [13, 14], the relative contributions of these two pathways to net ionic fluxes vary from proximal to distal bowel. The "shunt" pathway exhibits maximal permeability in the proximal bowel.

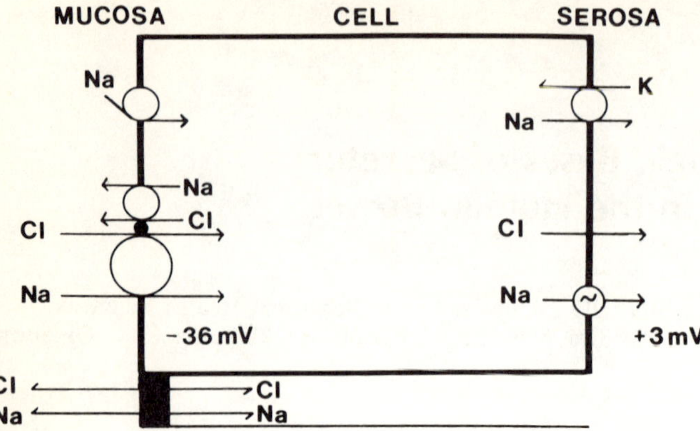

Figure 1 Model for electrolyte transport across intestinal epithelium. (Modified from Nellans et al. [10].)

Fluxes through this pathway are determined by electrochemical and osmotic forces. Therefore, the proximal bowel is relatively more permeable to passive diffusion than the distal bowel. On the other hand, transport through the transcellular route becomes increasingly effective in determining net fluxes as the intercellular permeability decreases progressively toward the distal bowel.

Sodium seems to move across the apical membrane via two different mechanisms. One is a Cl-coupled influx process, which conforms with the properties of carrier-mediated transport. It is freely reversible and probably responsible for the Na-coupled anion efflux process in ileal epithelium. As shown in Figure 2, this Cl-coupled Na transport is inhibited by cAMP. The other Na influx process is Cl-independent. Its nature is not clear yet, but a carrier-mediated cationic exchange mechanism has been suggested [15]. This transport function is not influenced by cAMP.

Obviously, a variety of factors not included in Figure 1 also influence ion movement through the intestinal mucosa. In fact, as recently discussed by Field [16], there is compelling evidence indicating that the model presented by Nellans et al. does not satisfactorily explain active Cl secretion by ileal mucosa, as observed under the influence of cAMP in vitro [10]. Building upon evidence presented first by Hendrix and Bayless [17], Field [16] has proposed a two-site model for cAMP-stimulated Cl efflux (Fig. 3). In this model, the nucleotide, in addition to inhibiting the Na-coupled influx process in the villus cells, would also stimulate the active secretion of Cl in the crypt cells. This model is consistent with the results of measurements of unidirectional ion fluxes on short-circuited intestinal epithelium [18, 19] and with observations on the effect of cAMP stimulation on net fluid production in vivo [20].

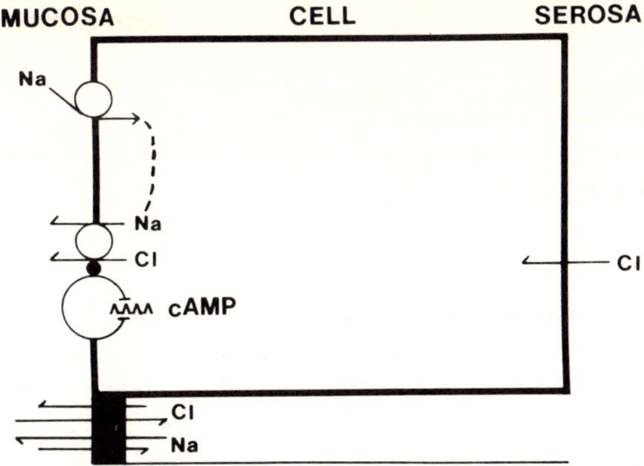

Figure 2 Model illustrating effect of cAMP rise on Na and Cl transport across intestinal epithelium. (Modified from Nellans et al. [10].)

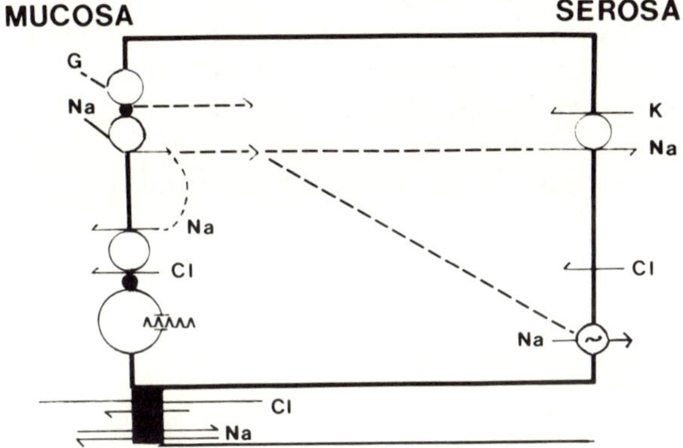

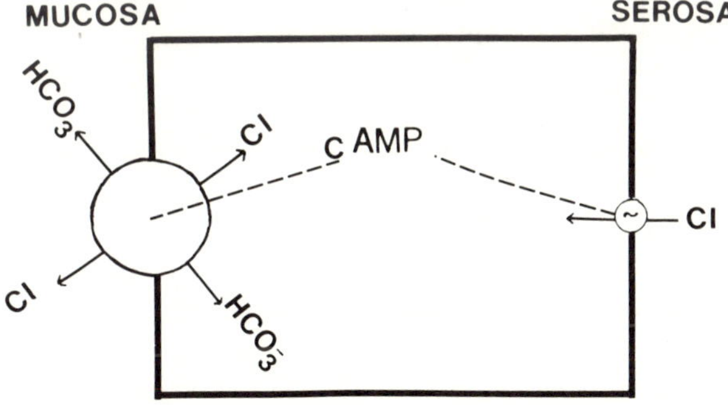

Figure 3 Model for two-site action of cAMP on Cl and Na transport ion intestinal epithelium. The broken lines on the villus cell diagram (top) represent the effect of glucose added to the luminal fluid. (Modified from Field [16] and Nellans et al. [10].)

II. Regulation of Intestinal Fluid Secretory Activity

A number of endogenous and exogenous agents are known to influence ion and water movement in the small and large bowel (Table 1).

A. Antidiuretic Hormone (ADH)

Soergel et al. [20] showed that ADH blocks the absorption of NaCl in intestinal mucosa. Subsequently Field et al. [21] extended this observation, demonstrating that the effect of ADH was due to inhibition of Na and Cl influx without alteration of the Na-anion efflux process. Therefore ADH elicited a net secretion of NaCl by a mechanism similar to that of theophylline and cAMP.

B. Catecholamines

The effect of the catecholamines on NaCl transport seems to be opposite to that described above for ADH. This was first demonstrated by Field and McColl [22] on short-circuited ileal mucosa. The short-circuit current in such preparation showed a residual component independent of the Na and Cl fluxes. Such a residual component was attributed to HCO_3 flux from cell to lumen. The catecholamines (epinephrine and norepinephrine) were shown to inhibit this

Table 1 Endogenous and Exogenous Stimulators of Intestinal Fluid Secretion

Alterations in tissue fluid dynamics
Increased mucosal capillary pressure
Impaired lymphatic drainage
Decreased colloid osmotic pressure
Secretagogues associated with cAMP rise in intestinal mucosa
Vasoactive intestinal peptide
Prostaglandins
Bacterial enterotoxins (*V. cholerae, E. coli, Shigella, Salmonella?*)
Methylxanthines (e.g., theophylline)
Deoxycholic and other dihydroxy bile acids
Secretin
Secretagogues nonassociated with cAMP rise in intestinal mucosa
Glucagon
Gastric inhibitory peptide
Acetylcholine
Serotonin
Calcitonin
Antidiuretic hormone
Laxatives

transport process with a decrease in SCC and increase in net Na and Cl absorptive fluxes. After these observations, Field et al. [23] investigated the effect of epinephrine on cAMP levels in rabbit ileal mucosa. Epinephrine did not affect the base-line levels or significantly antagonize the effect of theophylline on cAMP level. On the other hand, epinephrine and norepinephrine almost completely reversed the effect of cholera toxin on cAMP level and partially reversed that of prostaglandin E_1. Next, the effect of epinephrine on ion fluxes was measured after the addition of theophylline, cholera toxin, or cAMP. Epinephrine inhibited the theophylline-enhanced Cl secretion, but had no significant effect on the cAMP- or cholera toxin-induced secretion. To explain the observed discrepancies between catecholamine effects on cAMP and ion fluxes, the authors offered the following alternative possibilities: (1) that only a small fraction of the mucosal cAMP pool is related to the ion transport process; (2) that cAMP-mediated ion secretion is slowly reversible; and (3) that the effect of α-adrenergic stimulation on the fluxes is independent of that on cAMP.

In contrast to the action of α-adrenergic stimulators, cholinergic drugs elicit active Cl secretion in the jejunum. This was first shown by Tidball [24], using Thiry Vella loops in dog jejunum, and subsequently was shown in vitro by Turnberg and co-workers [25]. Recently, Browning and collaborators [26] designed experiments to localize the site of action of acetylcholine on rat jejunal and colonic mucosa in vivo. Their results suggested that acetylcholine acts at the level of the intestinal crypt cells, but has no effect on transport in the villus cells.

C. Glucocorticoids

The glucocorticoids administered in pharmacologic doses have been shown to enhance salt and water absorption in the rat in vivo [27]. It has been suggested that the effect of these agents could be mediated by the activation of (Na^+-K^+)-ATPase.

D. Vasoactive Intestinal Peptide (VIP)

The isolation of the VIP from the upper small intestine of the pig by Said and Mutt [28, 29] and its subsequent synthesis by Bodanszky, Klausner, and Said [30] opened the way to investigations of the role of this peptide on intestinal transport. Schwartz et al. [31] demonstrated that VIP added to rabbit ileal mucosa stimulated adenylate cyclase, causing a rapid increase of cAMP level. These changes correlated with increases in SCC and net secretory fluxes of Na and Cl. The observed effects of VIP on ion fluxes and conductance were similar to those previously described for cAMP [17], theophylline [17], and cholera enterotoxin [32]. More recently, a similar action of VIP has been demonstrated on rat colonic mucosa in vitro [33] and on dog jejunum in vivo [34].

E. Prostaglandins

The prostaglandins constitute another group of powerful stimulators of adenyl cyclase and secretory activity in the bowel. Pierce et al. [35] showed that the prostaglandins PGE, PGA, and $PGF_{2\alpha}$ reversed the net fluxes of water and ions from net absorption to net secretion in dog jejunum. Subsequently, Maturchansky and Bernier [36], using the intestinal perfusion technique, found a similar effect of PGE in human jejunum. Also, PGE_1 was shown to induce simultaneous increases in SCC and on cAMP in rabbit ileal mucosa [37a]. The similarity between this effect of PGE and that of cholera enterotoxin suggested that perhaps the prostaglandins acted as intermediates between toxin and adenylate cyclase. This possibility was dismissed, however, after the observation that PGE and cholera enterotoxin had additive effects on cAMP levels. Moreover, the elevation of cAMP levels by cholera enterotoxin was not influenced by indomethacin, which is a powerful inhibitor of mucosal prostaglandin synthesis. These findings were subsequently confirmed by Wald et al. [37b], who showed that indomethacin decreased the cholera enterotoxin-induced secretion in vivo, probably by inhibition of a prostaglandin-mediated step beyond cAMP. Further information about the characteristics of PGE-induced secretion and its site of action in intestinal epithelium was recently provided by the studies of Gerencser et al. [38] on isolated bullfrog small intestine. The authors examined the effect of PGE_1 added to either the serosal or the mucosal side in a short-circuited preparation. An increase in transepithelial PD and SCC was elicited only upon addition to the serosal side. Furthermore, this effect was enhanced in the presence of indomethacin, probably through removal of the competitive action of endogenous prostaglandin. It was concluded that the site of PGE_1 action was at the basolateral membrane of the epithelial absorptive cells, its effect being mediated either through a series of metabolic reactions or by direct stimulation of the Na pump.

F. Secretin and Glucagon

Secretin and glucagon are peptides structurally related to VIP. Likewise, both hormones have been shown to stimulate fluid secretion in the small and large bowel [39]. It was, therefore, assumed that their mechanism of action was similar to that of VIP. This, however, seems to be true only for secretin. This hormone, like VIP, stimulates adenylate cyclase and raises the mucosal level of cAMP in vitro. Makhlouf et al. [40] have suggested that secretin shares with VIP the same receptor sites in intestinal mucosa. In contrast to secretin, glucagon does not stimulate adenylate cyclase in vitro, and its effect on secretory activity in vivo is additive to that of VIP and theophylline [40]. Moreover, Mailman and MacFerran [41] have recently reported that glucagon induces a rise in mucosal capillary pressure in dog intestine. These observations led Makhlouf to postulate a hemodynamic action of glucagon on transmucosal fluid movement. The mechanism could be an increase in passive diffusion through the "shunt" pathway.

G. Deoxycholic Acid

Deoxycholic acid (DCA) is another agent capable of inducing cAMP-mediated stimulation of secretion in the colon. Taub et al. [42] were the first to show that the DCA effect on cAMP probably differed from other agents in its organ, as well as receptor, specificity. The authors compared cholera enterotoxin (CE) and DCA. Cholera enterotoxin stimulated adenylate cyclase in the small bowel, but not in the colon, whereas DCA did the opposite. Also, in the same studies it was shown that the DCA stimulation of adenylate cyclase in the colon was significantly decreased by propranolol, whereas this agent had no effect on the CE-stimulated adenylate cyclase. This result suggested different receptor specificities for DCA and CE.

III. Disturbances of Fluid Secretion in the Human Bowel

Enhanced intestinal fluid secretion is known to occur in a variety of diseases in children and adults (Table 2). Several types of tumors have been reported to be associated with secretory diarrhea. Verner and Morrison [43] were the first to report the association between certain pancreatic tumors and severe diarrhea. They provided a detailed clinical description of two patients who died from extremely profuse, watery diarrhea, and in whom pancreatic neoplasms were found at autopsy. The authors considered the possibility of a hormone-induced diarrhea, but the VIP was not known at the time of their observation. Subsequently, after the VIP was discovered, there were several reports of VIP-synthesizing pancreatic tumors associated with cholera-like diarrhea [44-46]. Other tumors known to be associated with the watery-diarrhea syndrome include carcinoid tumors, medullary carcinoma of the thyroid, and neoplasms arising in the sympathetic nervous system. Some of the endogenous agents discussed in the preceding section are probably implicated in these types of secretory diarrhea.

There is no doubt that knowledge about secretory phenomena in the human bowel is owed in large measure to the intensive research conducted on bacterial enterotoxins, especially on cholera toxin. It is now well known that some bacterial enterotoxins are powerful stimulators of adenylate cyclase. In the small bowel, this leads to enhanced anion secretion by the cAMP-mediated mechanism.

Leitch et al. [47] were the first to demonstrate that cell-free filtrates of *Vibrio cholerae* cultures promoted fluid accumulation in isolated intestinal

Table 2 Causes of Enhanced Fluid Secretion in Human Bowel

Causes
Functional disturbances of epithelial fluid transport
Bacterial (enterotoxic) diarrheas
Pancreatic cholera (non-B-islet cell tumor, other)
Ganglioneuroma, pheochromocytoma
Villous adenoma
Medullary carcinoma of thyroid
Carcinoid tumor
Laxative poisoning or abuse
Mucosal morphologic damage
Celiac disease
Tropical sprue
Bacterial (enteroinvasive) enteritis
Viral enteritis
Inflammatory bowel disease
Intestinal lymphoma and lymphosarcoma
"Allergic" enteropathy
Radiation injury
Other
Paralytic ileus
Intestinal obstruction

loops without causing significant mucosal damage. This led first to isolation of the enterotoxin [48, 49] and then to a description of its biological effects on different types of cells [50-54]. Researchers have studied extensively the effect of cholera enterotoxin on adenylate cyclase [55-60] and on cAMP levels in intestinal mucosa [61], as well as the resulting alterations of ion and water transport [16, 62-65]. The molecular structure of the toxin [66-69], the nature of its receptor sites in the membrane surface [70-74], and the cellular events that follow the toxin-receptor interaction [75-78] are areas of current investigations. Following the discoveries on cholera diarrhea, investigations of *Escherichia coli* diarrhea demonstrated that certain strains of *E. Coli* also produced enterotoxins with qualitatively identical effects on the bowel [79-90]. Whether enterotoxins are always involved in *E. Coli* diarrhea is not clear at present. Invasion of the intestinal mucosa by some strains is frequently implicated as an alternate mechanism. Invasiveness has been well documented in colonic epithelium. However, it is indeed possible that, as shown recently for shigella dysentery [91], the mechanism of fluid loss in enteroinvasive *E. Coli* infections is also mediated by the adenylate cyclase-cAMP system.

As indicated before, the overall effect of cholera enterotoxin on fluid production in the small bowel can be satisfactorily explained on the basis of a two-site action of cAMP- and Cl-transport: namely, a stimulation of Cl outflux in the crypt cells and a simultaneous inhibition of the Na-coupled Cl influx in the mature villus cells. This explanation, however, has been challenged by DeJonge [92], who measured the unidirectional fluxes of Na and Cl after short and prolonged exposure to cholera toxin in rats and guinea pigs in vivo. From such measurements he concluded that the toxin increased the outflux of Na and Cl in both the villus and crypt cells, depending on time of exposure. He found no toxin effect on the Na and Cl influx process. Nevertheless, the two-site model for cAMP-stimulated secretion, as proposed by Field, provides a cohesive explanation for a variety of secretory disturbances in human bowel in which either functional (cAMP-mediated) or anatomic imbalance between crypt and villus cells could occur.

Increased fluid secretion into the bowel is probably a significant factor in the diarrheal disturbance of celiac disease. Using the intraluminal perfusion technique, Fordtran et al. [93] have shown a net loss of Na, Cl, and water into the jejunum in patients with active celiac disease. Normal individuals absorbed fluid under identical perfusion conditions. The mucosal secretory losses are probably due to a break in the normal equilibrium between crypt and villus cell compartments.

Finally, we have recently shown [94] using the perfusion technique, that soy protein intolerance in infants is characterized by enhanced secretion of Na, Cl, and water into the jejunum. Further investigations are needed to elucidate the mechanisms involved in this type of secretory diarrhea.

References

1. S. G. Schultz, R. A. Frizzell, and H. N. Nellans. Ion transport by mammalian small intestine. *Annu. Rev. Physiol. 36,* 51-91 (1974).
2. R. C. Rose and S. G. Schultz. Studies on the electrical potential profile across rabbit ileum: Effects of sugars and amino acids on transmural and transmucosal electrical potential differences. *J. Gen. Physiol. 57,* 639-663 (1971).
3. J. F. White and W. McD. Armstrong. Effect of transport solutes on membrane potentials in bullfrog small intestine. *Am. J. Physiol. 221,* 194-201 (1971).
4. R. A. Frizzell and S. G. Schultz. Ionic conductances of extracellular shunt pathway in rabbit ileum: Influence of shunt on transmural sodium transport and electrical potential differences. *J. Gen. Physiol. 59,* 318-346 (1972).
5. M. Fujita, H. Matsui, K. Nagano, and M. Nakao. Asymmetric distribution of ouabain-sensitive ATPase activity in rat intestinal mucosa. *Biochim. Biophys. Acta 233,* 404-458 (1971).

6. M. Fujita, H. Ohta, K. Kawai, H. Matsui, and M. Nakao. Differential isolation of microvillus and baso-lateral plasma membranes from intestinal mucosa: Mutually exclusive distribution of digestive enzymes and ouabain-sensitive ATPase. *Biochim. Biophys. Acta 274*, 336-347 (1972).
7. W. Koopman and S. G. Schultz. The effect of sugars and amino acids on mucosal Na and K concentrations in rabbit ileum. *Biochim. Biophys. Acta 173*, 338-340 (1969).
8. S. G. Schultz, R. E. Fuisz, and P. F. Curran. Amino acid and sugar transport in rabbit ileum. *J. Gen. Physiol. 49*, 849-866 (1966).
9. R. A. Frizzell, H. N. Nellans, R. C. Rose, L. Markscheid-Kapsi, and S. G. Schultz. Intracellular Cl concentrations and influxes across the brush border of rabbit ileum. *Am. J. Physiol. 224*, 328-337 (1973).
10. H. C. Nellans, R. A. Frizzell, and S. G. Schultz. Coupled sodium-chloride influx across the brush border of rabbit ileum. *Am. J. Physiol. 225*, 467-475 (1973).
11. B. G. Munck. Effects of sugar and amino acid transport on transepithelial fluxes of sodium and chloride of short circuited rat jejunum. *J. Physiol. (Lond.) 223*, 699-717 (1972).
12. S. G. Schultz and R. Zalusky. Ion transport in isolated rabbit ileum. I. Short-circuit current and Na fluxes. *J. Gen. Physiol. 47*, 567-584 (1964).
13. J. S. Fordtran, F. C. Rector, Jr., and N. W. Carter. The mechanisms of sodium absorption in the human small intestine. *J. Clin. Invest. 47*, 567-584 (1964).
14. J. S. Fordtran, F. C. Rector, Jr., M. F. Ewton, N. Soter, and J. Kinney. Permeability characteristics of the human small intestine. *J. Clin. Invest. 44*, 1935-1944 (1965).
15. L. A. Turnberg, F. A. Bieberdorf, S. G. Morawski, and J. S. Fordtran. Interrelationships of chloride, bicarbonate, sodium and hydrogen transport in the human ileum. *J. Clin. Invest. 49*, 557-567 (1970).
16. M. Field. *Regulation of Active Ion Transport in the Small Intestine* (K. Elliott and J. Knight, Eds.). *CIBA Foundation Symposium* (new series). Elsevier North-Holland, Amsterdam, 1976, pp. 109-127.
17. T. R. Hendrix and T. M. Bayless. Digestion: Intestinal secretion. *Annu. Rev. Physiol. 32*, 139-164 (1970).
18. D. W. Powell, H. J. Binder, and P. F. Curran. Active electrolyte secretion stimulated by choleragen in rabbit ileum in vitro. *Am. J. Physiol. 225*, 781-787 (1973).
19. M. Field. Ion transport in rabbit ileal mucosa. II. Effects of cyclic 3′,5′-AMP. *Am. J. Physiol. 221*(4), 992-997 (1971).
20. K. H. Soergel, G. E. Whalen, and J. A. Harris. Effect of antidiuretic hormone on human small intestine water and solute transport. *J. Clin. Invest. 47*, 1071-1082 (1968).
21. M. Field, G. R. Plotkin, and W. Silen. Effects of vasopressin, theophylline and cyclic adenosine monophosphate on short-circuit current across isolated rabbit ileal mucosa. *Nature 217*, 469-471 (1968).

22. M. Field and I. McColl. Ion transport in rabbit ileal mucosa. III. Effects of catecholamines. *Am. J. Physiol. 225,* 852-857 (1973).
23. M. Field, E. S. Harland, A. Henderson, and P. L. Smith. Catecholamine effects on cyclic AMP levels and ion secretion in rabbit ileal mucosa. *Am. J. Physiol. 229*(1), 86-92 (1975).
24. C. S. Tidball. Active Cl transport during intestinal secretion. *Am. J. Physiol. 200,* 309-312 (1961).
25. L. A. Turnberg, P. E. T. Isaacs, C. L. Corbett, and A. K. Riley. In *Intestinal Ion Transport* (R. W. L. Robinson, Ed.). MTP, Lancaster, England, 1976, pp. 339-344.
26. J. G. Browning, J. Hardcastle, P. T. Hardcastle, and J. S. Redfern. Site of action of acetylcholine in regulating intestinal epithelial ion transport in the rat (Proceedings). *J. Physiol. (Lond.) 270*(1), 78P-79P.
27. A. N. Charney, M. D. Kinsey, L. Myers, R. A. Giannella, and R. E. Gotts. Na^{+}-K^{+}-Activated adenosine triphosphatase and intestinal electrolyte transport. Effect of adrenal steroids. *J. Clin. Invest. 56,* 653-660 (1975).
28. S. I. Said and V. Mutt. Polypeptide with Broad biological activity: Isolation from small intestine. *Science 169*: 1217-1218 (1970).
29. S. I. Said and V. Mutt. Isolation from porcine-intestinal wall of a vasoactive octacosapeptide related to secretin and to glucagon. *Eur. J. Biochem. 28,* 199-204 (1972).
30. M. Bodanszky, Y. S. Klausner, and S. I. Said. Biological activities of synthetic peptides corresponding to fragments of and to the entire sequence of vasoactive intestinal peptide. *Proc. Natl. Acad. Sci. USA 70,* 382-384 (1973).
31. C. J. Schwartz, D. V. Kimberg, H. E. Sheerin, M. Field, and S. I. Said. Vasoactive intestinal peptide stimulation of adenylate cyclase and active electrolyte secretion in intestinal mucosa. *J. Clin. Invest. 54,* 536-544 (1974).
32. M. Field, D. Fromm, Q. Al-Awqati, and W. B. Greenough. Effect of cholera enterotoxin on ion transport across isolated ileal mucosa. *J. Clin. Invest. 51,* 796-804 (1972).
33. L. C. Racusen and H. J. Binder. Alteration of large intestinal electrolyte transport by vasoactive intestinal polypeptide in the rat. *Gastroenterology 73,* 790-796 (1977).
34. G. J. Krejs, R. M. Barkley, N. W. Read, and J. S. Fordtran. Intestinal secretions induced by vasoactive intestinal polypeptide: A comparison with cholera toxin in the canine jejunum in vivo. *J. Clin. Invest. 6*(5), 1227-1245.
35. N. G. Pierce, C. C. J. Carpenter, H. L. Elliott, and W. B. Greenough. Effects of prostaglandins, theophylline and cholera exotoxin upon transmucosal water and electrolyte movement in the canine jejunum. *Gastroenterology 60,* 22-32 (1971).
36. C. Matarchanski and J. J. Bernier. Effect of prostaglandin E_1 on glucose, water, and electrolyte absorption in the human jejunum. *Gastroenterology 64,* 1111-1118 (1973).

37a. D. V. Kimberg, M. Field, E. Gershon, and A. Henderson. Effects of prostaglandins and *Cholera* enterotoxin on intestinal mucosal cyclic AMP accumulation: Evidence against an essential role for prostaglandins in the action of toxin. *J. Clin. Invest. 53,* 941-949 (1974).

37b. A. Wald, G. S. Gotterer, G. R. Rajendra, N. A. Turjman, and T. R. Effect of indomethacin on cholera-induced fluid movement, unidirectional sodium fluxes, and intestinal cAMP. *Gastroenterology 72,* 106-110 (1977).

38. G. A. Gerencser, T. Tyler, and S. Cassin. Sodium transport by isolated bull-frog small intestine. Effect of prostaglandin E_1. *Biochim. Biophys. Acta 509,* 159-169 (1978).

39. D. B. Waldman, J. D. Gardner, A. M. Zfass, and G. M. Makhlouf. Effects of vasoactive intestinal peptide, secretin, and related peptides on rat colonic transport and adenylate cyclase activity. *Gastroenterology 73,* 518-523 (1977).

40. G. M. Makhlouf. Distinct mechanisms for stimulation of intestinal secretion by vasoactive intestinal peptide (VIP) and glucagon. *N. Engl. J. Med. 72,* 386-392 (1977).

41. D. Mailman and S. MacFerran. Effects of glucagon on canine ileal Na and H_2O fluxes and regional blood flow. *Physiologist 19,* 281 (1976).

42. M. Taub, G. Bonorris, A. Chung, M. J. Coyne, and L. J. Schoenfield. Effect of propranolol on bile acid- and cholera enterotoxin-stimulated cAMP and secretion in rabbit intestine. *Gastroenterology 72,* 101-105 (1977).

43. J. V. Verner and A. B. Morrison. Islet cell tumor and a syndrome of refractory watery diarrhea and hypokalemia. *Am. J. Med. 25,* 374-380 (1958).

44. S. R. Bloom, J. M. Polak, and A. G. E. Pearse. Vasoactive intestinal peptide and watery-diarrhoea syndrome. *Lancet 2,* 14-16 (1973).

45. J. V. Verner and A. B. Morrison. Non-islet tumours and the syndrome of watery diarrhoea, hypokalemia and hypochlorhydria. *Clin. Gastroenterol. 3,* 595-605 (1974).

46. A. M. Ebeid, P. D. Murray, and J. E. Fischer. Vasoactive intestinal peptide and the watery diarrhea syndrome. *Ann. Surg. 187,* 411-416 (1978).

47. G. J. Leitch, W. Burrows, and L. C. Stolle. Experimental cholera in the rabbit intestinal loop: Fluid accumulation and sodium pump inhibition. *J. Infect. Dis. 117,* 197-202 (1967).

48. R. A. Finkelstein and J. J. LoSpalluto. Session III production, purification and assay of cholera toxin. *J. Infect. Dis. 121,* S63-S72 (1970).

49. R. A. Finkelstein, J. Boesman, S. H. Noeh, M. K. LaRuse, and R. Delaney. Dissociation and recombination of the subunits of the cholera enterotoxin (choleragen) *J. Immunol. 113,* 145-150 (1974).

50. R. A. Finkelstein. Cholera. *CRC Crit. Rev. Microbiol. 2,* 553-623 (1973).

51. B. M. Sultzer and J. P. Craig. Cholera toxin inhibits macromolecular synthesis in mouse spleen cells. *Nature New Biol. 244,* 178-180 (1973).

52. W. B. Greenough. Titration of cholera enterotoxin and antitoxin in isolated fat cells. *J. Infect. Dis. 121,* S11-113 (1970).

53. J. Davies, D. A. J. Tyrrel, D. B. Ramsden, L. N. Louis, and R. G. Milner. Some inhibitors of the effect of cholera toxin on HeLa cells. *Exp. Mol. Pathol. 18,* 1-9 (1973).
54. D. M. Gill and C. A. King. Mechanism of action of cholera toxin in pigeon erythrocyte lysates. *J. Biol. Chem. 20,* 6424-6432 (1975).
55. G. W. G. Sharp and S. Hynie. Stimulation of intestinal adenyl cyclase by *Escherichia coli* enterotoxin: Comparison of strains from an infant and an adult with diarrhea. *Nature 229,* 266-269 (1971).
56. L. D. Chen, J. D. Rhode, and G. W. G. Sharp. The effect of calcium and other salts upon the release of glucagon-like immunoreactivity from the gut. *J. Clin. Invest. 51,* 731-740 (1972).
57. G. W. G. Sharp, S. Hynie, H. Ebel, D. G. Parkinson, and P. A. Witkum. Properties of adenylate cyclase in mucosal cells of the rabbit ileum and the effect of cholera toxin. *Biochim. Biophys. Acta 309,* 339-348 (1973).
58. D. V. Kimberg, M. Field, J. Johnson, A. Henderson, and I. Gershaw. Stimulation of intestinal mucosal adenyl cyclase by cholera enterotoxin and prostaglandins. *J. Clin. Invest. 50,* 1218-1230 (1971).
59. N. F. Pierce, W. G. Greenough, and C. C. J. Carpenter. Vibrio Cholera enterotoxin and its mode of action. *Bacteriol. Rev. 35,* 1-13 (1971).
60. R. J. Gand, F. M. Torti, and S. Jaksina. Development of intestinal adenyl cyclase and its response to cholera enterotoxin. *J. Clin. Invest. 52,* 2053-2059 (1973).
61. D. E. Schafer, W. D. Lust, B. Sircar, and N. D. Goldberg. Elevated concentration of adenosine 3′:5′-cyclic monophosphate in intestinal mucosa after treatment with cholera toxin. *Proc. Natl. Acad. Sci. USA 67,* 851-856 (1970).
62. M. Field. Intestinal secretion: Effect of cyclic AMP and its role in cholera. *N. Engl. J. Med. 284,* 1137-1144 (1971).
63. M. Field, D. Fromm, and Q. Al-Awquati. Effect of cholera enterotoxin on ion transport across isolated ileal mucosa. *J. Clin. Invest. 51,* 796-804 (1972).
64. S. A. Rudolph, D. E. Schafer, and P. Greengard. Effects of cholera enterotoxin on catecholamine-stimulated changes in cation fluxes, cell volume, and cyclic AMP levels in the turkey erythrocyte. *J. Biol. Chem. 252,* 7132-7139 (1977).
65. J. G. Banwell, N. F. Pierce, R. C. Mitra, K. L. Brigham, G. J. Caranasos, R. I. Keimowitz, D. S. Fedson, J. Thomac, S. L. Gorbach, R. B. Sack, and A. Mondal. Intestinal fluid and electrolyte transport in human cholera. *J. Clin. Invest. 49,* 183-195 (1970).
66. G. W. G. Sharp. Action of cholera toxin on fluid and electrolyte movement in the small intestine. *Annu. Rev. Med. 24,* 19-28 (1973).
67. J. W. Jacobs, H. D. Niall, and G. W. G. Sharp. The amino terminal sequence of cholera toxin subunits. *Biochem. Biophys. Res. Commun. 61,* 391-395 (1974).

68. J. J. LoSpalluto and R. A. Finkelstein. Chemical and physical properties of cholera exo-enterotoxin (choleragen) and its spontaneously formed toxin (choleragenoid). *Biochim. Biophys. Acta 257,* 158-166 (1972).
69. J. Holmgren and I. Lonnrotti. Oligomeric structure of cholera toxin characteristics of the H and L subunits. *J. Gen. Microbiol. 86,* 49-65 (1975).
70. V. Bennett, X. O'Keefe, and P. Cuatrecasas. Mechanism of action of cholera toxin and the mobile receptor theory of hormone receptor-adenylate cyclase interactions. *Proc. Natl. Acad. Sci. USA 72,* 33-37 (1975).
71. P. Cuatrecasas. Interaction of vibrio Cholera enterotoxin with cell membrane. *Biochemistry 12,* 3547-3558 (1973).
72. P. Cuatrecasas. Gangliosides and membrane receptors for cholera toxin. *Biochemistry 12,* 3558-3566 (1973).
73. J. Holmgren, I. Lonnroth, and L. Svennerholm. Tissue receptor for cholera endotoxin: postulated structure from studies with G_{ml} ganglioside and related glycolipids. *Infect. Immun. 8,* 208-214 (1973).
74. C. A. King and W. E. Van Heyningen. Evidence for the complex nature of the ganglioside receptor for cholera toxin. *J. Infect. Dis. 131,* 643-648 (1975).
75. S. Van Heyningen. Cholera toxin: Interaction subunits with ganglioside G_{ml}. *Science (Wash. D.C.) 138,* 656-657 (1974).
76. J. Flores and G. W. G. Sharp. Effects of cholera toxin on adenylate cyclase. Studies with guanylylimidodiphosphate. *J. Clin. Invest. 56,* 1345-1349 (1975).
77. J. Flores and G. W. G. Sharp. *The Activation of Adenylate Cyclase by Cholera Toxin: Possible Interaction with Nucleotide Regulatory Site.* (K. Elliott and J. Knight, Eds.). *CIBA Foundation Symposium* (new series). Elsevier North-Holland, Amsterdam, 1976, pp. 89-108.
78. D. M. Gill and C. A. King. Properties of adenyl cyclase human jejunal mucosa during naturally acquired cholera and convalescence. *J. Biol. Chem. 250,* 6424-6432 (1975).
79. H. L. Dupont, S. B. Formal, R. B. Hornick, M. J. Snyder, J. P. Libonati, D. G. Sheaham, E. H. LaBree, and J. P. Kalas. Pathogenesis of *Escherichia coli* diarrhea. *N. Engl. J. Med. 285,* 1-9 (1971).
80. R. C. Sack. Enterotoxigenic *Escherichia coli* isolated from patients with severe cholera-like disease. *J. Infect. Dis. 123,* 378-385 (1971).
81. D. J. Evans, K. S. Chen, and G. T. Curling. Technology message springs few surprises. *Nature New Biol. 236,* 137-138 (1972).
82. S. Etking and S. L. Gorgach. Studies on enterotoxin from *Escherichia coli* associated with acute diarrhea in man. *J. Lab. Clin. Med. 78,* 81 (1971).
83. G. D. Dean, Y. C. Ching, R. G. Williams, and L. B. Harden. Test for *Escherichia coli* enterotoxin using infant mice application in a study of diarrhea in children in Honolulu. *J. Infect. Dis. 125,* 407-411 (1972).
84. J. S. Kantor, P. Tao, and C. Wisdom. Action of *Escherichia coli*

enterotoxin adenylate cyclase behavior of intestinal epithelial cells in culture. *Infect. Immun. 9,* 1003-1010 (1974).

85. H. S. Kantor, P. Tao, and S. L. Gorbach. Stimulation of intestinal adenyl cyclase by *Escherichia coli* enterotoxin: Comparison of strains from an infant and an adult with diarrhea. *J. Infect. Dis. 129*, 1-9 (1974).
86. D. G. Evans, D. J. Evans, and N. F. Pierce. Differences in the response of rabbit small intestine to heat-labile and heat-stable enterotoxins of *Escherichia coli. Infect. Immun. 7,* 873-880 (1973).
87. S. L. Gorbach and C. M. Khurana. Toxigenic *Escherichia coli.* A cause of infantile diarrhea in Chicago. *N. Engl. J. Med. 287,* 791-795 (1972).
88. S. L. Gorbach, B. H. Kean, D. G. Evans, D. J. Evans, and D. Bessudo. Traveler's diarrhea and toxigenic *Escherichia coli. N. Engl. J. Med. 292,* 933-936 (1975).
89. R. L. Guerrant, U. Ganguly, G. T. Casper, E. J. Moore, N. F. Pierce, and C. C. G. Carpenter. Effect of *Escherichia coli* on fluid transport across canine small bowel. Mechanism and time-course with enterotoxin and whole bacterial cells. *J. Clin. Invest. 52,* 1707-1714 (1973).
90. H. W. Moon, S. C. Whipp, and A. L. Baetz. Comparative effects of enterotoxins *Escherichia coli* and *Vibrio cholerae* on rabbit and swine small intestine. *Lab. Invest. 25,* 133-140 (1971).
91. J. G. Banwell and H. Sherr. Effect of bacterial enterotoxins of the gastrointestinal tract. *Gastroenterology 65,* 467-497 (1971).
92. H. R. DeJonge. The response of small intestinal villous and crypt epithelium to choleratoxin in rat and guinea pig. Evidence against a specific role of the crypt cells in choleragen-induced secretion. *Biochim. Biophys. Acta 381,* 128-143 (1975).
93. J. S. Fordtran, F. C. Rector, T. W. Locklear, and M. F. Ewton. Water and solute movement in the small intestine of patients with sprue. *J. Clin. Invest. 46,* 287-298 (1967).
94. G. K. Donovan and R. Torres-Pinedo. Effect of D-galactose on the fluid loss in soybean protein (SBP) intolerance. *Pediatr. Res. (Program Issue) 12,* (1978).

20
Viral Gastroenteritis

D. GRANT GALL / The University of Calgary, Calgary, Alberta, Canada

I. Introduction

Gastroenteritis remains one of the most common disorders of childhood. It is estimated that 18 million infants and children die each year from acute infectious enteritis. The majority of these deaths occur in underdeveloped areas, but even in temperate climates infectious diarrhea remains a serious problem in terms of morbidity and mortality [1].

The etiology of acute gastroenteritis has been the subject of extensive research for many years. Bacterial agents, even with the recognition of newer pathogens such as *Yersinia* and *Campylobacter,* account for only 10-20% of cases of acute infectious diarrhea in temperate climates. Improved techniques for the identification of viral pathogens has led to the recognition that the majority of cases of acute nonspecific gastroenteritis are caused by viral agents. However, earlier work in the late 1940s had already provided strong evidence for a viral etiology of infectious diarrhea. Light and Hodes, studying nursery epidemics, were able to consistently induce diarrhea in newborn calves by feeding bacteria-free filtrates of feces from sick infants. Dr. Hodes fortunately saved samples from these studies, and they were recently shown to contain particles resembling human rotavirus [1]. Studies to identify viral agents over the next two decades drew a virtual blank. These studies of fecal viral flora in gastroenteritis by means of tissue culture techniques showed the same frequency of viral isolation in controls as in patients. Then in the early 1970s the Norwalk agent [2] was described. This agent was obtained from an outbreak of gastroenteritis in an elementary school in Norwalk, Ohio, and was proved to be a pathogen by transmission studies in human volunteers.

II. Rotavirus

The long-overdue application of electron microscopic techniques to the examination of stool specimens led to the identification of a specific virus responsible for a significant proportion of diarrhea in young children. The virus was first demonstrated by Bishop and her co-workers in duodenal biopsy specimens from young children, by means of electron microscopy [3]. Shortly thereafter, in Melbourne, Birmingham, Washington, and Toronto, the same viral particles were identified in feces from children with acute diarrhea [4]. Identification depends on electron microscopy of stools, since the virus has not been successfully maintained in tissue culture. It is a double strand of RNA virus with a capsid diameter of 64-70 nm. The human virus is morphologically identical and antigenically similar to viral agents causing diarrhea in the young of many mammalian species: for example, calves, piglets, foals, and infant mice, rabbits, monkeys, and sheep. There is still controversy over the naming of this virus, but the agent described by many centers throughout the world is identical. The virus has been variously named orbivirus, duovirus, rotavirus, reovirus-like agent, and infantile gastroenteritis virus by different workers. At present, the name favored is rotavirus.

Proof that rotavirus is a true pathogen comes from a number of observations [5]. In acute cases, virus is found in stools in massive quantities, but not in convalescent patients. It is rarely seen in stools of asymptomatic controls; the only exception is the frequent recovery of virus in stools from asymptomatic newborns. The virus is found in the duodenal mucosa and intestinal juice of children with acute enteritis, and there is a significant rise of antibody titer in convalescent sera. Finally, an adult volunteer has been infected.

A. Epidemiology

The virus has been recognized in all parts of the world and in all races. In temperate climates it is responsible for 40-50% of yearly hospital cases of acute enteritis, with the incidence rising as high as 80% in the cooler months [6]. Regardless of location, the peak incidence occurs in the colder months of the year: December to April in Toronto, May to August in Melbourne. It is highly contagious and spreads with ease from patient to patient in institutions and households. Approximately 10-15% of cases of viral enteritis identified in our institution are of nosocomial origin. Infection occurs primarily in young infants between 6 months and 3 years of age and rarely causes significant illness in children over 6 years old. Kapikian and co-workers [6] have demonstrated that by 36 months of age 90% of the population has complement fixation antibodies to rotavirus. This pattern of rapid acquisition of antibody is comparable to that seen with respiratory syncytial and parainfluenza viruses.

B. Pathology

Rotavirus invades the mucosal epithelium of the small bowel with localization in the cytoplasm of mature villus cells. Infection may cause little structural change; however in the majority of patients there is mucosal damage ranging from spotty subtotal atrophy of surface epithelium to severe flattening of villi and derangement of surface epithelium. Mucosal disaccharidase activities are usually depressed [7, 8].

C. Clinical Features

The incubation period is brief: 24-48 hr. Vomiting and fever occur early, even before diarrhea in many cases, and subside in a day or two, while the diarrhea usually persists for 3-5 days. The diarrhea is relieved by fasting, aggravated by feeding. Rotavirus enteritis is usually a self-limited disease, but it can kill and kill quickly. In our metropolitan area all coroner's cases involving children are autopsied at The Hospital for Sick Children, and each year we identify five fatal cases from this infection. Many patients die quickly, even before receiving medical attention in some cases [7, 8].

In a study of 27 patients with rotavirus infection we found that diarrhea was associated with vomiting in all cases and with fever in most. Vomiting was always short-lived, but preceded the onset of diarrhea in half the patients. Many had an associated respiratory infection, which is unexplained, since there is no evidence that rotavirus replicates in respiratory epithelium. Physical signs of dehydration were present in less than half the patients at the time of diagnosis. Laboratory studies demonstrated mild compensated metabolic acidosis with decreased plasma bicarbonate levels in most of the patients. Serum sodium concentrations were normal in most, byt hypo- or hypernatremia did occur. Potassium levels were decreased and chloride levels increased in many patients. Stool losses were significantly increased in the acute phase as compared to the convalescent period, and the increase in fecal losses was associated with significantly increased concentrations of stool Na^+ and Cl^-. These concentrations, however, were considerably less than those seen in enterotoxigenic diarrhea. There was no evidence of escess loss of sugar or fat. In the household of index cases there was evidence of gastrointestinal upset, virus shedding, and serological conversion, in both children and adults. Of the 57 household contacts, 12 individuals (8 adults and 4 children) suffered a diarrheal illness within 1 week of the index case, and in 6 cases rotavirus was identified in stool specimens. A rise in serum antibody titer occurred in 12 adults, and 7 children demonstrated seroconversion. This finding and other data indicate that reinfection can occur with rotavirus and suggest that there may be a number of serotypes.

III. Other Viruses

The examination by electron microscopy of stools from patients with acute diarrhea has led to "sightings" of a number of particles and probable viruses which are associated with diarrhea in children [9]. However, the relationship between these particles and disease is not clear, and their frequency is also unknown. Like rotavirus, these agents have not been successfully isolated in tissue culture. The inability to grow viral enteric pathogens in vitro continues to be the main obstacle in studying and identifying etiologic agents of acute viral gastroenteritis.

The role of adenovirus in acute diarrhea remains controversial. Earlier studies using isolation techniques demonstrated similar numbers of isolates from controls as from patients. But by electron microscopy adenovirus can be found in feces in the acute stage of diarrhea in enormous numbers, and these disappear during convalescence. Moreover, adenovirus can be seen by electron microscopy in duodenal juice during the acute phase. Despite the finding of viral particles–in enormous numbers–in feces, isolation by tissue culture is usually unsuccessful. Additional evidence that adenoviruses are true pathogens comes from hospital outbreaks in which the virus breeds true; the same viral particles are seen in secondary and tertiary cases. The evidence to date, while not conclusive, strongly supports a role for adenovirus in acute childhood diarrhea.

Picorna parvoviruses are small (22-28 nm) particles which are associated with the Norwalk agent. These agents are true pathogens. Morphologically similar particles have been observed in epidemics of diarrhea in Hawaii and Montgomery County, Maryland. In cross-challenge studies in human volunteers, Kapikian and co-workers have demonstrated that the Norwalk and Hawaii agents are distinct, but that the Norwalk and Montgomery agents are related. These studies suggest that, as seen with rotavirus, there are several serotypes in this family of viruses.

Other "candidate" viral particles thought to be associated with acute gastroenteritis include minireo- and calicivirus; and while not yet conclusive, the evidence to date strongly suggests that these agents are also true pathogens. For example, they are found in feces from children with diarrhea in the acute stage but not during convalescence, and they breed true in single-room hospital epidemics. In a recent 12-month survey by Dr. Middleton and co-workers using direct electron microscopy of stools from patients with acute diarrhea, rotavirus, as expected, was the most commonly identified etiologic agent. Minireovirus was the next most common agent, with a frequency slightly greater than that for adenovirus and picorna parvovirus. Particles resembling calicivirus were seen infrequently, while particles resembling coronavirus were not identified.

IV. Pathophysiology

The ability to identify viral agents responsible for diarrhea has provided important clinical and epidemiologic data but has not answered the question as to how a virus actually causes diarrhea. In an attempt to identify the mechanisms by which viral agents cause diarrhea, we have been studying an animal model of viral enteritis in piglets–transmissible gastroenteritis (TGE) [10]. The causative agent in TGE is a coronavirus which differs structurally from human rotavirus, but the disease in piglets is remarkably similar to that seen in human infants. The TGE virus, like human rotavirus, invades small-bowel epithelium only, is mainly a disease of the young, and has a short incubation period. Transmissible gastroenteritis has proved to be a consistently reproducible model, with the onset of diarrhea occurring 16-24 hr after infection, accompanied by fever and vomiting. As with the human disease, fever and vomiting subside quickly while the diarrhea persists–peaking at 40 hr and then settling over the next 2-3 days. Early studies in TGE demonstrated that stool volumes were massive, with increased concentration of electrolytes. There was no evidence of steatorrhea or excess sugar loss, despite the finding of decreased disaccharidase activities in intestinal mucosa. Marker perfusion studies demonstrated Na^+, K^+, Cl^-, and water secretion in the upper gut.

To define the interaction of virus with the intestinal epithelium and to identify the timing of the infection, we examined intestinal tissue by immunofluorescence for viral antigen at intervals after infection. In serial studies we found that fluorescence for viral particles occurred only in the small bowel and was maximal within 6-12 hr after oral challenge. Viral antigen was virtually absent by 24 hr when diarrhea was just beginning, and this absence persisted at 40, 72, and 144 hr after infection. The data suggest that diarrhea is occurring at a time when the virus is no longer present in the intestinal epithelium.

To more specifically define the transport abnormalities and to correlate the timing of these abnormalities with epithelial infection, we looked at Na^+ transport in stripped intestinal tissue in Ussing chambers under short-circuited conditions. Tissue was obtained at intervals following infection. The Na^+ flux under basal conditions, that is, in the absence of glucose, was not significantly altered and was secretory in tissue from both control and infected animals. In the intestine the presence of glucose normally stimulates active Na^+ absorption. In tissue from infected animals the response of Na^+ transport to glucose was blunted, and this effect became significant 40 and 72 hr after infection.

We also monitored the relative maturity of the epithelium at the same intervals by measuring the activity of marker enzymes in cells isolated exclusively from villus tips. We looked at the activities of thymidine kinase, an enzyme involved in DNA replication and normally confined to crypts, and of sucrase, an enzyme normally found in the brush border of mature cells on villi. As expected, in control tissue thymidine kinase activity was low and sucrase activity high. After infection, thymidine kinase activity increased, reaching significant levels at 25 and 40 hr post infection. Sucrase activity showed the opposite effect of the thymidine kinase data; levels decreased after infection, reaching significantly depressed levels at 40 hr and then gradually recovering. The data indicate that at the time of diarrhea the mucosa is composed of enterocytes with crypt cell characteristics. When the timing of changes in Na^+ transport and thymidine kinase levels is compared with the presence of epithelial infection and the occurrence of severe diarrhea, it becomes apparent that diarrhea occurs during that period when villus enterocytes show enzymatic characteristics of immaturity, and when abnormalities of transport are most prominent, and not when the virus is present in the epithelium.

Recently, we have successfully infected 14-16-day-old piglets with human rotavirus produces abnormalities of function similar to those seen with TGE virus. Watery diarrhea occurs 60-72 hr after infection, at a time when few or no viral particles are seen in the epithelium by immunofluorescence and when light microscopy demonstrates decreased villus height and increased crypt depth in the upper small bowel. When diarrhea is present, as seen in TGE, glucose-stimulated Na^+ transport is blunted in tissue from rotavirus-infected animals, and villus enterocytes in the upper small bowel show enzymatic characteristics of cryptlike cells with increased thymidine kinase activity and decreased sucrase activity.

V. Final Considerations

In summary, we are suggesting that the virus invades mature epithelial cells on villi and that these infected cells are shed, resulting in an increased turnover rate with accelerated migration of cells from the crypt onto villi. These cells fail to mature in time and result in functionally immature cells clothing villi. It is these uninfected but immature cells that are responsible for the diarrhea.

While there still remains much to be learned, research to date has provided some practical information. Our knowledge of the pathophysiology suggests that treatment will remain supportive. The short incubation period and the nature of the infection, with symptoms occurring only after the virus has already invaded and initiated the pathophysiologic state, make it unlikely that a specific mode of therapy will be found. Development of a vaccine, especially with the identification of human rotavirus, now appears feasible. Unfortunately, preventive therapy remains a distant possibility because of our inability to successfully maintain these viral agents in tissue culture.

References

1. F. Lifshitz. Etiology, pathology and treatment of acute gastroenteritis. In *Proc. 73rd Ross Conference on Pediatric Research, Ponte Vedra Beach, Florida, March 20-22, 1977.* Ross Labs, Columbus, Ohio.
2. A. Z. Kapikian. Identificational serology of rotavirus, Norwalk and Norwalk-like agent. In *Proc. 73rd Ross Conference on Pediatric Research, Ponte Vedra Beach, Florida, March 20-22, 1977.* Ross Labs, Columbus, Ohio.
3. R. F. Bishop, G. P. Davidson, I. H. Holmes, and B. J. Ruck. Detection of a new virus by electron microscopy of fecal extract from children with acute gastroenteritis, *Lancet 1,* 149-151 (1974).
4. Rotavirus of man and animals. (Editorial). *Lancet 1,* 257-259 (1975).
5. J. R. Hamilton, D. G. Gall, B. Kerzner, D. G. Butler, and P. J. Middleton. Recent developments in viral gastroenteritis. *Pediatr. Clin. North Am. 22,* 747-755 (1975).
6. A. Z. Kapikian, H. W. Kim, R. G. Wyatt, W. L. Cline, J. O. Arrobio, C. O. Brandt, W. J. Rodriguez, D. A. Sack, R. M. Chanock, and R. H. Parrott. Human reovirus-like agent as the major pathogen associated with winter gastroenteritis in hospitalized infants and young children. *N. Engl. J. Med. 294,* 965-972 (1976).
7. J. R. Hamilton, D. G. Gall, D. G. Butler, and P. J. Middleton. Viral gastroenteritis: Recent progress, remaining problems. *CIBA Foundation Symposium 42 (New Series). Acute Diarrhea in Childhood.* Elsevier North-Holland, Amsterdam, 1976, pp. 209-222.
8. S. Tallet, C. MacKenzie, P. J. Middleton, B. Kerzner, and J. R. Hamilton. Clinical, laboratory and epidemiologic features of a viral gastroenteritis in infants and children. *Pediatrics 60,* 217-222 (1977).
9. P. J. Middleton, M. T. Szymanski, and M. Petric. Viruses associated with acute gastroenteritis in young children. *Am. J. Dis. Child. 131,* 733-737 (1977).
10. G. P. Davidson, D. G. Gall, M. Petric, D. G. Butler, and J. R. Hamilton. Human rotavirus enteritis induced in conventional piglets. *J. Clin. Invest. 60,* 1402-1409 (1977).

21 Bacterial Diarrhea: Pathogenesis and Principles for Control and Chemotherapy

GERALD T. KEUSCH / Mount Sinai School of Medicine, New York, New York

I. Introduction

The past two decades have produced a renaissance in the study of the bacterial diarrheas [1]. Not only have new pathophysiologic mechanisms been revealed, with some understanding of the biochemical pathways involved, but also new pathogens have been discovered and old pathogens have been redefined. This explosive increase in knowledge makes it possible at last to view current therapy in a rational way and to project into the future the probable nature of therapy to come [2].

II. Pathogenesis

Two principal virulence mechanisms have been defined [1]. These are: first, the production by certain microorganisms of protein toxins which cause active salt and water secretion by the small intestine; and, second, the ability of other pathogens to invade intestinal epithelial cells and to multiply within them and within the lamina propria–resulting in an acute inflammatory enteritis. This basic classification fits very well with observations on the infectious dose for human adults of several bacterial species [3-6], as determined experimentally by Hornick, DuPont, Levine, Snyder, and colleagues. When the infectious doses are graphed on a linear scale (Fig. 1.), the organisms can be divided into two groups. One, including *Vibrio cholerae* and *Escherichia coli,* requires large

Present Affiliation:
Tufts University School of Medicine, and New England Medical Center Hospital, Boston, Massachusetts

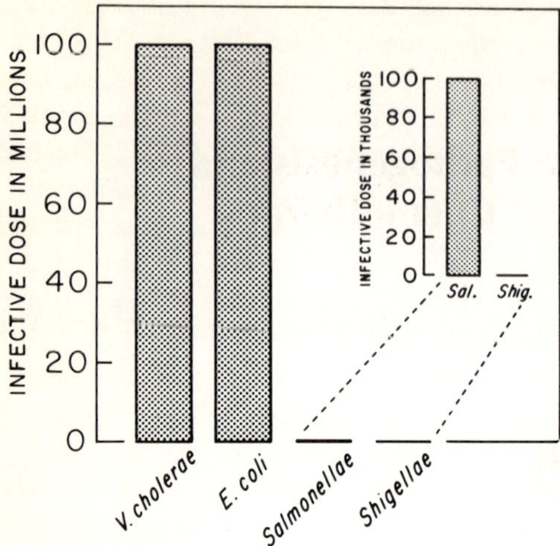

Figure 1 Oral infective dose of enteric pathogens.

numbers of bacteria to cause disease (in excess of 100 million organisms). The other, including species of *Salmonella* and *Shigella* requires so few bacteria relative to the first group that the inoculum does not even show on the vertical scale of the graph. When this scale is expanded (Fig. 1., inset), it can be seen that about 100 thousand salmonellae suffice, while for virulent shigellae, such as the strain of the 1969 epidemic of Mexico and Central America where as few as 10-100 organisms will cause clinical disease. As it turns out, group 1, the high-inoculum species, are noninvasive and cause disease primarily through the production of an enterotoxin mediator. Large numbers of organisms are in some way necessary to establish intestinal colonization, so that toxin can be locally elaborated in the small bowel. Group 2, the relatively low-inoculum pathogens, are the invasive organisms. By this means they are more efficiently able to overcome host defenses and find a suitable ecosystem in which to multiply. At the same time they cause the bowel inflammation which characterizes the pathology of the disease.

A. Enterotoxins

The enterotoxins of noninvasive enteric pathogens are the actual virulence factors which induce diarrhea. However, these toxins are metabolic products of bacterial growth, and therefore gut colonization is a necessary prerequisite. Because the gastrointestinal tract resists the establishment of residence by new strains, and because the proximal small bowel, the site of isotonic fluid secretion in both cholera and *E. coli* diarrhea, is normally free of significant numbers of bacteria (less than 10^3/cc succus entericus), pathogens would be aided by virulence attributes which serve to overcome normal host defenses. That this is indeed the case was first clearly shown by veterinary scientists studying fatal *E. coli* diarrhea in newborn piglets—a disease known as colibacillosis. In this illness, it was observed that pathogenic *E. coli* colonized the proximal small intestine of the affected pigs, reaching very high densities, whereas avirulent strains failed to take hold and thence to multiply [7]. When these strains were examined in greater detail, it was found that the virulent strains possessed a distinctive surface antigen, K-88, known to mediate agglutination of erythrocytes [8], whereas the avirulent strains were K-88-negative. These observations suggested that K-88 might be an adherence factor for virulent *E. coli* in pigs [9]. The discovery that the genetic information for production of K-88, as for enterotoxin in these same strains, was present in plasmids (nonchromosomal segments of DNA transferable from one bacterium to another during conjugation) allowed direct testing of the hypothesis. Beginning with a toxin-negative/K-88-negative avirulent strain, Williams-Smith and Linngood [10] inserted the plasmids for toxin and K-88 individually and together. The presence of K-88 allowed intestinal colonization by organisms and multiplication in proximal bowel to high numbers, but did not result in illness. A strain containing enterotoxin alone, without K-88, neither colonized nor exhibited virulence, although the toxin itself produced in vitro from the same organism could cause diarrhea if placed directly in the small bowel. But the combination of the two factors in the same organism resulted in a colonizing and virulent disease-inducing strain. More recent studies have demonstrated analogous colonizing factors in *E. coli* pathogenic for other animals [11] and for humans [12]. Many, but not all, strains of *E. coli* virulent in the human possess the same antigenic colonization factor, called Cf by Evans et al. [13].

B. Adherence

The ability of bacteria to adhere to surfaces appears to be a property common to many microorganisms [9]. Because adhesion is probably the initial stage in the colonization of many diverse habitats, this mechanism is of undoubted ecological significance, and certainly this is obvious for the pathogenic *E. coli* discussed above. The chemical basis for the adherence phenomenon and for the specificity of the interaction between bacterium and intestinal brush border is not known. However, it has been proposed [2] that an appropriate conceptual model is the interaction between mammalian cells and lectins, plant proteins which are capable of "recognizing" certain cell surface sugars with remarkable specificity. Many lectins possess multiple binding sites and thus can cause agglutination of cells with the proper surface characteristics to permit binding; while some lectins induce remarkable physiologic changes in cells bearing the appropriate receptor, such as phytohemagglutinin or *Concanavalin A*-induced mitogenic responses in human T-lymphocytes. The binding of *E. coli* to immature intestinal cells from weanling rat gut or to human fetal intestinal cells in culture is sugar inhibitable by monosaccharides—a finding consistent with the lectin model [14, 15].

C. Receptor

In no instance is the cell surface receptor well characterized. A complex heterosaccharide layer, called the glycocalyx, coats the intestinal epithelial cell brush border. There is sufficient variation in sugar composition, chain length, degree of branching, and linkage within the carbohydrates of the glycocalyx to account for receptor activity for a number of distinct substances. For K-88 antigen, receptor activity has been shown to be present in a still-undefined carbohydrate-rich fraction of the brush border [9]. The gut of certain pigs appears to lack receptor activity, and these animals are not affected by K-88-positive, toxin-producing organisms [16]. Such animals may be selected out by judicious breeding experiments. Consistent with the model, the brush borders from "receptorless" pigs do not have the analogous carbohydrate containing K-88-binding membrane component. Receptors for other enteric pathogens are even less well defined, but Thaler et al. [14], Bergman et al. [15], and Jones and Freter [17] have respectively described D-mannose, neuraminic acid, and L-fucose: inhibitable receptors on intestinal cells, for *E. coli* in the first two instances, and for *V. cholerae* in the third.

D. Sequence of Events

The sequence of events in pathogenesis thus would be, first, ingestion of a sufficient inoculum of the causative organism to ensure survival through the stomach and into the proximal small bowel. Then a specific adherence phenomenon would facilitate colonization, overcoming the usual and efficient clearance mechanisms of duodenum and jejunum [1]. Subsequent multiplication to high numbers would be accompanied by enterotoxin synthesis, which initiates the actual process of fluid secretion. Not surprisingly, toxins, like the producing microorganisms, interact with the cell surface membranes in specific receptor-ligand relationships. Cholera and *E. coli* toxins appear to bind to G_{M1} ganglioside in the membrane [18]. Several lines of evidence support this. Free or insoluble G_{M1} ganglioside acts as a potent competitive inhibitor of binding of cholera toxin [19]. Increasing the membrane content of G_{M1} ganglioside results in increased binding and in increased sensitivity to biological effects of the toxins [20, 21]. Indeed, the number of binding sites for cholera toxin correlates directly with the content of G_{M1} ganglioside in the membrane [20]. Shigella enterotoxin binds to a distinct and different receptor, demonstrated to be present on HeLa and normal rat liver cell membranes [22]. This receptor appears to contain oligomeric $\beta 1 \rightarrow 4$ linked *N*-acetylglucosamine (GlcNAc), based on the ability to competitively inhibit toxin binding with trimeric or tetrameric GlcNAc, destruction of the receptor by lysozyme which uses GlcNAc oligosaccharides as a substrate, and receptor blockade by the GlcNAc-specific lectin, wheat germ agglutinin [22].

E. Types of Toxins

Enterotoxins are actually defined by their capacity to induce secretion of isotonic fluid into the lumen of the bowel [1]. When the rate of secretion exceeds the capacity of the rest of the gut to reabsorb the water, diarrhea results. A number of types of toxins have been described, but this discussion will be limited to just three types: the antigenically similar heat-labile toxins (LT) of *V. cholerae* and *E. coli,* the heat-stable toxin (ST) of *E. coli,* and the cytotoxic enterotoxin of *Shigella dysenteriae* 1 (SdT). Selected properties of these molecules are compared in Table 1. Both LT and SdT are relatively large, capable of inducing neutralizing antibodies, whereas ST is small and apparently nonantigenic. The LT clearly acts through its capacity to stimulate adenylate cyclase, causing an increase in the intracellular content of cyclic AMP, the signal for intestinal cells to secrete [18, 23]. Some evidence suggests that SdT may act on proximal intestine by the same basic mechanism [24]; however the data are not nearly as conclusive as for LT. Recently, studies have demonstrated that ST activates guanylate cyclase, resulting in increased cyclic GMP levels within the cell—which also seems to turn on a secretory response in rabbit intestine [25]. How these cyclic nucleotides accomplish this, however, is not yet known.

F. Shigella

Shigellae, which, as already noted, produce an enterotoxin, are among the low-inoculum invasive pathogens. New data suggest that these two properties may be important in disease pathogenesis, but at distinct sites in the gastrointestinal tract: namely, the proximal small and large bowel respectively. The information, summarized in Ref. 2, indicates that clinical shigellosis is a combination of a noninvasive, possibly enterotoxin-induced proximal secretory diarrhea and an inflammatory invasive bacterial colitis which results in the dysentery syndrome. The latter is, of course, the classic hallmark of shigellosis, an infection traditionally known as bacillary dysentery. However, it has long been known, yet conveniently overlooked, that watery diarrhea is the first, if not the only, manifestation of shigella infection. Nevertheless, while invasion cannot explain the whole of shigellosis [2], noninvasive toxigenic variants of fully virulent strains cannot produce even a secretory diarrhea [26]; such strains are, in fact,

Table 1 Comparison of Properties of Three Classes of Enterotoxins

Property	LT[a]	ST[b]	SdT[c]
Heat lability	Yes	No	Intermediate
Receptor	G_{M1} Ganglioside	?	Oligomeric *N*-acetyl-D-glucosamine
Antigenicity	Yes	No	Yes
Molecular weight	84000	<10,000	~86,000
Mechanism	↑ Adenylate cyclase	↑ Guanylate cyclase	?↑ Adenylate cyclase ? ↓ Protein synthesis

[a]Heat-labile toxin of *Vibrio cholerae* and *Escherichia coli.*
[b]Heat-stable toxin of *E. coli.*
[c]Cytoenterotoxin of *Shigella dysenteriae* 1.

avirulent in the intact animal. This observation is still unexplained. However it is possible, if not probable, that the nonmotile shigella organism must have some mechanism enabling it to first stick to the colonic mucosa which it ultimately will invade. Otherwise it is difficult to see how the introduction of as few as 100-1000 microorganisms into a gut already colonized by more than 100 billion bacteria per gram of colonic contents could lead to a sufficient number of random contacts to permit invasion and development of clinical disease. A simple speculative extension of this hypothesis would be to suggest that the same adherence mechanism acts in the proximal bowel, where, for some reason inherent to the tissue, invasion fails to take place thereafter. Thus a strain which loses invasive properties, such as the opaque colonial mutants described by Formal and colleagues [26], would simultaneously lose adherence properties and be unable to colonize the proximal gut. The speculative nature of this discussion is, of course, due to the dearth of real information about these properties. While the specifics of the process of invasion remain a secret known to the bacterium alone, several surface features of the organisms are clearly relevant, including colonial morphology, the nature of the lipopolysaccharide, and the chemical composition of the O-repeat unit [27].

G. Salmonella

Nontyphoid salmonellae are another clear example of invasive pathogens. In fact, and in contrast to the shigellae (perhaps because most are sensitive to the complement-dependent serum bactericidal reaction), salmonellae are so adept at invasion that they frequently produce bacteremia early in the course of infection [1]. In most instances, bacteremia during salmonella gastroenteritis is asymptomatic, and it clears spontaneously. Experimental studies in animals have firmly demonstrated that virulent salmonellae must invade and multiply in the gastrointestinal mucosa [28]. This process occurs predominantly in the ileum. However, not all invasive strains cause experimental diarrhea; disease-producing strains must also provoke an inflammatory response in the gut. Moreover, some data suggest that, additionally, a toxin may be involved as the final mechanism [29]. Thus an invasive, inflammation-provoking strain may not necessarily cause fluid secretion [28]. Whatever the specific stimulus involved, the elevation of intracellular cyclic AMP levels appears to mediate it [28].

H. E. coli

Certain *E. coli* of distinct O-antigen serogroups (including 028ac, 0112, 0124, 0136, 0143, 0144, 0152, 0164) are invasive—much like the shigellae [30], to which many of these *E. coli* strains are antigenically related [27]. They do not produce either ST or LT, nor are they known to produce an SdT-like toxin [31].

To complicate matters even more, Cantey and associates have studied a rabbit-virulent *E. coli* (RDEC-1) which is adherent but noninvasive, does not produce ST or LT, causes damage to the underlying intestinal epithelial cells, and elaborates very small amounts of SdT-like material, active as a HeLa cytotoxin which is neutralized by antibody to the *S. dysenteriae* 1 product [32].

III. Clinical-Anatomic-Pathophysiologic Correlates

Within the limits of our current knowledge, summarized above, it appears that watery diarrhea due to bacterial agents is a small-bowel disease, involving an active secretory process, probably mediated by a cyclic nucleotide (either cAMP or cGMP). Activation of the appropriate cyclase enzyme by pathogens acting on the proximal small bowel is through a toxin, whereas those involving the distal small bowel are at least invasive, if not toxigenic as well. The resulting clinical syndrome is a watery diarrhea of mild to severe degree, producing—at the extreme—marked dehydration, acidosis, and death. The latter type of syndrome is exemplified by cholera, whereas the other agents tend to produce a mild to moderate disease. Toxigenic *E. coli* appear to be one of the principal causes of travelers' diarrhea, as well as of a considerable number of cases of infantile diarrhea in both highly sanitized industrialized nations and developing countries, with little or no effective control of water and waste disposal [34].

Invasive pathogens of the large bowel cause an inflammatory lesion which, if extensive enough, results in the dysentery syndrome. Rather than a dehydrating watery diarrhea, dysentery is a painful, frequent evacuation of scant quantities of stool, largely composed of blood and mucus. The triad of mucosanguineous ejecta, cramps, and tenesmus defines the latter clinical picture. Endoscopy reveals the inflamed colonic mucosa, with punctate or extensive hemorrhages and ulcerations present when symptoms are marked.

IV. Therapeutic Implications

With the very real advances in understanding of the pathogenesis of bacterial diarrheas detailed in this chapter, we can speculate on a number of possible intervention points to control these infections. These have been recently presented [2] under six headings shown in Table 2, only two of these strategies (antibacterial therapy and physiologic antagonism) are currently available to clinicians. We are all familiar with antimicrobial drugs as therapeutic agents for bacterial diarrheas, with the exception of gastroenteritis due to *Salmonella* sp.; the drugs to which these bacteria are susceptible fail to shorten the course of acute illness and may prolong convalescent carriage. The trouble is that, even where successful, many organisms have developed resistance to commonly employed drugs and continue to acquire resistance factors for new compounds being introduced. Currently available and reasonable-choice antimicrobials are shown in Table 3 [35, 36]; however, local epidemiologic differences makes it mandatory to determine the susceptibility of strains isolated in each geographic region, and indeed within regions, to define the pattern in individual institutions or neighborhoods. No drug is recommended for *E. coli* enteritis because supporting data are not yet available, or for use against *Salmonella* because studies show no benefit in treatment of uncomplicated gastroenteritis [1, 36]. Systemic infection, more common with *Salmonella typhimurium* than other nontyphoid salmonellae, may require therapy, and it is reasonable to treat these problems in the same manner currently useful for typhoid fever itself.

Listed under the heading *Physiologic antagonism* are (1) the highly effective oral rehydration regimen employing a glucose-electrolyte solution, a tested and proven therapy available now [37], and (2) steroid activation of intestinal (Na^+-K^+)-ATPase, a nonrecommended therapy tested only under experimental conditions in the laboratory [38]. Even if steroids are similarly effective in humans, it is unlikely that the risk entailed will balance the benefit to justify their use. However the principle has been established that activation of the intestinal absorption mechanism for electrolyte, mediated by (Na^+-K^+)-ATPase, can balance the fluid loss due to a potent enterotoxin. Other means to activate this mechanism may be found with less potential risk than steroids, making it possible to carry out a clinical trial in the future.

The category *Physiologic pharmacology* entails specific reversal of the biochemical pathway involved in pathogenesis by drugs. While a number of

Table 2 Scientific Strategies for Control of Bacterial Diarrheas

Technique	Principle	Example
		Antimicrobial Agents
Antibacterial therapy and prophylaxis	To kill the pathogen or to immunologically inactivate virulence mechanisms	Antibody Complement-dependent bactericidal Opsonic Antitoxin (neutralizing antibinding) Antiestablishment (antiadherence factor)
Receptor megatherapy	To provide an excess of a suitable receptor for toxin or bacterium in the bowel lumen, to successfully compete with the natural receptor	G_{M1} Ganglioside cholera toxin receptor Chitotriose shigella toxin receptor Surface receptor (chemically undefined) on swine intestinal epithelium for K-88
Receptor blockade	To provide a biologically inactive molecule with affinity for the natural toxin, or bacterial receptor to compete successfully for the receptor site and, by so occupying it, to prevent binding of the toxin or bacterium	Free binding portion of cholera toxin (B subunit) Wheat germ agglutinin with binding affinity for chitotriose (shigella toxin receptor)
Elution therapy	To provide in great excess the specific saccharide of the receptor site—which may serve to dislodge or displace the toxin or bacterium from the natural receptor	Use of *N*-acetylglucosamine to remove shigella toxin Displacement of *Vibrio cholerae* from intestinal brush border membranes by *L*-fucose Displacement of *Escherichia coli* from intestinal epithelium by D-mannose
Physiologic pharmacology	To pharmacologically inhibit or reverse the specific biochemical process involved in the pathophysiology of the disease: e.g., cholera or *E. coli* toxin-induced activation of intestinal adenylate cyclase	Ethacrynic acid or nicotine acid reversal of cholera toxin stimulation of adenylate cyclase Indomethacin inhibition of post-adenylate cyclase secretory events for cholera toxin or intact salmonellae
Physiologic antagonism	To abrogate the secretory fluid loss by means of independent stimulation of an equal and opposite transport of water and electrolytes (absorption) through a totally unrelated mechanism	Oral glucose-electrolyte rehydration therapy based on glucose-facilitated sodium absorption in proximal small bowel Enhancement of sodium absorption from the bowel lumen by methyl prednisolone activation of intestinal $(Na^{+}-K^{+})$-ATPase

Source: Taken from G. T. Keusch [2].

Table 3 Currently Available and Reasonable-Choice Antimicrobials

Microbial agent	Drug of first choice	Alternate
Escherichia coli		
Toxigenic	None proven effective	–
	? Doxycycline for turista strains	–
Invasive	Not evaluated	–
Salmonella sp. (Nontyphoid)	None indicated unless systemic invasion	
	Ampicillin	Trimethoprim-sulfamethoxazole Chloramphenicol
Shigella sp.	Ampicillin	Trimethoprim-sulfamethoxazole Nalidixic acid
Vibrio cholerae	Tetracycline	Trimethoprim-sulfamethoxazole

possibilities are presented, no drug is available for use in clinical trials, and so this approach as well remains for the future.

The remaining three categories deal with the specific receptor mechanisms for bacteria and/or bacterial products (e.g., enterotoxins) described above. Receptors can be used as competitive inhibitors of binding, can be blocked (this is already a valid clinical approach to prevention of adrenergic disease mechanisms, inhibition of the histamine receptor mediating gastric acid secretion, and antagonism or reversal of narcotic effects), or can be stripped of the ligant by an excess of the critical recognition determinant in soluble form (elution) [39]. These approaches to the bacterial diarrheal diseases are novel and untested, but have merit and promise for the future. Resistance, as we know it with respect to antimicrobial agents, is unlikely to occur. However it will be necessary to be certain that interaction with the receptor does not turn on some physiologic process which would adversely affect the host. While the time has not yet arrived to clinically employ these therapeutic options, it is clear that we may anticipate their development in the next few years into potent and effective measures.

References

1. G. E. Grady and G. T. Keusch. Pathogenesis of bacterial diarrheas. *N. Engl. J. Med. 285,* 831-845; 891-900 (1971).

2. G. T. Keusch. Ecologic control of the bacterial diarrheas. A scientific strategy. *Am. J. Clin. Nutr. 31*, 2208-2218 (1978).
3. H. L. DuPont, R. B. Hornick, M. J. Snyder, J. P. Libonati, D. G. Sheahan, E. H. LaBrec, and J. P. Kalas. Pathogenesis of *Escherichia coli* diarrhea. *N. Engl. J. Med. 285,* 1-9 (1971).
4. R. W. Armstrong, T. Fodor, G. T. Curlin, A. B. Cohen, G. K. Morris, W. T. Martin, and J. Feldman. Epidemic salmonella gastroenteritis due to contaminated imitation ice cream. *Am. J. Epidemiol. 91,* 300-307 (1970).
5. M. M. Levine, H. L. DuPont, S. B. Formal, R. B. Hornick, A. Takeuchi, E. J. Gangarosa, M. J. Snyder, and J. P. Libonati. Pathogenesis of *Shigella dystenteriae* 1 (Shiga) dysentery. *J. Infect. Dis. 127,* 261-270 (1973).
6. S. I. Music, J. P. Libonati, R. P. Wenzel, M. J. Snyder, R. B. Hornick, and T. E. Woodward. Induced human cholera. In *Antimicrob. Agents Chemother. 1970* (G. R. Hobby, Ed.). American Society for Microbiology, Washington, D.C., 1971, pp. 462-466.
7. H. Williams-Smith and J. E. T. Jones. Observations on the alimentary tract and its flora in healthy and diseased pigs. *J. Pathol. Bacteriol. 86,* 387-412 (1963).
8. J. Ørskov and F. Ørskov. Episome-carried surface antigen K88 of *Escherichia coli. J. Bacteriol. 91,* 69-75 (1966).
9. G. W. Jones. The attachment of bacteria to the surfaces of animal cells. In *Microbial Interactions–Receptors and Recognition* (J. L. Reissig, Ed.), Series B, Vol. 3. Chapman & Hall, London, 1977, pp. 141-176.
10. H. Williams-Smith and M. A. Linggood. Observations on the pathogenic properties of the K88, HLY and ENT plasmids of *Escherichia coli* with particular reference to porcine diarrhea. *J. Med. Microbiol. 4,* 467-493 (1971).
11. M. R. Burrows, R. Sellwood, and R. A. Gibbons. Haemagglutinating and adhesive properties associated with the K99 antigen of bovine strains of *Escherichia coli. J. Gen. Microbiol. 96,* 269-275 (1976).
12. D. G. Evans, R. P. Silver, D. J. Evans, Jr., D. G. Chase, and S. L. Gorbach. Plasmid controlled colonization factor associated with virulence in *Escherichia coli* enterotoxigenic for humans. *Infect. Immun. 12,* 656-667 (1975).
13. D. G. Evans, D. J. Evans, Jr., W. S. Tjoa, and H. L. DuPont. Dectection and characterization of colonization factor of enterotoxigenic *Escherichia coli* isolated from adults with diarrhea. *Infect. Immun. 19,* 727-736 (1978).
14. M. Thaler, M. Hirschberger, and D. Mirelman. Adherence of *Escherichia coli* to immature intestine is mediated by mucosal receptors of mannose-specific bacterial lectins. *Clin. Res. 25,* 469A (1977).
15. M. J. Bergman, E. G. Evans, J. Sullivan, G. L. Mandell, I. E. Salit, and R. L. Guerrant. Attachment of *E. coli* to human intestinal epithelial cells. A functional in vitro test for intestinal colonization factor. *Clin. Res. 26,* 558A (1978).
16. R. Sellwood, R. A. Gibbons,) (W. Jones, and J. M. Rutter. Adhesion of

enteropathogenic *Escherichia coli* to pig intestinal brush borders: The existence of two pig phenotypes. *J. Med. Microbiol. 8,* 405-411 (1975).
17. G. W. Jones and R. Freter. Adhesive properties of *Vibrio cholerae:* Nature of the interaction with isolated rabbit brush border membranes and human erythrocytes. *Infect. Immun. 14,* 240-245 (1976).
18. J. Holmgren and A. M. Svennerholm. Mechanisms of disease and immunity in cholera: A review. *J. Infect. Dis. 136,* S105-S112 (1977).
19. J. Holmgren, I. Lönnroth, and L. Svennerholm. Tissue receptor for cholera exotoxin: Postulated structure from studies with G_{M1} ganglioside and related glycolipids. *Infect. Immun. 8,* 208-214 (1973).
20. J. Holmgren, I. Lönnroth, J.-E. Mansson, and L. Svennerholm. Interaction of cholera toxin and membrane G_{M1} ganglioside. *Proc. Natl. Acad. Sci. USA 72,* 2520-2524 (1975).
21. P. Cuatrecasas. Gangliosides and membrane receptors for cholera toxin. *Biochemistry 12,* 3558-3566 (1973).
22. G. T. Keusch and M. Jacewicz. Pathogenesis of shigella diarrhea. VII. Evidence for a cell membrane toxin receptor involving $\beta 1 \rightarrow 4$ linked *N*-acetyl-D-glucose amine oligomers. *J. Exp. Med. 146,* 535-546 (1977).
23. M. Field. Intestinal secretion: Effect of cyclic AMP and its role in cholera. *N. Engl. J. Med. 284,* 1137-1144 (1971).
24. A. N. Charney, R. E. Gots, S. B. Formal, and R. A. Giannella. Activation of intestinal mucosal adenylate cyclase by *Shigella dysenteriae* 1 enterotoxin. *Gastroenterology 70,* 1085-1090 (1976).
25. J. M. Hughes, F. Murad, B. Chang, and R. L. Guerrant. Role of cyclic GMP in the action of heat-stable enterotoxin of *Escherichia coli. Nature 271,* 755-756 (1978).
26. P. Gemski, A. Takeuchi, O. Washington, and S. B. Formal. Shigellosis due to *Shigella dysenteriae* 1: Relative importance of mucosal invasion versus toxin production in pathogenesis. *J. Infect. Dis. 126,* 523-530 (1972).
27. P. Gemski and S. B. Formal. Shigellosis: An invasive infection of the gastrointestinal tract. In *Microbiology–1975* (D. Schlessinger, Ed.). American Society for Microbiology, Washington, D.C., 1975, pp. 165-169.
28. R. A. Giannella, S. B. Formal, G. J. Dammin, and H. Collins. Pathogenesis of salmonellosis. Studies of fluid secretion, mucosal invasion, and morphologic reaction in the rabbit ileum. *J. Clin. Invest. 52,* 441-453 (1973).
29. P. D. Sandefur and J. W. Peterson. Neutralization of salmonella toxin-induced elongation of Chinese hamster ovary cells by cholera antitoxin. *Infect. Immun. 15,* 988-992 (1977).
30. F. Orskov. Virulence factors of the bacterial cell surface. *J. Infect. Dis. 137,* 630-633 (1978).
31. E. F. Tulloch, Jr., K. J. Ryan, S. B. Formal, and F. A. Franklin. Invasive enteropathic *Escherichia coli* dysentery. *Ann. Int. Med. 79,* 13-17 (1973).
32. J. R. Cantey and R. K. Blake. Diarrhea due to *Escherichia coli* in the rabbit: A novel mechanism. *J. Infect. Dis. 135,* 454-462 (1977).
33. A. D. O'Brien, M. R. Thompson, J. R. Cantey, and S. B. Formal. Production of *Shigella dysenteriae*-like toxins by pathogenic *Escherichia coli.*

Abstract. Proceedings at the American Society for Microbiology, 1977, p. 32.

34. R. B. Sack. The epidemiology of diarrhea due to enterotoxigenic *Escherichia coli. J. Infect. Dis. 137,* 639-640 (1978).
35. The choice of antimicrobial drugs. *The Medical Letter 22*, 5-12 (1980).
36. H. F. Conn (Ed.). *Current Therapy–1978.* Saunders, Philadelphia, 1978, pp. 13-17, 19-21, 26-29, 65-67.
37. N. F. Pierce and N. Hirschhorn. Oral fluid–A simple weapon against dehydration in diarrhea. How it works and how to use it. *WHO Chron. 31,* 87-93 (1977).
38. A. N. Charney and M. Donowitz. Prevention and reversal of cholera enterotoxin-induced intestinal secretion by methylprednisolone: Induction of Na^+-K^+ATPase. *J. Clin. Invest. 57,* 1590-1599 (1976).
39. G. T. Keusch. Specific membrane receptors: Pathogenetic and therapeutic implications in infectious diseases. *Rev. Infect. Dis. 1,* 517-529 (1979).

22 Protozoan Diarrheas: Dientamoebiasis and Giardiasis

MURRAY WITTNER / Albert Einstein College of Medicine, Bronx, New York

I. Introduction

Diarrhea can be caused by a number of protozoans that inhabit the intestinal tract of man. While it is widely agreed that infection with such organisms as *Entamoeba histolytica* and *Balantidium coli* can be responsible for severe tissue pathology, intestinal symptoms, and sometimes fatal disease, infections with such organisms as *Dientamoeba fragilis* and *Giardia lamblia* have often been regarded as relatively benign, with mild or sometimes moderate symptoms that often could be ignored. Events of the past several years, however, suggest that infections with *Dientamoeba* and *Giardia* are not as benign as we once believed, since experience has taught us that many individuals can be severely affected as a result of infection with these organisms. This chapter, therefore, will be devoted to considerations of recent information regarding *Dientamoeba* and *Giardia* as important causes of protozoan diarrhea.

II. Dientamoeba fragilis

While usually considered to be an amoeba by many protozoologists, *D. fragilis* has most recently been shown to be properly classified among the flagellates, with close affinities to such flagellate genera as *Trichomonas* and *Histomonas*. However, in *Dientamoeba*, only the ameboid stage has been described: quite small, averaging 6-12 μm in diameter. Among its characteristic features is the presence of pointed, leaf-shaped pseudopodia. When properly stained, about 60% of the organisms reveal two characteristic nuclei that have a fine nuclear membrane and a karyosome consisting of a group of four to six chromatin granules. No cyst or resistant stage has been described.

It is not clear how *D. fragilis* is transmitted, but a number of investigators have suggested that this organism is transmitted with the egg of the pinworm, *Enterobius vermicularis,* in a manner similar to that which has been shown for the transmission of *Histomonas meleagridis* within the egg of the nematode. *Heterakis gallinae.* In a recent report by Yang and Scholten [1], *D. fragilis* and enterobius infections were found associated about nine times more often than expected on the basis of random distribution of these parasites. Similar observations were reported by Burrows et al. [17], who also found the association between *D. fragilis* and pinworm to occur about "20 times more frequently than would be expected on the basis of random and independent distribution of these two parasites." These data are also supported by the observations of others [2]. A variety of other epidemiological data also tends to support this hypothesis. For example, *D. fragilis* is found more frequently in young females than in older individuals and males. Moreover, the fact that attempts to infect volunteers orally with *D. fragilis* have consistently failed and that these organisms live for only a very short time in fresh water makes oral transmission in the usual fashion appear unlikely.

The protozoan *D. fragilis* has been found, inhabiting the large bowel, in most parts of the world. The incidence varies widely from about 1 to 20%. Surveys of inmates in mental institutions and Indians from Arizona show a very high incidence of 19-47%. In New York City, our experience indicates an incidence of just under 4%.

Many years ago Wenrich [18], at the University of Pennsylvania, found that students with *D. fragilis* infection had many more gastrointestinal complaints than those free of infection. Patients with *D. fragilis* may have frank diarrhea with soft, mushy, or normally formed stools. They may complain most frequently of mild to severe diarrhea and abdominal pain, anal pruritis, abdominal distension, and flatulence (Table 1). It is unusual to find blood in the stools, although this has been reported. These organisms have not been reported to invade the colonic mucosa, although we have aspirated and isolated these parasites from the base of a rectal ulcer in one patient from whom no other parasite was ever obtained, despite repeated attempts. After therapy the ulcer healed and the patient became entirely well. Some authors have reported low-grade eosinophilia with this infection, but in our experience it is not often found. It should be emphasized that many individuals harbor this protozoan in their colon and have few if any complaints.

The diagnosis of *D. fragilis* infection depends upon finding this parasite in a stool specimen that has been properly collected and promptly examined. If the latter policy cannot be adhered to, then the entire stool specimen should be preserved in polyvinyl alcohol (PVA) fixative and examined at a later time. It is sometimes difficult to properly identify this parasite if, as occasionally may occur, most of the trophozoites are uninucleate; it is then possible to

Table 1 Reported Occurrence of Symptoms Associated with *Dientamoeba fragilis* Infection Only[a]

Symptoms	% of Patients
Abdominal pain	47
Diarrhea	43
Unformed stools	21
Nausea and/or vomiting	21
Flatulence	20
Lassitude	14
Weight loss	11
Constipation	8
Eosinophilia	5
Other	20

[a]There were 113 patients diagnosed and treated at the Tropical Disease Clinic Bronx Municipal Hospital Center from 1970 to 1975.

mistakenly diagnose a *D. fragilis* infection as due to *Endolimax nana*—a harmless commensal ameba of the large bowel. It is important that a reliable laboratory with highly skilled personnel be available if this difficult diagnosis is to be made with confidence.

Treatment with diiodohydroxyquin is recommended: for adults, 650 mg t.i.d. for 20 days, for children, 40 mg/kg body weight per day in 3 divided doses for 20 days. Alternatively, adults may receive tetracycline 500 mg q.i.d. for 10 days and children 10 mg/kg body weight q.i.d. for 10 days (maximum 2 g).

III. Giardia lamblia

Infection with the flagellate protozoan *G. lamblia* is often associated with diarrhea and a myriad of other abdominal complaints. This organism is highly characteristic in both its trophozoite and cyst stages. The trophozoite is about 10-20 μm long by 5-15 μm wide and appears bilaterally symmetrical with four pairs of flagella and two nuclei. It is dorsally convex, and there is a slightly anteroventral concavity, presumably a sucking disk or holdfast structure. The ovoid cysts are 8-10 μm by 7-10 μm and have two nuclei when immature; whereas the mature cyst contains an organism that has four nuclei and a double set of cytoplasmic organelles. When excystment occurs, the cell divides immediately, producing two motile organisms.

Giardia is usually found in the duodenum and proximal jejunum, but occasionally it has been reported to have been isolated from the biliary system, including the gallbladder. Examination of duodenal and jejunal biopsy specimens has demonstrated that trophozoites adhere to the mucosal surface by the ventral sucking disk. It is not clear whether they obtain nutriment in this fashion or whether they absorb food solely from the luminal contents.

The transmission of *Giardia* is believed to be accomplished by the ingestion of mature cysts in food and water contaminated by sewage, as well as by fecal-oral transmission of the cyst in institutional and family settings [3]. In recent years, the National Center for Disease Control reports that *Giardia* is the most frequently diagnosed intestinal parasitic pathogen in public health laboratories in the United States. Outbreaks of giardial epidemics have been reported with increasing frequency throughout the United States–having occurred at Aspen and Boulder, Colorado; Utah; and Camas, Washington. In the Rome, New York, epidemic an attack rate of 10.6% of the city's residents was reported. In a well-documented study by Black et al. [3] child-to-child transmission in three day-care centers was demonstrated. Moreover, family members of those children in the day-care centers also acquired the infection, an occurrence suggesting that close personal contact with an infected person could lead to secondary infection. The carrier rate of *Giardia* in the United States is believed to be between 1.5 and 20%, depending upon the community and age group surveyed. The occurrence of giardiasis in the Soviet Union, especially in Leningrad, is well recognized–having been reported on a number of occasions by tourists and groups visiting that city. In most of these reports, infection was water-borne [4], and in one instance (Aspen, Colorado) sewage was found leaking into the community water supply [5]. Thus, giardiasis is found throughout the world wherever sanitary sewage facilities are absent and water supplies are not properly treated or safeguarded. Moreover, several outbreaks in rural parts of the United States have been reported, suggesting that *Giardia* sp. from a variety of feral animals can successfully infect man.

Most surveys indicate that children are more frequently infected and symptomatic than adults. Many individuals, however, gradually become asymptomatic as they reach adolescence–although they may continue to maintain the infection, while others evidently eliminate the infection spontaneously. It has been suggested, but not proved, that immunological mechanisms play a decisive role in this process.

A number of investigators have shown convincingly that *G. lamblia* infection is an important cause of diarrheal diseases in man. The most frequent symptoms encountered are flatulence, abdominal pain, tenderness to palpation, midepigastric distress, weight loss, nervousness, constipation, and diarrhea. Small-intestinal mucosal abnormalities have been described in a number of studies; but these findings in clinically ill patients have not been uniform. In some cases small-bowel biopsies have demonstrated mild-to-severe blunting or flattening of the villi, with round cell infiltration of the lamina propria. These morphologic findings resemble those reported in sprue. Many of these ptients have had malabsorption symptoms similar to those usually associated with gluten-sensitive sprue. Moreover, during the past decade patients with immune deficiency states have been reported to have an increased frequency of giardiasis. Initially, Hermans et al. [6] reported a group of patients with giardial infection associated with nodular lymphoid hyperplasia of the small intestine, low serum IgA, diarrhea, and steatorrhea. Several of their patients had "sprue-like" biopsy specimens. Since this report appeared, a number of other studies have confirmed the association of giardial infection and a variety of dysgammaglobulinemic states. It is clear, however, that many patients suffering with hypogammaglobulinemia and sprue and sprue-like symptoms do not necessarily have giardiasis. Further, it is not clear whether patients with low mucosal IgA are at special risk with regard to giardial infection, although patients with achlorhydria are often found with this infection.

For many years, *Giardia* has been regarded as a luminal parasite, although, as early as 1913, Fairise and Jacquot [7] reported mucosal invasion by this flagellate. More recently Morecki and Parker [8], Brandborg et al. [9], and Saha and Ghosh [10] have clearly demonstrated that trophozoites of *Giardia* may invade the intestinal mucosa. Wright et al. [11] were able to show that in 12 patients, all having steatorrhea, parasites were found to have penetrated the surface epithelium and to have entered the lamina propria. All of these patients had what was regarded as "heavy infections" and were clinically ill. Similarly, in studies on giardiasis with malabsorption reported by Wright and others, the more severe clinical symptoms were associated with more marked histological abnormalities as judged by examination of jejunal biopsy material. Moreover, D-xylose, fat, and vitamin B_{12} malabsorption was commonly found. The precise cause of malabsorption, however, remains obscure—although the large number of parasites in the small intesitne, bacterial colonization of the upper small bowel by various species of Enterobacteriaceae [12], parasitogenic injury to the mucosa, as well as tissue invasion, are variously thought to be responsible.

Few studies have been done regarding the antibody response of patients to giardial infection. However, in a recent study by Ridley and Ridley [13], there was, in general, a positive correlation between the presence of a significant antibody titer and the severity of jejunal lesions. In this study, early infection was associated with the production of IgM. Circumstantial evidence derived from epidemiologic data and from the murine model [14] suggests that acquired immunity to giardiasis occurs; nevertheless, reinfection is said to take place.

Following experimental infection, the onset of clinical disease averages about 9 days [15] although the prepatent period can vary widely. In this study 40 volunteers ingested as few as 10 cysts, and some became infected, although infection could be assured if 100 or more cysts were consumed. Despite infection, clinical manifestations vary widely from completely asymptomatic to severe diarrhea with malabsorption (Table 2). In many patients, even when

Table 2 Symptoms Reported by 168 Patients with *Giardia lamblia* Infection

Symptom	Number of patients
Flatulence	112
Midepigastric tenderness and pain	62
Diarrhea	77
Constipation	62
Loose stools (not diarrhea)	89
Alternating periods of diarrhea and Constripation	43
Weight loss	39
Right upper quadrant pain	11

Note: Age of patients ranged from 18 months to 69 years.

a history of diarrhea cannot be obtained, their stools are never really formed but assume a soft grumous consistency. Bloody diarrhea or melena is not seen as a result of giardial infection.

The acute onset of a giardial infection can be severe, with frequent, explosive watery stools, often foul-smelling, together with flatulence, midepigastric pain, nausea, and vomiting. These acute symptoms are usually short-lived, e.g., 2 or 3 days, but can persist for months. The clinical disease usually becomes less troublesome, with the patient having episodes of soft, grumous stools, at times alternating with constipation. Many patients compalin only of abdominal distension and flatulence with midepigastric distress, especially after meals. Right upper quadrant pain with fatty-food intolerance and belching is sometimes encountered, suggesting gallbladder disease. In those giardiasis patients in whom evidence of lactose intolerance is found, proper treatment to eliminate *Giardia* often alleviates the disaccharidase deficiency, and abnormal jejunal biopsy results may return to normal.

Diagnosis of a *Giardia* infection is usually made by examination of a stool specimen. Trophozoites can be found in diarrheic stools, while cysts are encountered in formed or semiformed fecal specimens. A concentration technique should be employed to enhance the chances of discovering the cysts. Trophozoites, however, do not survive zinc sulfate or formol-ether methods and must be found on direct smear examination.

It should be appreciated that the diagnosis of a giardial infection can be elusive even after multiple stool examinations. There have been a number of reports demonstrating that some infected individuals have periods when few if any parasites may be found in their stools. These intervals purportedly may alternate with periods of relatively higher parasite excretion. In other individuals, many parasites are present all the time. Danciger and Lopez [16] characterized three patterns of giardial excretion: (1) high excreters, with the parasite abundant in all stools; (2) low excreters, with the parasite detectable in only 40% of stools and being scarce even then; and (3) mixed excreters, with periods of 1-3 weeks of high excretion alternating with usually shorter periods of low excretion (i.e., 60% of the stools being positive). It is evident, therefore, that the standard three-stool examination may not be sufficient to successfully diagnose a giardial infection. It seems reasonable to conclude that, if the parasite cannot be found after a number (four or five) correctly performed stool examinations, it may be necessary to resort to duodenal aspiration or small-bowel biopsy. Our own experiences, moreover, as well as those of others, have shown that the use of purgatives has not been found helpful in increasing the number of positive stools or increasing the number of parasites per stool [15, 16]. The use of a weighted duodenal gelatin capsule containing 140 cm of 3-ply white nylon yarn* has been found to be an effective method for aiding in the diagnosis of giardiasis.

Serological tests are not generally available. Ridley and Ridley [13], however, have shown a general correlation between an immunofluorescent antibody titer and the severity of jejunal histologic lesions as well as of gastrointestinal symptoms.

Therapy for giardiasis should be provided for all individuals, whether asymptomatic or not, inasmuch as infection evidently can be readily transmitted to family members, and food handlers may serve as a source of infection to restaurant patrons. For adults, quinacrine 100 mg after meals t.i.d. for 5 days, or for children, 2 mg/kg body weight (maximum 300 mg daily) after meals t.i.d. for 5 days, is the recommended treatment. Rarely, quinacrine may provoke toxic psychosis, but this is usually encountered only in patients with past psychiatric history. This drug is also contraindicated in patients with psoriasis. Quinacrine is very bitter-tasting, so it must be disguised for young children by being suspended in a sweet vehicle such as chocolate or cherry syrup. Occasionally, quinacrine will stain the sclera or skin yellow. This should not be of concern as the discoloration will disappear shortly after therapy has been completed. Metronidazole 250 mg t.i.d. for 10 days for adults or 5 mg/kg body weight t.i.d. for 10 days for children is a satisfactory alternative treatment, although the cure rate is somewhat lower. However, metronidazole has been reported to be carcinogenic and mutagenic, which makes its use somewhat questionable. There is no chemoprophylactic agent for giardiasis. Therefore, caution should be followed when traveling especially where there is risk of waterborne infection. Water should be boiled, since treatment

*Entertest HEDECO Co., Palo Alto, California.

with "cysticidal" tablets that have as their active ingredient tetraglycine hydroperiodide (Globaline) has proven to be ineffective. Cysts of *Giardia* are killed instantly at 50-55°C, and they resist 0.5% chlorinated water for several days. Raw contaminated fruits and vegetables are a frequent source of infection. Such fresh fruits and vegetables as strawberries, lettuce, and cucumbers should be avoided unless blanched, peeled, or treated in water containing suitable concentrations of iodine or chlorine.

References

1. J. Yang and T. Scholten. *Dientamoeba fragilis:* A review with notes on its epidemiology, pathogenicity, made by transmission and diagnosis. *Am. J. Trop. Med. Hyg. 26,* 16-22 (1977).
2. G. Ockert and U. Schultz. Pathogenetischen Rolle von *Dientamoeba fragilis. Dtsch. Gesundheitses. 27,* 1156-1158 (1972).
3. R. E. Black, A. C. Dykes, S. P. Sinclair, and J. G. Wells. Giardiasis in day-care centers: Evidence of person to person transmission. *Pediatrics 60*:486-490.
4. P. K. Shaw, R. E. Brodsky, D. O. Tyman, B. T. Wood, C. P. Hibler, G. R. Healy, K. I. E. Macheod, W. Stahl, and M. Schultz. A community-wide outbreak of giardiasis with evidence of transmission by a municipal water supply. *Ann. Int. Med. 87,* 426-432 (1977).
5. G. T. Moore, W. M. Cross, D. McGuire, C. S. Mollohan, N. N. Gleason, G. R. Healy, L. H. Newton. Epidemic giardiasis at a ski resort. *N. Engl. J. Med. 281,* 402-407 (1969).
6. P. E. Hermans, K. A. Huizenga, H. N. Hoffman, A. L. Brown, and H. Markowitz. Dysgammaglobulinemia associated with nodular lymphoid hyperplasia of the small intestine. *Am. J. Med. 40,* 78-89 (1966).
7. C. Fairise and C. Jacquot. Colite ulcereuse due à un parasite flagellate le *Lamblia intestinalis* (Lamble): Perforation puis occlusion intestinale mort. Étude des lesions produites per le parasite. *Arch. Mal. App. Dig. Mal. Nutr. 7,* 301-307 (1913).
8. R. Morecki and J. G. Parker. Ultrastructural studies of the human *Giardia lamblia* and subjacent jejunal mucosa in a subject with steatorrhea. *Gastroenterology 52,* 151-164 (1967).
9. L. Brandborg, C. B. Tankersley, S. Gottlieb, M. Baranicik, and V. E. Sartor. Histological demonstration of mucosal invasion by *Giardia lamblia* in man. *Gastroenterology 52,* 143-150 (1967).
10. T. K. Saha and T. K. Ghosh. Invasion of small intestinal mucosa by *Giardia lamblia* in man. *Gastroenterology 72,* 402-405 (1977).
11. S. G. Wright, A. M. Tomkins, and D. S. Ridley. Giardiasis: Clinical and therapeutic aspects. *Gut 18,* 343-350 (1977).
12. A. M. Tomkins, S. G. Wright, B. S. Drasar, and W. P. T. James. Bacterial colonization of jejunal mucosa in giardiasis. *Trans. R. Soc. Trop. Med. Hyg. 72,* 33-36 (1978).
13. M. J. Ridley and D. S. Ridley. Serum antibodies and jejunal histology in giardiasis associated with malabsorption. *J. Clin. Pathol. 29,* 30-34 (1976).

14. I. C. Roberts-Thomson, D. P. Stevens, A. Mahmoud, and K. Wanen. Giardiasis in the mouse: An animal model. *Gastroenterology 71,* 57-61 (1976).
15. R. C. Rendtorff and O. J. Holt. The experimental transmission of human intestinal parasites IV. Attempts to transmit *Endamoeba coli* and *Giardia lamblia* by water. *Am. J. Hyg. 60,* 327-338 (1954).
16. M. Danciger and M. Lopez. Numbers of *Giardia* in the feces of infected children. *Am. J. Trop. Med. Hyg. 24,* 237-242 (1975).
17. R. B. Burrows and M. A. Swerdlow. *Enterobius vermicularis* as a probable vector of *Dientamoeba fragilis. Am. J. Trop. Med. Hyg. 5,* 258-265 (1956).
18. D. H. Wenrich, R. M. Stabler, and J. H. Arnett. *Entamoeba histolytica* and other intestinal protozoa in 1060 college freshmen. *Am. J. Trop. Med. 15,* 331-345 (1935).

PART V

Consequences of Gastrointestinal Disorders

23
Secondary Carbohydrate Intolerance in Infancy

FIMA LIFSHITZ / Cornell University Medical College, New York, New York, and North Shore University Hospital, Manhasset, New York

I. Introduction

Alterations in the digestion and absorption of carbohydrates may lead to carbohydrate intolerance in patients of all age groups. This may be due to primary inborn alterations in absorptive ability, such as congenital lactase or sucrase-iso maltase deficiencies [1], or may be due to ethnic patterns of lactose malabsorption which affect the majority of the world's population, such as ontogenetic lactase deficiency (Chapter 16 of this volume and Refs. 2-4). Carbohydrate malabsorption may also occur as a result of secondary alterations in the absorptive capacity in a variety of clinical disorders [5-7].

Secondary carbohydrate intolerance was first recognized at the beginning of this century in infants with transient lactose intolerance following gastroenteritis [8]. A more prolonged and more severe illness was related to the presence of this complication, which could be reduced when the offending carbohydrate, lactose, was eliminated from the diet. It is known that secondary carbohydrate intolerance may be associated with any one of several diverse systemic and/or intestinal disorders [7]. Secondary carbohydrate intolerance is usually related to a depression of small-intestinal oligosaccharidase activity as a result of mucosal damage induced by the primary disease process [5-7]. The lesion may affect lactase and/or one or all of the other mucosal oligosaccharidases [9]. It may also alter the intestinal transport processes, and at times even intestinal permeability.

Some of the current concepts concerning the consequences of secondary transient carbohydrate malabsorption in children are reviewed here. This complication plays an important role in the pathophysiologic alterations of the primary disease, as well as in the eventual fate of the patient. Lactase may be the target enzyme for the rotavirus which produces infantile gastroenteritis, frequently leading to lactase deficiency [10]. The carbohydrate intolerance which therefore occurs may be the cause and consequence of the many alterations occurring in infants with diarrhea [6].

II. Pathophysiology of Carbohydrate Intolerance

Carbohydrate malabsorption from any cause may result in diarrhea and further carbohydrate intolerance. The major cause of diarrhea in carbohydrate malabsorption is the presence of osmotically active carbohydrate and fermentative products within the lumen of the bowel. The osmotic load of the unabsorbed carbohydrate results in secretion of fluid and electrolytes into the small intestine and colon until osmotic equilibrium is reached [11, 12]. The local osmotic gradients that ensue when there are unabsorbed solutes in the small intestine may also augment the losses of intestinal epithelial cells and enzymes into the lumen of the bowel. It has been found that exposure of rat jejunal lumen to a hyperosmolar mannitol load produces significant loss of mucosal epithelial cells and a washing-off of intestinal disaccharidases from the mucosal surface [13]. There is accumulation in the lumen of protein, [^{3}H] thymidine-labeled DNA, and disaccharidases; therefore morphological alterations are induced: i.e., the microvilli of some cells are shortened and fused at their bases.

A part of the unabsorbed carbohydrate is secreted unaltered in the feces, while a greater portion may be hydrolyzed by intestinal bacteria in the lower segments of the intestine into smaller carbohydrate molecules and into other fermentative products. These include short-chain organic acids, such as lactic acid, and large quantities of hydrogen gas [14]. The concentration of carbohydrates within the luminal content is thus reduced, and the pH decreases. The organic acids produced are poorly absorbed by the colon, and they further increase the osmotic pressure within the lumen. In addition, they interfere with the absorption of water and electrolytes. Furthermore, a more rapid intestinal motility may develop from the increased intraluminal volume, contributing to diarrhea [12]. The stools are therefore characterized by an acid pH due to organic acids and by the presence of unabsorbed carbohydrates. The elimination of the unabsorbed sugar from the diet very often breaks the cycle, and a lessening of the diarrhea results—regardless of the etiology of the disease [6].

III. Carbohydrate Intolerance in Diarrheal Disease

The principal cause of acquired carbohydrate malabsorption in infancy is diarrheal disease. Carbohydrate malabsorption was observed in 78% of a large group of infants with severe gastroenteritis [6]. Carbohydrate intolerance and diarrheal disease was frequently specific for lactose, but often involved other disaccharides, and at times it even included all carbohydrates [6]. The alteration in carbohydrate absorption was seen during the initial stages of the illness, after a prolonged clinical course, or intermittently throughout the duration of the disease. In all instances, the disturbance was temporary, with complete recovery 3-4 months after improvement of the disease. The alterations in the absorption of carbohydrates were more prevalent and more severe in children with underlying malnutrition [6].

For quite some time many have wondered whether the usually well baby with mild diarrhea would also have carbohydrate intolerance, as seen in the malnourished child with severe gastroenteritis. Kumar et al. studied 90 well babies prospectively during an outbreak of mild gastroenteritis which did not lead to dehydration [15]. They showed that the percentages of well-nourished children with mild gastroenteritis who developed secondary lactose malabsorption as a complication of the disease were similar to those reported previously in malnourished and severely dehydrated patients. The peak incidence of lactose intolerance in gastroenteritis was during the first 2 years of life, whereas it was very unusual in older children with this illness. However, the incidence of multiple disaccharide intolerances was less in well-nourished children with mild diarrhea than has been reported by others in patients with severe diarrhea and malnutrition [6, 16].

Carbohydrate malabsorption in diarrheal disease is probably due to small-intestinal injury. This could be due to infection or local physiological alterations in the small intestine, including alterations in luminal pH and increased osmolality [13]. The hyperosmolality within the intestinal lumen may produce a washing-off of intestinal disaccharidases, as mentioned above. In addition, the systemic complications of the diarrheal process, such as dehydration, shock, or malnutrition, may also produce intestinal injury and secondary carbohydrate malabsorption [5-7]. Intestinal infection may lead to carbohydrate malabsorption by mucosal damage and disruption of the enterocyte; such mucosal damage results from either tissue invasion with resultant inflammation or from cell injury caused by products of bacterial metabolic activity acting upon foodstuffs and host secretions [17]. Among the bacteria-generated factors which are injurious to the small intestine are deconjugated bile salts, short-chain organic acids, hydroxy fatty acids, and alcohol. Once intestinal mucosal integrity is altered, the result is depression of brush border oligodisaccharidases and intestinal transport derangements.

Certain enteric viruses (e.g., rotavirus, Norwalk agent) also induce morphologic and functional changes in the small intestine by penetration of the enterocyte [8, 19]. Rotaviruses seem to be the principal cause of diarrhea and carbohydrate intolerance in infancy (Chapter 20 of this volume and Refs. 18, 18). It has been postulated that intestinal lactase is the receptor and uncoating enzyme for these enteritis viruses. Before diarrhea is seen, the virus must infect gut epithelium rich in lactase. This hypothesis is consistent with the high prevalence of lactose intolerance in gastroenteritis in infancy. It also has implications for the epidemiology of gastroenteritis. Infants are more susceptible to the disease, and its incidence may be decreased in lactase-deficient individuals. Perhaps lactase deficiency is an evolutionary device that arose in defense against this lethal disease, which occurs in the greater part of the world's population [10].

The type of enzyme deficiencies secondary to diarrheal disease may also be the result of dietary manipulations that such patients receive during their illness. Under the experimental conditions of chronic hyperosmotic stress in rats, the intestinal oligosaccharidases were altered in relation to the specific disaccharide represented in the diet [11]. Chronic force-feedings of unabsorbable hyperosmotic mannitol were associated with significant decreases in the intestinal mucosal levels of only lactase and sucrase when the diet contained starch, whereas maltase, the enzyme with dietary substrate representation, remained unchanged. When sucrose was the only carbohydrate in the diet the sucrase levels were maintained, while lactase and maltase, not represented by disaccharides in the diet, were significantly reduced by osmotic diarrhea. Analogous results were obtained when no sucrose was present in the diet. When all disaccharides were eliminated and replaced by glucose feedings, all three intestinal oligosaccharidases tested were found to be depressed by osmotic diarrhea. Thus, a magnified substrate dependency of intestinal oligodisaccharidases during stress seems evident.

IV. Carbohydrate Intolerance in Hypoxia

In addition to enteritis and diarrheal disease, carbohydrate intolerance can also be induced by other pathophysiologic stresses. Hypoxia is known to lead to derangements in glucose transport by the small intestine. In rats, fish, guinea pigs, and other animals, following hypoxia there is malabsorption of glucose, as well as histologic damage [20-22]. In the human fetus and newborn infants there may be a relationship between monosaccharide intolerance, following neonatal hypoxia, and necrotizing enterocolitis [23-25]. The effects on carbohydrate metabolism may continue beyond the duration of the hypoxia. These effects may be seen as metabolic abnormalities in response to a glucose oral load during convalescence from hypoxia in newborn babies. We recently performed glucose tolerance tests on 15 infants who had respiratory difficulties and hypoxia in the neonatal period [26]. They all had a diminished absorption of oral glucose loads early in their convalescence from hypoxia (Fig. 1). Concomitantly they had metabolic acidosis with a drop in serum bicarbonate and blood pH levels after glucose intake. These data suggest that carbohydrate intolerance in these

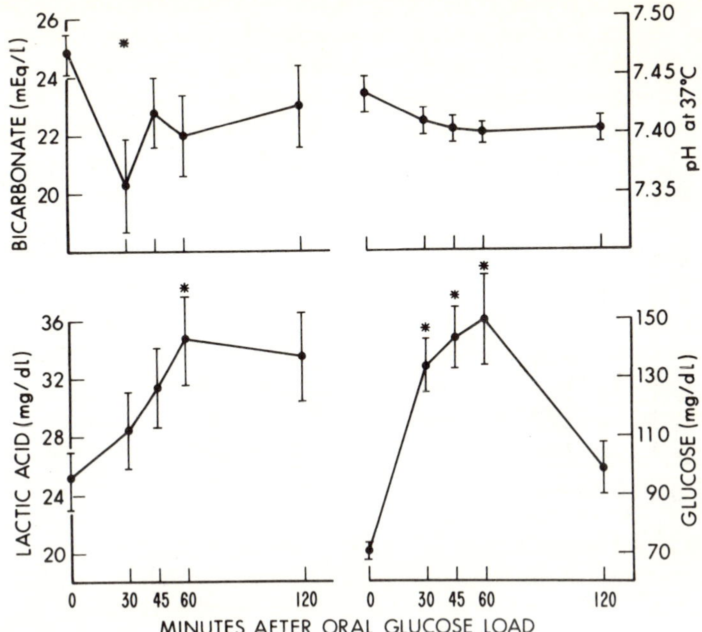

Figure 1 Metabolic changes in response to an oral glucose load during convalescence from hypoxia in newborn infants. Changes in blood bicarbonate, blood pH, plasma lactic acid, and plasma glucose are shown. All data ±SD; asterisk indicates $P < 0.05$. Further details are published elsewhere [26].

patients may be a most important complication hindering recovery once the principal illness has already abated. Furthermore, in premature infants this complication of neonatal hypoxia could lead to carbohydrate intolerance and necrotizing enterocolitis [23-25].

The mechanism of impaired transport capacity during hypoxia has been studied in rats. Experimental hypoxia in rats results in a rapid decrease in the intestinal (Na^+-K^+)-ATPase activity, which is currently believed to be involved in the transport of glucose (Fig. 2). There was a significant decrease in sodium- and potassium-activated ATPase activity of the jejunal mucosa after only 4 hr of exposure to an atmosphere of 93% N_2/7% O_2. A more marked alteration of the ATPase activity of the jejunum occurred after 48 hr of continuous hypoxia in rats. The (Na^+-K^+)-ATPase activity was markedly reduced, whereas the magnesium-activated portion of mucosal ATPase was increased. The reduction in jejunal K^+- activated ATPase activity was accompanied by a marked alteration

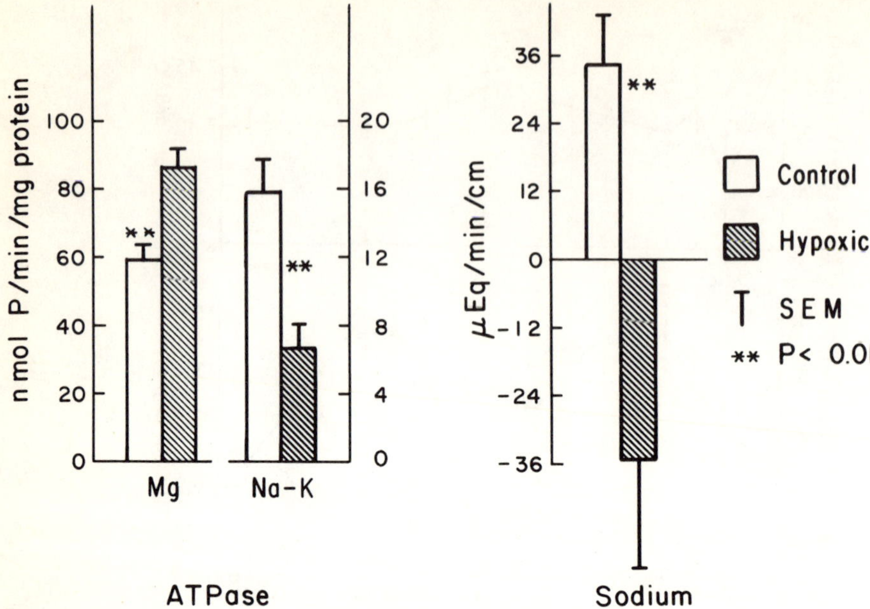

Figure 2 Effects of hypoxia on intestinal ATPase and sodium transport. Hypoxia was induced in rats by exposure to nitrogen-air atmosphere in concentrations of 93% nitrogen for 48 hr in acrylic chambers kept at atmospheric pressure. Controls were kept in similar conditions exposed to compressed air. At time of study, rats had following arterial blood gas means ±SD.

Group	pH	Arterial pO_2 (mmHg)	$pHCO_3$ (mmHg)	Arterial pCO_2 (mmHg)
Controls	7.32 ± 0.02[a]	146.0 ± 3.0	20.8 ± 2.0	32.5 ± 12.5
Hypoxic	7.14 ± 0.01	43.6 ± 21.2	9.9 ± 3.1	32.8 ± 19.1

[a] $P < 0.05$.

The $(Na^+\text{-}K^+)$-dependent ATPase of the jejunum was measured by method of Kramer et al. [39] : subtracting ouabain-insensitive ATPase activity from total ATPase activity. Jejunal segment studied was 20 cm long, from ligament of Treitz.

in the transport of sodium across the small intestine. There was a decreased absorption of sodium in rats subjected to an atmosphere of 93% N_2 for up to 4 hr. Moreover, there was secretion of Na into the jejunal lumen with hypoxia more than 4 hr in duration.

Hypoxia also interfered with the intestinal transport of glucose. Rats exposed to an atmosphere of 93% N_2 for more than 4 hr showed a reduced absorption of

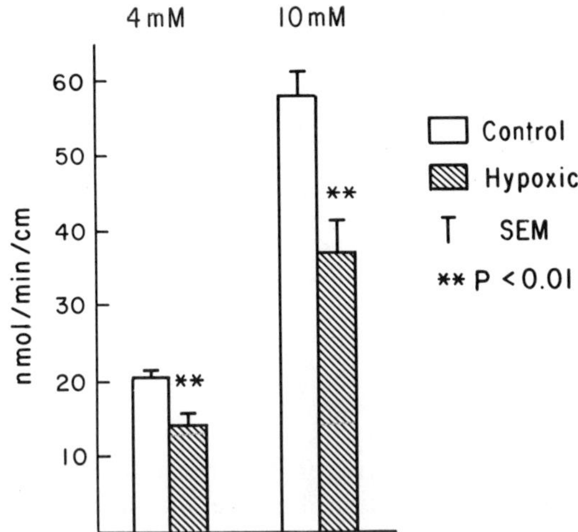

Figure 3 Effects of hypoxia on jejunal glucose transport. Intestinal transport of glucose was studied by in vivo perfusion technique described in detail elsewhere [40]. Krebs-Henseleith bicarbonate buffer was perfused at rate of 0.2 ml/min into jejunum for 2 hr while rats were kept in acrylic chambers under atmospheres of N_2/O_2, described in Figure 2.

glucose across the jejunum. Hypoxia maintained for 48 hr was associated with an even more severe alteration in the intestinal transport of this carbohydrate (as shown in Fig. 3). Both 4-mM and 10-mM perfusions resulted in decreased glucose transport. Moreover, hypoxia also interfered in the intestinal absorption of other actively transported solutes, such as amino acids (e.g., phenylalanine and tyrosine) and carbohydrates (e.g., galactose and 3-O-methylglucose), which are actively dependent on Na for their transport across the small-intestinal mucosa [27]. The reduced intestinal transport capacity was evident despite the fact that there were no alterations in intestinal disaccharidase levels in jejunal tissue or the ultrastructure of epithelial cells. These experimental findings suggest that hypoxia per se may play an important role in inducing alterations in intestinal transport—which could result in carbohydrate malabsorption as seen in several animal species [21, 22] and newborn infants [23-26].

V. Clinical Consequences of Carbohydrate Intolerance

The clinical consequences of carbohydrate intolerance are listed in Table 1. The most frequent complications of carbohydrate intolerance are dehydration and

Table 1 Consequences of Carbohydrate Intolerance

Prolongation of diarrhea
Increased severity of diarrhea
Dehydration and metabolic acidosis
Malnutrition
Bacterial proliferation in small bowel
Aggravation of intestinal malabsorption
Pneumatosis intestinalis
Macromolecular absorption

electrolyte deficits. Fluid losses in diarrhea are triggered by the initial insult (usually infection), but the severity may be influenced by the intestinal osmotic gradients induced by unabsorbed carbohydrates. It has long been known that fasting often reduces fluid losses in diarrhea, and the volume of water excreted by these patients may be up to three times that of an isotonic solution of the sugar present in the bowel [12]. In addition, there may be other smaller molecules of high osmotic potential, which result from carbohydrate fermentation and which contribute to fluid losses.

The duration of the disease may be related to carbohydrate intolerance more than to the infective agent which triggered the initial illness. For example, diarrhea in acute gastroenteritis may persist for as long as lactose is present in the diet; when this carbohydrate is eliminated, a prompt recovery may ensue [6].

Carbohydrate malabsorption can also lead to metabolic acidosis, which is a prominent feature of severe diarrhea. It has been shown that the most important source of excess hydrogen ions in children with diarrhea is bacterial carbohydrate fermentation [28]. In addition, the presence of organic acids within the intestinal lumen may stimulate the secretion and loss of large quantities of bicarbonate from serum to neutralize the luminal acid load.

The general nutritional status of an infant may be profoundly affected by carbohydrate malabsorption. Fifty percent of the total calorie requirements of children are derived from dietary carbohydrates. Therefore, losses of carbohydrates would account for considerable calorie deficits, even when diarrhea is mild. The presence of unabsorbed carbohydrates in the intestinal lumen also enhances protein and nitrogen losses [29]. In addition, it may lead to dilution of bile acid to concentrations below the critical micellar level for efficient fat absorption [30].

The presence of unabsorbed carbohydrates and of fermentative products in the small-bowel lumen during acute diarrhea may facilitate the colonization and proliferation of enteric bacteria in the upper segments of the intestine–an effect which may directly aggravate the intestinal function alterations [31]. It has been postulated that the initial infection that triggers acute diarrhea may induce a disturbed bowel function, with subsequent overgrowth of host colonic and fecal flora in the upper segments of the small intestine–a process that leads to a chronic diarrhea. Among the factors that may influence enteric bacterial dissemination are altered motility, presence of free carbohydrates in the lumen, and other metabolic alterations (e.g., luminal pH) resulting from carbohydrate intolerance [17]. Intestinal function might deteriorate further because of bacterial overpopulation of the upper bowel, which may generate additional injurious factors such as deconjugated bile salts, hydroxy fatty acids, and alcohol [17]–leading to aggravation of the intestinal malfunction and worsening of the diarrhea. When diarrhea persists for more than 2 weeks there is a higher incidence of generalized disaccharide intolerance, and, at times, even intolerance to all carbohydrates, including monosaccharides such as glucose and fructose. The intensification of intestinal malabsorption usually results when dietary therapy is delayed for 2-3 weeks [6]. Monosaccharide intolerance is present in up to 16% of patients who have diarrhea for more than 3 weeks [6, 32].

Continuing dietary intolerance and nutrient losses may also impair the infant's ability to recover from the initial illness and increase the susceptibility to other conditions. Pneumatosis intestinalis may result from carbohydrate intolerance [33], since unabsorbed carbohydrates generate large quantities of gas within the intestinal lumen [14]. The volume of the gas itself may, therefore, be sufficient to produce local intestinal abnormalities and pneumatosis intestinalis. The quantity of lactose contained in 30 ml of milk may produce 50 ml of gas in a normal person. Under abnormal circumstances, the bowel flora may increase the hydrogen production more than 100-fold. When the production of gas in the intestinal lumen exceeds the ability of the bowel to expel it, distension of the gut with increasing pressure results. If severe, it may lead to ischemia or necrosis of the intestinal mucosa, possibly providing access for the gas to the tissue space, resulting in pneumatosis intestinalis. This complication often occurs in infants with lactose intolerance secondary to diarrheal disease [33] and to neonatal hypoxia [23, 24, 26]. In both instances there is a process producing gas under pressure, namely, carbohydrate malabsorption–resulting from different mechanisms but leading to equivalent and often fatal complications.

It has long been known that macromolecular permeability might be altered in gastroenteritis, since there is measurable absorption of egg albumin, and frequently there are milk antibodies present in serum following diarrhea [34]. An increased macromolecular absorption with the development of hypersensitivity and allergy to foodstuffs could be related to malabsorption of monosaccharides and disaccharides, and to the severe hyperosmotic gradients which

Table 2 Serum HRP Levels in Rats Given Chronic Disaccharide Lactose Loads

Group	Serum HRP (μmol/min/cm)[a]
Controls	0.138 ± 0.005
Lactose	0.210 ± 0.020[b]
Maltose	0.115 ± 0.016

[a]Corrected for 0.2 ml/min perfusion rates/1 cm of intestine perfused.
[b]$P < 0.05$ versus controls.
Note: Male, albino Wistar rats, weighing about 100-150 g were used. The controls were fed a saline gavage, whereas the experimental groups were gavaged with a 60% carbohydrate solution. The forced feedings of any one of these solutions were administered at a dose of 5 ml/100 g body weight, twice daily, for 6 days. After the specific stress, the intestinal absorption of the macromolecular tracer HRP was studied 12 hr after the last dose of carbohydrate. The HRP was quantitated enzymatically by measuring serum concentrations after 1 hr of perfusion (0.2 ml/min) of jejunum with an isotonic glucose-saline solution, pH 6.9, containing 0.5 g% HRP type II.
Source: From Ref. 41.

result within the small intestine. Recent experimental studies in our laboratories [35] have indicated that elevated luminal osmolality due to a nonabsorbable agent, mannitol, leads to an enhanced rate of transport of a macromolecular tracer, horseradish peroxidase (HRP, molecular weight 40,000), across the intestinal epithelium. After 60 min of a hypertonic mannitol perfusion, transport of the tracer across the epithelium into the lamina propria of the villi was very marked. The HRP may be absorbed across the tight junctions which normally are a barrier to the leakage of macromolecules. Our data suggest that this barrier may be damaged by high luminal osmotic gradients.

An enhanced rate of HRP absorption is also demonstrable when rats are fed a diet high in lactose [36]. Rats are normally lactase deficient and therefore do not absorb lactose well after weaning. In Table 2 there are quantitative data on the absorption of HRP into serum following different disaccharide feedings. Lactose provoked an enhanced rate of HRP absorption even after only 1 day of such stress. This was associated with severe diarrhea. In contrast, feedings with another disaccharide which did not provoke diarrhea did not enhance HRP absorption over that seen in saline-fed controls, even after 1 week of maltose feedings. The possible clinical implications of these experimental findings were noted recently in a patient with carbohydrate intolerance and diarrhea, who developed soy protein sensitivity [37]. Other possible implications and findings regarding macromolecular transport across the intestine are reviewed in Chapter 13 of this volume.

VI. Therapeutic Considerations

The treatment of carbohydrate malabsorption by elimination of the offending carbohydrate from the diet usually results in prompt improvement. Dietary therapy should be instituted as soon as the diagnosis of carbohydrate intolerance is made. In the congenital forms of disaccharidase deficiency and of glucose-galactose malabsorption, prolonged adherence to the dietary regimen is necessary, although a gradual increase in tolerance of the offending carbohydrate might be observed. The disaccharides or monosaccharides involved should always be restricted in the diet to the quantities needed to keep the patient symptom-free and growing at a normal rate. Ultimately, a full diet might be tolerated. However, most patients require some limitations throughout life, with respect to their specific intolerances.

The dietary treatment of secondary carbohydrate intolerance in diarrheal disease has been published in detail elsewhere [38]. Since lactose intolerance occurs frequently in patients with short courses of diarrhea, the administration of feedings that contain disaccharides other than lactose is recommended in the early recovery period. Those patients who have had prolonged diarrheal courses usually have more generalized disaccharide intolerances and should, therefore, be treated with disaccharide-free, glucose-containing formulas. These diets are commercially available and may be routinely offered as the starting formulas for all infants hospitalized for severe diarrheal disease, provided that the glucose concentration is limited to 5% or less. The use of carbohydrate-free formulas should be reserved only for those patients who continue to have diarrhea and demonstrate glucose intolerance on such a regimen. Carbohydrate-free feedings are not without danger; hypoglycemia may ensue as a severe complication during the acute stage or after recovery. Utmost care should be exercised to provide parenteral glucose to these infants throughout the time they are not fed carbohydrates.

The capacity to tolerate all carbohydrates is rapidly recovered after the diarrhea ceases. Once glucose is tolerated, the disaccharides may be introduced. Maltose should be used initially, followed by sucrose and, ultimately, lactose. Even patients with severe forms of carbohydrate intolerance following gastroenteritis tolerate lactose within a few weeks of the acute stage of the illness. An attempt should be made to diagnose other alterations if carbohydrate intolerance persists. The elimination of dietary carbohydrates for prolonged periods may, of itself, perpetuate altered carbohydrate absorption [11] or other nutritional aberrations.

References

1. F. Lifshitz. Inborn errors of carbohydrate absorption. In *Metabolism and Disease* (T. K. Murray, Ed.). Food and Drug Directorate, Department of National Health and Welfare, Ottawa, 1971.
2. N. Kretchmer. Lactose and lactase. *Sci. Am. 227,* 70-78 (1972).
3. J. D. Johnson, N. Kretchmer, and F. J. Simoons. Lactose malabsorption: Its biology and history. *Adv. Pediatr. 21,* 197-237 (1974).
4. A. D. Newcomer, D. B. McGill, P. S. Thomas, and A. F. Hofmann. Tolerance to lactose among lactase deficient American Indians. *Gastroenterology 74,* 44-46 (1978).
5. J. J. Herbst, P. Sunshine, and N. Kretchmer. Intestinal malabsorption in infancy and childhood. *Adv. Pediatr. 16,* 11-64 (1969).
6. F. Lifshitz, P. Coello-Ramirez, G. Gutierrez-Topete, and M. C. Cornado-Cornet. Carbohydrate intolerance in infants with diarrhea. *J. Pediat. 79,* 760-767 (1971).
7. F. Lifshitz. Carbohydrate problems in pediatric gastroenterology. *Clin. Gastroenterol. 6,* 415-429 (1977).
8. H. Finkelstein and L. F. Meyer. Zur technik und Indikation der Ernährung mit Eiweissmilch. *Munch. Med. Wochenschr. 58,* 340-345 (1911).
9. G. M. Gray. Carbohydrate digestion and absorption. Role of the small intestine. *N. Engl. J. Med. 292,* 1225-1230 (1975).
10. I. H. Holmes, R. D. Schnagi, S. Rodger, B. J. Ruck, I. D. Gust, R. F. Bishop, and G. L. Barnes. Is lactase the receptor and uncoating enzyme for infantile enteritis (rota) viruses? *Lancet 1,* 1387-1388 (1976).
11. R. Pergolizzi, F. Lifshitz, S. Teichberg, and R. A. Wapnir. Interaction between dietary carbohydrates and intestinal disaccharidase in experimental diarrhea. *Am. J. Clin. Nutr. 30,* 482-489 (1977).
12. K. Launialia. The effect of unabsorbed sucrose and mannitol on the small intestinal flow rate and mean transit time. *Scand. J. Gastroenterol. 39,* 665-671 (1968).
13. S. Teichberg, F. Lifshitz, R. Pergolizzi, and R. A. Wapnir. Response of rat intestine to a hyperosmotic feeding. *Pediatr. Res. 12,* 720-725 (1978).
14. F. J. Ingelfinger. Malabsorption: The clinical background. *Fed. Proc. 26,* 1388-1390 (1967).
15. V. Kumar, R. Chandrasekaran, and R. Bhaskar. Carbohydrate intolerance associated with acute gastroenteritis. *Clin. Pediatr. 16,* 1123-1127 (1977).
16. W. P. T. James. Effects of protein-calorie malnutrition on intestinal absorption. *Ann. N.Y. Acad. Sci. 176,* 244-261 (1971).
17. F. Lifshitz. The enteric flora in childhood disease–Diarrhea. *Am. J. Clin. Nutr. 30,* 1811-1818 (1977).
18. Editorial. Rotavirus of man and animals. *Lancet 1,* 257-259 (1975).

19. A. Z. Kapikian, H. W. Kim, R. G. Wyatt, W. L. Cline, J. O. Arrobio, C. O. Brandt, W. J. Rodriguez, D. A. Sack, R. M. Chanock, and R. H. Parrott. Human reovirus-like agent as the major pathogen associated with winter gastroenteritis in hospitalized infants and young children. *N. Engl. J. Med. 294,* 965-972 (1976).
20. D. R. DeVillers. Ischaemia of the colon: An experimental study. *Br. J. Surg. 53,* 497-503 (1966).
21. D. W. Northrup and E. J. Van Liere. Effect of anoxia on absorption of glucose and glycine from small intestine. *Am. J. Physiol. 134,* 288-291 (1941).
22. J. E. Guthrie and J. H. Quastrel. Absorption of sugars and amino acids from isolated surviving intestine after experimental shock. *Arch. Biochem. Biophys. 62,* 485-496 (1956).
23. F. Akesode, F. Lifshitz, and M. Hoffman. Transient monosaccharide intolerance in a newborn infant. *Pediatrics 51,* 891-897 (1973).
24. L. S. Book, J. J. Herbst, and A. L. Jung. Carbohydrate malabsorption in necrotizing enterocolitis. *Pediatrics 57,* 201-204 (1976).
25. G. L. Bunton, G. M. Durbin, N. McIntosh, D. G. Shaw, A. Taghizadeh, E. O. R. Reynolds, R. P. A. Rivers, and G. Urman. Necrotizing enterocolitis: Controlled study of three years experience in a neonatal intensive care unit. *Arch. Dis. Child. 52,* 772-777 (1977).
26. N. Tejani, F. Lifshitz, and R. G. Harper. The response to an oral glucose load during convalescence from hypoxia in newborn infants. *J. Pediatr. 94,* 792-796 (1979).
27. F. Lifshitz, R. A. Wapnir, R. Pergolizzi, S. Teichberg, and A. Lipkin. Alterations in intestinal transport and Na^+-K^+ ATPase in hypoxia. *Fed. Proc. 35,* 464 (1976).
28. C. Lugo-de-Rivera, H. Rodriguez, and R. Torres-Pinnedo. Studies on the mechanism of sugar malabsorption in infantile infectious diarrhea. *Am. J. Clin. Nutr. 25,* 1248-1253 (1972).
29. D. C. Darrow. The retention of electrolyte during recovery from severe dehydration due to diarrhea. *J. Pediat. 28,* 515-539 (1946).
30. R. E. Ringrose, J. B. Thompson, and J. D. Walsh. Lactose malabsorption and steatorrhea. *Am. J. Dig. Dis. 17,* 533-538 (1972).
31. P. Coello-Ramirez and F. Lifshitz. Enteric microflora and carbohydrate intolerance in infants with diarrhea. *Pediatrics 49,* 233-242 (1972).
32. F. Lifshitz, P. Coello-Ramirez, and G. Gutierrez-Topete. Monosaccharide intolerance and hypoglycemia in infants with diarrhea. I. Clinical course of 23 cases. *J. Pediatr. 77,* 595-603 (1970).
33. P. Coello-Ramirez, G. Gutierres-Topete, and F. Lifshitz. Pneumatosis intestinalis. *Am. J. Dis. Child. 120,* 3-9 (1970).
34. F. L. Gruskay and R. E. Cooke. The gastrointestinal absorption of unaltered protein in normal infants and in infants recovering from diarrhea. *Pediatrics 16,* 763-769 (1955).
35. M. Cooper, S. Teichberg, and F. Lifshitz: Alterations in rat jejunal permeability to a macromolecular tracer during a hyperosmotic load. *Lab. Invest. 38,* 447-454 (1978).

36. F. Lifshitz, U. Fagundes-Neto, S. Teichberg, and M. A. Bayne. Enhanced macromolecular absorption in lactose-induced diarrhea. *Proceedings of the Eleventh International Congress of Nutrition,* Rio de Janeiro, Brazil, Aug. 1978. pp. 230.
37. K. Goel, F. Lifshitz, E. Kahn, and S. Teichberg. Monosaccharide intolerance and soy-protein hypersensitivity in an infant with diarrhea. *J. Pediatr. 93,* 617-619 (1978).
38. F. Lifshitz. Current therapy of the malabsorption syndrome and intestinal disaccharidase deficiencies. In *Current Pediatric Therapy,* 6th Ed. (S. Gellis and B. M. Kagan, Eds.). Saunders, Philadelphia, 1973, pp. 236-247.
39. H. J. Kramer, A. Backer, and F. Kruck. Inhibition of intestinal sodium potassium ATPase in experimental uremia. *Clin. Chim. Acta 50,* 13-18 (1974).
40. F. Lifshitz, R. A. Wapnir, H. J. Wehman, S. Diaz-Bensussen, and R. Pergolizzi. The effects of small intestinal colonization by fecal and colonic bacteria on intestinal function in rats. *J. Nutr. 711,* 1913-1923 (1978).
41. Peroxidase (horseradish). In *Worthington Enzyme Manual,* Worthington Biochemical Corp., Freehold, N.J., 1972, pp. 43-45.

24

Intestinal Enzyme Adaptation in Health and Disease

NORTON S. ROSENSWEIG / Cornell University Medical College, New York, New York, and North Shore University Hospital, Manhasset, New York

I. Introduction

Traditional teaching emphasizes the role of intestinal enzymes in the digestion and metabolism of the food that one eats. Studies in the past decade have called attention to the fact that the food one eats can alter the enzymes which act upon the food: i.e., the principle of adaptation to diet. These studies have dealt extensively with dietary sugars and the adaptive response of enzymes of carbohydrate digestion and metabolism. Accordingly, this review will focus on dietary sugars and the carbohydrate enzymes. In addition to clarifying normal physiologic mechanisms, these studies of adaptation and intestinal enzymes have helped to further our understanding of certain intestinal disorders.

II. Adaptive Properties of Intestinal Disaccharidases

A. Dietary Carbohydrates

The common dietary disaccharides are lactose, sucrose, and maltose. In the small intestine these disaccharides are poorly absorbed as intact molecules and must be hydrolyzed by their respective disaccharidases to their component monosaccharides in order for proper absorption to take place. The resulting monosaccharides are well absorbed. Lactose, or milk sugar, is hydrolyzed by lactase to glucose and galactose; sucrose, or table sugar, is split by sucrase to glucose and fructose; and maltose, the breakdown product of starch digestion, is

Present Affiliation:
Columbia University College of Physicians and Surgeons, and St. Luke's Hospital Center, New York, New York

hydrolyzed by maltase to two molecules of glucose. This hydrolysis takes place at the epithelial brush border of the villus. The subject of carbohydrate malabsorption is reviewed in detail in Chapter 16 of this book.

B. Adaptive Properties in Health

In many of the early studies, attempts were made to alter or increase lactase activity by feeding lactose [1-4]. In humans, these attempts have been based on the supposition that lactase activity was low as a result of failure to ingest adequate amounts of lactose in the diet. These attempts have all been singularly unsuccessful, demonstrating that human lactase does not adapt to dietary lactose and appears to be under genetic control [5].

Although the feeding of large amounts of lactose to humans failed to alter lactase activity, a series of subsequent investigations demonstrated that the feeding of selected dietary sugars can regulate human sucrase and maltase activities [2, 6, 7]. In these studies, performed under metabolic-ward conditions, normal human volunteers, with no history of disaccharide intolerance, were fed isocaloric liquid diets containing only one carbohydrate. Sucrose, glucose, fructose, maltose, lactose, and galactose were tested.

Specifically, sucrose feeding, as compared to glucose feeding, significantly increased jejunal sucrase and maltase activities but not lactase activity. The other sugars, lactose, galactose, and maltose, failed to increase activities above those seen with glucose. However, fructose, the end product of sucrose hydrolysis, produced an increase in sucrase and maltase activities similar to that seen with sucrose. This suggests that fructose is the active principle in the sucrose molecule and demonstrates that a specific substrate is not necessary for the adaptive response. When the results were expressed as sucrase-to-lactase and maltase-to-lactase ratios for each biopsy, a significant increase in both ratios was seen with sucrose and fructose feedings. It is felt that the use of the ratios minimizes variability in results due to the depth of the biopsy.

The adaptive increase in disaccharidase activity with sucrose feeding occurs in 2-5 days and falls in 2-5 days when sucrose feeding is discontinued [6]. This time response is similar to the estimated renewal or turnover time of the human small-intestinal epithelium. It suggests that the sucrose effect occurs at the crypt cell level and manifests itself as the crypt cell matures, migrates up the villus, and expresses the increase in disaccharidase activity.

Additional studies have demonstrated a dose-related response of sucrase and maltase activities to increasing doses of sucrose and glucose [7]. The increase in sucrose feeding produced a greater increase in the slope of the sucrase dose-response curve than did glucose feeding alone.

C. Adaptive Properties in Disease

The demonstration that fructose, a nonsubstrate, can regulate sucrase activity led to the speculation that fructose might be used to treat sucrase-isomaltase deficiency because fructose dose not require prior hydrolysis and is readily absorbed. Greene et al. tested this speculation [8]. A 7-year-old girl with almost lifelong diarrhea and a failure to gain weight was shown to have sucrase-isomaltase deficiency. With fructose feedings the sucrase and isomaltase activities increased fourfold, and the sucrose tolerance test changed from "flat" to a rise of 25 mg%. The child was next treated with a sucrose-restricted, 20% fructose diet. When fed this diet, the child became asymptomatic, gained weight, and could tolerate small amounts of sucrose.

Before any general conclusions can be offered, it will be necessary to treat other such patients with fructose, in order to determine if this is an effect seen in all such patients or is an effect limited only to this patient. Nonetheless, the above study shows that dietotherapy is a potentially effective treatment in selected enzyme deficiency states.

In diarrheal disease, there may be secondary alterations in the intestinal mucosa and a reduction in disaccharidase activities [9-12]. Thus, the ingestion of disaccharides during the acute stage of illness may lead to an increased severity of diarrhea, acidosis, and carbohydrate intolerance [13], all of which improve following elimination of the offending carbohydrate from the diet [13-16]. However, because of the possible relationship between dietary carbohydrate and intestinal disaccharidases, the enzyme deficiencies may be prolonged or even aggravated. Thus, the traditional method of dietary treatment in diarrhea [17], involving the removal of the offending carbohydrate, may itself give rise to subsequent intestinal enzyme deficiencies.

Recently it was suggested that all the jejunal disaccharidases are dependent upon their corresponding specific dietary substrates during diarrhea induced by a hyperosmotic load [18]. However complex the relationship between dietary carbohydrate intake and specific disaccharidases may be in normal rats, during osmotic diarrhea there is an enhanced dependence of disaccharidases on their specific substrates. The adaptive mechanisms by which these intestinal enzymes respond to the presence of their dietary substrates still remain to be resolved. The levels of disaccharidases may also be controlled by other factors, such as stress [19] or the release of gastrointestinal hormones (e.g., gastrin) that are known to be potent intestinal trophic hormones [20-22] and can directly stimulate intestinal disaccharidases.

The individual subunits of certain enzyme complexes appear to be independently regulated. Under osmotic diarrhea, dietary maltose (in the form of starch) prevented maltase activity from declining, but had no effect on sucrase activity [18]. The converse was also true; sucrose prevented sucrase reduction, but did not protect maltase. It is known that maltase activity is shared by several enzymes in the mammalian brush border, at least one of which has sucrase activity [23-25]. This enzyme complex has recently been fractionated into subunits with discrete activities [23-25]. Thus, it may turn out that the levels of particular subunits of such enzyme complexes or certain isozymes can be preferentially synthesized under particular conditions. Considerable work is obviously needed to make it possible to more fully understand this phenomenon.

The mechanisms of adaptation of the small intestine during stress and recovery, in an animal model, may help to provide an understanding of the best method of dealing with disaccharidase deficiencies and carbohydrate intolerance —conditions that are often present in patients with intestinal disease and diarrhea.

III. Adaptive Properties of Other Intestinal Enzyme Systems

Attention has been directed at investigating a possible adaptive response of other enzyme systems in addition to intestinal disaccharidases. A series of studies showed that these same dietary sugars, glucose and fructose, increased human and rat jejunal glycolytic enzyme activities [26-29]. Table 1 lists the enzymes evaluated in these studies of adaptation to dietary sugars.

There was a gradient of adaptive responses depending on the sugar fed and enzyme studied. All the enzyme activities were higher with high-carboyhydrate diets as compared with carbohydrate-free diets. Also, specific enzymes were highest with specific sugars. Glucose feeding produced the highest increase in hexokinase activity; fructose feeding led to highest increases in fructokinase, fructose-1-phosphate aldolase, and pyruvate kinase activities; and

Table 1 Glycolytic Enzymes Investigated in Dietary Adaptation Studies

Enzyme	Reaction
Hexokinase	Glucose + ATP → glucose-6-phosphate + ADP
Fructose-1,6-diphosphate aldolase	Fructose-1,6-diphosphate → glyceraldehyde-3-phosphate + dihydroxyacetone-phosphate
Fructokinase	Fructose + ATP → fructose-1-phosphate + ADP
Fructose-1-phosphate aldolase	Fructose-1-phosphate → glyceraldehyde + dihydro-hydroxyacetone-phosphate
Pyruvate kinase	Phosphoenol pyruvate + ADP → pyruvate + ATP

galactose feeding produced the highest activities of the galactose-metabolizing enzymes.

In contrast with the disaccharidases, glycolytic enzyme adaptation occurred in hours and was complete in 1 day [30-32]. This suggests that glycolytic enzyme adaptation occurs directly at the villus epithelial cell level, in contrast with disaccharidase adaptation, which occurs at the crypt cell level. The mechanism of the adaptive response is unknown.

The regulation of intestinal enzymes of carbohydrate metabolism is not limited to dietary sugars. Studies of glycolytic enzymes in patients with tropical sprue has led to the investigation of the effects of folic acid and other substances in patients and normal volunteers [32, 33]. Oral folic acid produces an increase in jejunal glycolytic enzyme activities but not in disaccharidase activity. The effect is not seen with tetracycline, vitamin B_{12}, or intramuscular folate. The mechanism is unknown. Subsequent studies have shown that certain drugs and hormones also regulate human jejunal glycolytic enzymes [29, 34-36].

In a preliminary report, the author and his colleagues have studied this adaptive response of jejunal glycolytic enzyme activities to dietary sugars in selected patients with chronic gastrointestinal complaints (such as diarrhea) and negative conventional gastrointestinal evaluation [37]. It was postulated that, if the dietary regulation of intestinal enzymes is a necessary physiologic mechanism, then a failure of this regulation should be associated with gastrointestinal disorders. In many of the patients, the high-carbohydrate diet failed to produce an adaptive increase in glycolytic enzyme activities. In addition, these high-carbohydrate diets often exacerbated symptoms in these patients, while the carbohydrate-free diets produced relief.

This association between the failure of enzyme adaptation to dietary sugars and the production of symptoms by these sugars has been terms an "intestinal maladaptation syndrome." Although the mechanism of this syndrome is not understood, these studies show that disorders of gastrointestinal function need not be related to an enzyme deficiency state. Possibly the defect is due to a failure of the proper regulation of enzyme activity (or metabolic process) by stimuli such as diet. Further studies of this syndrome are needed to define its specific role in clinical medicine.

References

1. N. S. Rosensweig. *A Review of Dietary Lactose and Its Varied Utilization by Man.* Whey Products Institute, Chicago, 1978.
2. N. S. Rosensweig and R. H. Herman. Control of jejunal sucrase and maltase activity by dietary sucrose or fructose in man. A model for the study of enzyme regulation in man. *J. Clin. Invest. 47,* 2253-2262 (1968).

3. T. Gilat, S. Russo, E. Gelman-Malachi, and T. A. M. Aldor. Lactase in man: A nonadaptable enzyme. *Gastroenterology 62,* 1125-1127 (1972).
4. G. T. Keusch, F. J. Troncale, B. Thararamara, P. Prinyaront, P. R. Anderson, and N. B. Bhamarapiarath. Lactase deficiency in Thailand: Effect of prolonged lactose feeding. *Am. J. Clin. Nutr. 22,* 638-641 (1969).
5. N. S. Rosensweig. Adult lactase deficiency: Genetic control or adaptive response? *Gastroenterology 60,* 464-467 (1971).
6. N. S. Rosensweig and R. H. Herman. Time response of jejunal sucrase and maltase activity to a high sucrose diet in normal man. *Gastroenterology 56,* 500-505 (1969).
7. N. S. Rosensweig and R. H. Herman. Dose response of jejunal sucrase and maltase activities to isocaloric high and low carbohydrate diets in man. *Am. J. Clin. Nutr. 23,* 1373-1377 (1970).
8. H. L. Greene, F. B. Stifel, and R. H. Herman. Dietary stimulation of sucrase in a patient with sucrase-isomaltase deficiency. *Biochem. Med. 6,* 409-418 (1972).
9. F. Lifshitz and G. H. Holman. Disaccharidase deficiencies with steatorrhea. *J. Pediatr. 64,* 34-44 (1964).
10. P. Sunshine and N. Kretchmer. Studies of small intestine during development. III. Infantile diarrhea associated with intolerance to disaccharides. *Pediatrics 34,* 38-50 (1964).
11. N. J. Hirschhorn, J. R. Saha, and A. Siddeque. Jejunal disaccharidase activities in acute diarrhea and convalescence. Abstract. *Gastroenterology 54,* 1244 (1968).
12. G. Aguss, R. Dolin, R. G. Wyatt, A. J. Tousimis, and R. S. Northrup. Acute infectious nonbacterial gastroenteritis: Intestinal histopathology. *Ann. Intern. Med. 79,* 18-25 (1973).
13. F. Lifshitz, R. Coello-Ramirez, G. Gutierrez-Topete, and M. C. Cornado-Cornet. Carbohydrate intolerance in infants with diarrhea. *J. Pediatr. 79,* 760-767 (1971).
14. F. Lifshitz, P. Coello-Ramirez, and G. Gutierrez-Topete. Monosaccharide intolerance and hypoglycemia in infants with diarrhea. I. Clinical course of 23 cases. *J. Pediatr. 77,* 595-603 (1970).
15. P. Coello-Ramirez, G. Gutierrez-Topete, and F. Lifshitz. Pneumatosis intestinalis. *Am. J. Dis. Child. 120,* 3-9 (1970).
16. M. D. Bowie, G. L. Brinkman, and J. D. L. Hansen. Acquired disaccharide intolerance in malnutrition. *J. Pediatr. 66,* 1083-1091 (1965).
17. F. Lifshitz. Current therapy of the malabsorption syndrome and intestinal disaccharidase deficiencies. In *Current Pediatric Therapy,* 6th Ed. (S. Gellis and B. M. Kagan, Eds.). Saunders, Philadelphia, 1973, pp. 236-248.
18. R. Pergolizzi, F. Lifshitz, S. Teichberg, and R. A. Wapnir. Interaction between dietary carbohydrates and intestinal disaccharidases in experimental diarrhea. *Am. J. Clin. Nutr. 30,* 482-489 (1977).
19. O. Koldovsky and F. Chytil. Postnatal development of β-galactosidase

activity in the small intestine of the rat. Effect of adrenalectomy and diet. *Biochem. J. 94,* 266-270 (1965).
20. L. R. Johnson and P. D. Guthrie. Secretin inhibition of gastrin-stimulated deoxyribonucleic acid synthesis. *Gastroenterology 67,* 610-616 (1974).
21. L. R. Johnson, L. M. Lichtenberger, E. M. Copeland, S. J. Dudrick, and G. A. Castro. Action of gastrin on gastrointestinal structure and function. *Gastroenterology 68,* 1184-1192 (1975).
22. G. A. Castro, E. M. Copeland, S. J. Dudrick, and L. R. Johnson. Alteration of mucosal enzymes in response to the absence of food in the gastrointestinal tract. *Gastroenterology 68,* 1177-1183 (1975).
23. H. Braun, A. Gogoli, and G. Semenza. Dissection of small intestinal sucrase-isomaltase complex into enzymatically active subunits. *Eur. J. Biochem. 52,* 475-480 (1975).
24. A. Quaroni, E. Gershon-Quaroni, and G. Semenza. Tryptic digestion of native small intestinal sucrase-isomaltase complex. Isolation of the sucrase subunit. *Eur. J. Biochem. 52,* 481-486 (1975).
25. J. Kolinska and J. Kramel. Separation and characteristics of sucrase isomaltase and of glucoamylase of rat intestine. *Biochim. Biophys. Acta 284,* 235-247 (1972).
26. N. S. Rosensweig, F. B. Stifel, R. H. Herman, and D. Zakim. The dietary regulation of the glycolytic enzymes. II. Adaptive changes in human jejunum. *Biochim. Biophys. Acta 170,* 228-234 (1968).
27. N. S. Rosensweig, R. H. Herman, and F. B. Stifel. Dietary regulation of glycolytic enzymes. VI. Effect of dietary sugars and oral folic acid on human jejunal pyruvate kinase, phosphofructokinase and fructose-diphosphatase activities. *Biochim. Biophys. Acta 208,* 373-380 (1970).
28. F. B. Stifel, N. S. Rosensweig, D. Zakim, and R. H. Herman. Dietary regulation of glycolytic enzymes. I. Adaptive changes in rat jejunum. *Biochim. Biophys. Acta 170,* 221-227 (1968).
29. F. B. Stifel, R. H. Herman, and N. S. Rosensweig. Dietary regulation of glycolytic enzymes. IV. *Biochim. Biophys. Acta 184,* 495-502 (1969).
30. N. S. Rosensweig, F. B. Stifel, D. Zakim, and R. H. Herman. Time response of human jejunal glycolytic enzymes to a high sucrose diet. *Gastroenterology 57,* 143-146 (1969).
31. N. S. Rosensweig, F. B. Stifel, R. H. Herman, and D. Zakim. Time response of diet-induced changes in human jejunal glycolytic enzymes. Abstract. *Fed. Proc. 28,* 323 (1969).
32. N. S. Rosensweig, R. H. Herman, F. B. Stifel, and Y. F. Herman. Regulation of human jejunal glycolytic enzymes by oral folic acid. *J. Clin. Invest. 48,* 2038-2045 (1969).
33. N. S. Rosensweig, R. H. Herman, F. B. Stifel, Y. F. Herman, A. Dreskin, and D. Chipman. Effect of folic acid on jejunal glycolytic enzyme activity in tropical sprue. Abstract. *Gastroenterology 56,* 1261 (1969).

34. E. G. Lufkin, F. B. Stifel, R. H. Herman, N. S. Rosensweig, and L. Hagler. Effect of testosterone on jejunal pyruvate kinase activities in normal hypogonadal males. *J. Clin. Endocrinol. Metab. 34,* 586-591 (1972).
35. N. S. Rosensweig, F. B. Stifel, and R. H. Herman. Effect of phenobarbital (PB) on human jejunal glycolytic, gluconeogenetic and pentose phosphate path enzymes. Abstract. *Clin. Res. 17,* 596, (1969).
36. D. Zakim, R. H. Herman, N. S. Rosensweig, and F. B. Stifel. Clofibrate-induced changes in the activity of human intestinal enzymes. *Gastroenterology 56,* 494-499 (1969).
37. N. S. Rosensweig, R. H. Herman, F. B. Stifel, L. Hagler, H. L. Greene, Jr., and Y. F. Herman. Gastrointestinal disease associated with a failure of adaptation of jejunal glycolytic enzymes. Abstract. *Gastroenterology 62,* 802 (1972).

25
Growth Failure in Intestinal Diseases

DREW G. KELTS* and RICHARD J. GRAND / Harvard Medical School, and The Children's Hospital Medical Center, Boston, Massachusetts

I. Introduction

Severe impairment of linear growth is a well-known complication of chronic disease in childhood and may serve as an important marker of the duration and activity of disease. Growth failure is often the major complication for which definitive treatment is sought by the patient, and restitution of normal growth often signals remission of disease. Of all the manifestations of chronic illness in childhood, none is as poorly understood or resistant to therapy as chronic growth failure. Recently, accumulating data have pointed to the nutritional basis for growth failure in many gastrointestinal disorders. Indeed, reversal of growth failure can be achieved in a number of intestinal disorders by purely nutritional means.

It is the purpose of this discussion to review available data concerning growth failure in gastrointestinal disorders, to highlight the metabolic implications of such complications, and to identify effective forms of therapy where available. This discussion is by no means encyclopedic, and for additional information the reader is referred to the recent monograph of Smity [1] and that of Cheek [2].

II. Normal Growth and Development

Under normal conditions, human growth is a dynamic and complex process whereby the young infant changes proportions, shape, size, and cell number in a carefully regulated pattern. Growth in childhood and adolescence is a smooth process which, when recorded on a growth chart, is usually

Present Affiliation:
*University of California Medical Center, San Diego, California.

"channeled." That is, it continues along a relatively narrow path, unchanged except for a slowing of the rate in the first two years of life and a rapid acceleration in adolescence. For the purposes of discussion, normal growth may be divided into four major periods.

A. Intrauterine Development

Until approximately 5 months of gestational age, there is a rapid increase in growth rate with almost concomitant development of weight and height. Thereafter, size at birth appears to be related primarily to maternal factors—uterine size and state of nutrition being primary. The smaller the mother's body habitus, the greater is the likelihood for a small newborn. Firstborn infants tend to be an average of 0.34 cm smaller and 0.18 kg lighter than subsequent siblings. Male fetuses grow faster than female, particularly after the 32nd week of gestation, and average 0.9 cm longer and 0.15 kg heavier than females at birth. The bone age of girls is often advanced over that of boys by about 2 weeks of age, and this trend in bone age advancement continues until approximately 1 year of age.

B. Birth and Infancy

If early nutrition is adequate, infants begin to seek their "genetic channel" for growth within the first 9-18 months of life. Depending on the genetic potential for size, one-third of infants appear to adjust their weight upward in percentiles, one-third remain stable, and one-third adjust their weight down in percentiles toward their predestined size. While birth weight appears to be governed by maternal factors, size after birth appears to be dictated by genetic factors which may be affected by environmental influences.

In the first year of life, rapid weight gain appears in excess of increase in linear growth. The normal linear growth of approximately double the birth length is usually reached by 1 year. Linear growth rate then begins to slow by age 2 years, and weight gain will continue to predominate throughout childhood. Head growth and brain growth attain peak velocity at birth and slow thereafter until age 2 years, when 90% of adult head size has been achieved. The remainder of body growth, however, continues, and the skull which was 20% of the body weight in the infancy period is only 3% of the body weight by age 16.

C. Childhood

Growth from age 2 to 10 years tends to remain remarkably constant, ranging between 5 and 7.5 cm per year, with a gradual slowing as the child approaches adolescence. Adiposity increases from midchildhood on, particularly as the child begins the adolescent growth spurt. During this period, growth tends to remain within the genetic channel. Boys appear to grow more rapidly at this stage than girls, but do not enter puberty as early.

D. Adolescence

Adolescence is a time of widely divergent growth patterns, determined primarily by genetic and nutritional factors. Parental growth patterns paly an important role in the expression of adolescent growth. Linear growth rate normally increases to an average of 9 cm per year at age 12 years. Menarche generally follows at age 13 years, but girls will often continue to show slowing growth rates for as long as 4 or 5 additional years. Boys appear to show a more predictable pattern, with the onset of puberty occurring between 9 and 12 years, paralleled by testicular enlargement. Linear growth increases steadily to a peak velocity of 10.3 cm per year at approximately 14 years. Although most linear growth is accomplished by 18 years in males, growth may continue until age 21 years or even after, with additional height accrued mostly in the trunk.

Both lean body mass and fat accumulate during the adolescent growth spurt, but the proportion of fat growth in girls is greater, resulting in approximately 25% of body weight as fat at maturity, as opposed to about 12-18% in boys. The larger the child before the adolescent growth spurt, the greater the tendency for early and rapid maturation. Likewise, the smaller the child, the longer and slower the process is likely to be. Against this background, one may begin to evaluate the impact of disease on growth. The wide variety of patterns and rates, as well as sex differences, must be analyzed if one is to decide whether altered growth truly represents the effects of illness or is merely an expression of variations in an individual's normal pattern.

Abnormalities in growth patterns induced by chronic disease are often accompanied by delays in sexual maturation, and an association between such developmental retardation and nutritional status has been cited repeatedly. This concept has led to the popularization of "critical weight" as a necessary precursor to normal sexual maturation [3], a theory which has received considerable criticism [4]. Nevertheless, abnormal height and weight patterns have been identified in numerous chronic diseases in childhood which are also associated with poor nutrition. Many of these diseases involve the gastrointestinal tract.

III. Nutritional Deprivation and "Catch-up" Growth

One of the criteria for reversal of a pathological process affecting growth is the pattern of growth during the healing process. That is, does growth continue along a lower channel as a result of permanent injury to the growth pattern, or does it "catch up" and return to the premorbid, genetically determined channel? Very often the nature of the insult, its time of onset, and its duration are the critical factors in the subsequent growth pattern.

The concept of catch-up growth deserves further comment. In 1963, in a study of chronically ill children with growth failure, Prader et al. demonstrated that the depressed growth velocity which accompanied clinical illness was rapidly recovered when the disease was cured or controlled [5]. The authors were thus able to demonstrate acceleration of growth velocity, at a rate well beyond normal, which occurred until the child's size more closely approximated its genetically determined premorbid level. Skeletal maturation also followed a similar pattern of catch-up growth.

Forbes [6] has recently developed a mathematical model describing catch-up growth, which shows that the velocity excess during the recovery period must at least equal the deficit previously present in order to correct the abnormal growth pattern. The mechanisms which control the onset and cessation of catch-up growth are unknown. Clearly, however, *energy supply* in the form of calories and other metabolic substrates and *energy utilization* for either growth or other metabolic needs must be critical factors.

Energy requirements may be conceptualized as follows: energy is necessary for catch-up growth, and food intake must meet the increased requirements during the entire recovery period if catch-up growth is to be achieved. The total energy required during the period of active growth in adolescence, if growth failure has previously occurred, can be considered in terms of the following formula:

Energy (total) = energy (maintenance) + energy (for growth) + energy (deficit)

Maintenance energy is that which supplies normal metabolic processes for a given body size. Energy for growth is a variable depending upon the maturational age of the child, being high during periods of rapid growth (infancy and adolescence) and less, but still present, during periods of slower growth. If demands for energy for growth are successfully met, maintenance energy requirements also rise as body mass increases. These two terms may be considered together in the normal child since they are inextricably bound during the growth process. Energy for deficit is that which would be required to return a child with subnormal growth to a body mass appropriate for height *before* subsequent growth would occur. Thus, in a growth-deprived child, energy deficits must be replaced before active catch-up growth begins.

In the normal state, appetite fulfills these energy demands. Indeed, during recovery from severe malnutrition, appetite is usually increased [7]. It is known that chronic disease markedly alters appetite; and the ability to ingest adequate calories may also be impaired in many gastrointestinal disorders associated with severe growth failure.

IV. Clinical Features of Growth Failure

The patterns of growth after the onset of clinical illness are quite similar, no matter what the etiology of the disease. Thus, patients with celiac sprue (gluten-sensitive enteropathy), chronic liver disease, inflammatory bowel disease, and numerous other disorders may present with a similar impact on growth. Figure 1 shows a 16-year-old girl with Crohn's disease which began when she was 12 years old. Menarche never appeared, secondary sex characteristics are absent, she is in the 10th percentile for height (having previously been in the 50th percentile), and, at the time she was first seen, she also showed the chronic stigmata of malnutrition.

A growth pattern for a child with cystic fibrosis and celiac disease is shown in Figure 2. This child, who has been reported upon previously [8], showed the marked reduction in weight quite typical of the onset of infantile celiac disease, as well as marked catch-up growth with the institution of a gluten-free diet.

A typical growth pattern for a patient with Crohn's disease is shown in Figure 3. This patient was in the 50th percentile for height and weight prior to the onset of illness, and, as can be readily seen, growth failure began prior to the onset of clinical symptoms, probably at about age 10½. It is obvious that, by the time symptoms appeared, severe impairment of linear growth and weight gain had occurred—which were not significantly improved by steroids. However, the total removal of affected bowel led to complete recovery, with catch-up growth; and the patient remained well after surgery. Note that both height and weight returned to slightly abobe the 50th percentile by age 18.

Figure 4 shows a similar patient, whose growth and development prior to the onset of illness had been in the 40th percentile. Note that a change in percentile growth occurred prior to the onset of symptoms; that steroid therapy achieved improvement in weight gain but not in linear growth; and that surgery with complete removal of the diseased segment was followed by catch-up growth and return to the premorbid growth channel. A recurrence which occurred at age 17, after puberty had been completed, had no effect on weight or linear growth.

By contrast, the patient shown in Figure 5 had a much more serious problem. This boy was in the 10th percentile for height and weight prior to the onset of Crohn's disease. He then had prolonged and severe growth failure despite medical and surgical intervention. A course of hyperalimentation at age 17½ stimulated improved weight gain but had no major effect on linear growth, although over the next several years linear growth did occur, with the slow appearance of puberty; and by age 20 he had reached a height of 62 in (now shown).

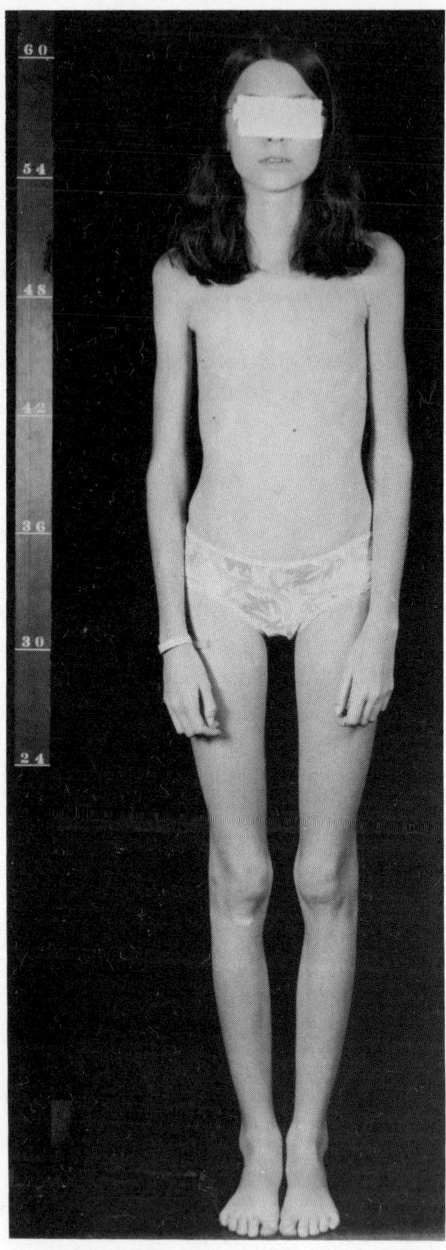

Figure 1 A 16-year-old girl with Crohn
disease which began at age 12 years. N
severe growth failure and malnutrition.

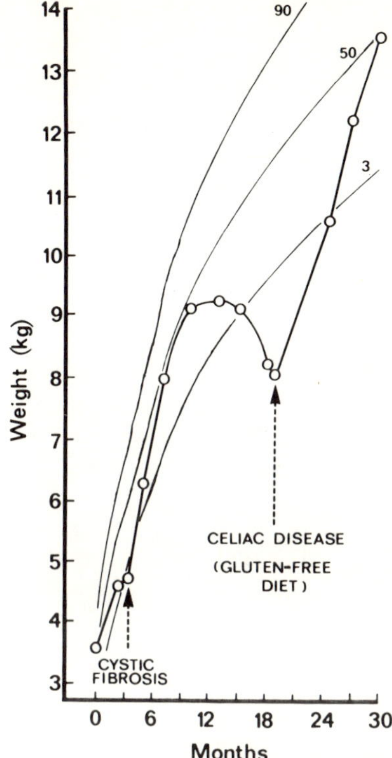

Figure 2 Growth pattern of child with cystic fibrosis and celiac sprue. (Reprinted from Ref. 8, with permission.)

A growth pattern from a patient with gylcogen storage disease (type IV) is shown in Figure 6. Note that the onset of serious liver disease clinically (shown by the arrow) was preceded by significant growth impairment. Despite attempts at adequate nutrition, the clinical course was complicated by anorexia, abdominal distension with ascites, and steatorrhea; prolonged and severe failure to thrive ensued. The growth pattern is quite similar to that presented above for the patients with Crohn's disease and celiac disease.

Since most of our data on growth failure and chronic disease are related to studies of Crohn's disease in the pediatric age range, the remainder of the present chapter will emphasize inflammatory bowel disease. Nevertheless, all of the mechanisms involved in the etiology of the growth failure and the nutritional impact on growth in inflammatory bowel disease can be applied to most other diseases of the gastrointestinal tract which affect growth. Therefore, inflammatory bowel diseases should be considered as prototype disorders—the information from which could be applied to chronic liver disease, celiac sprue, cystic fibrosis, and other chronic malabsorptive states, such as short small-bowel

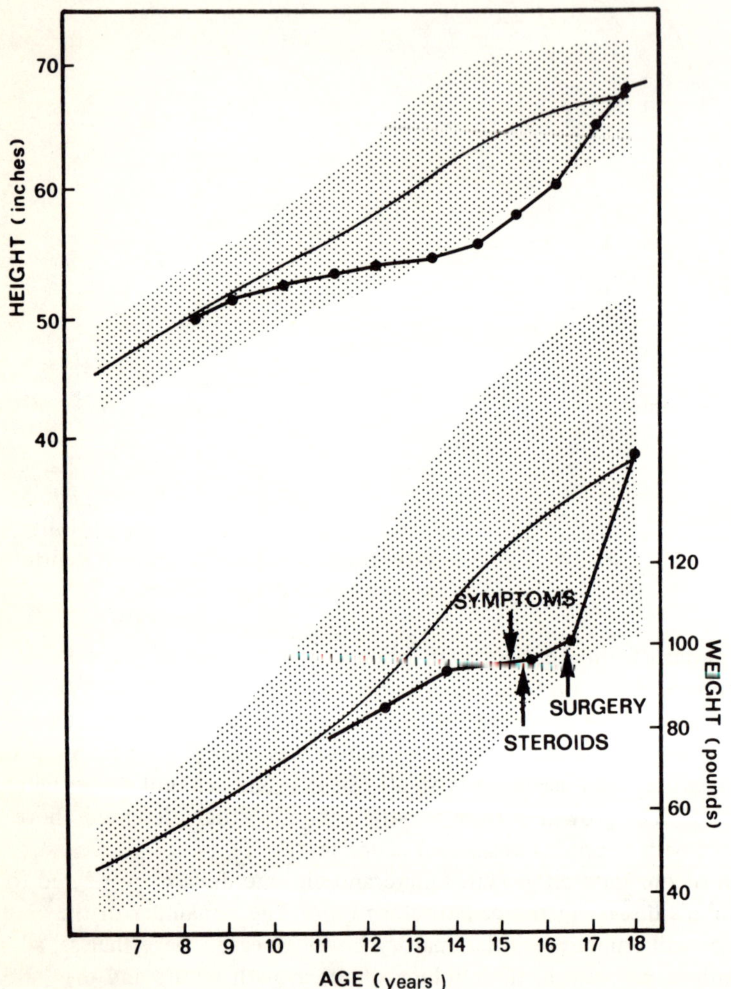

Figure 3 Growth pattern of child with Crohn's disease, who demonstrated "catch-up" growth after surgery.

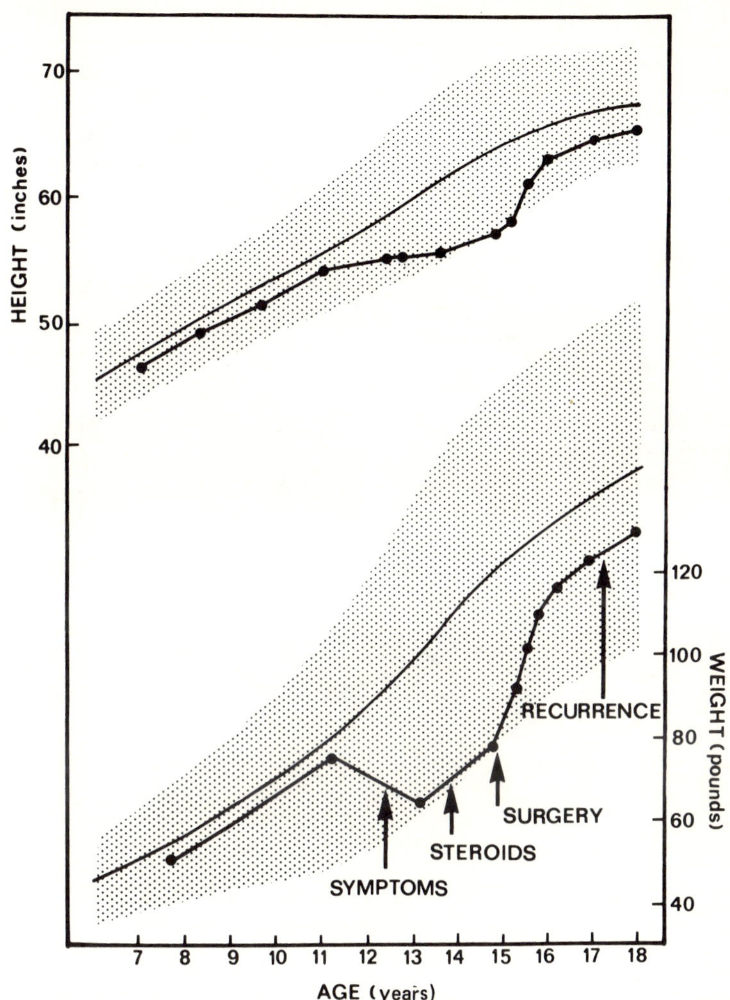

Figure 4 Growth pattern of child with Crohn's disease, who demonstrated "catch-up" growth after surgery and before onset of recurrence.

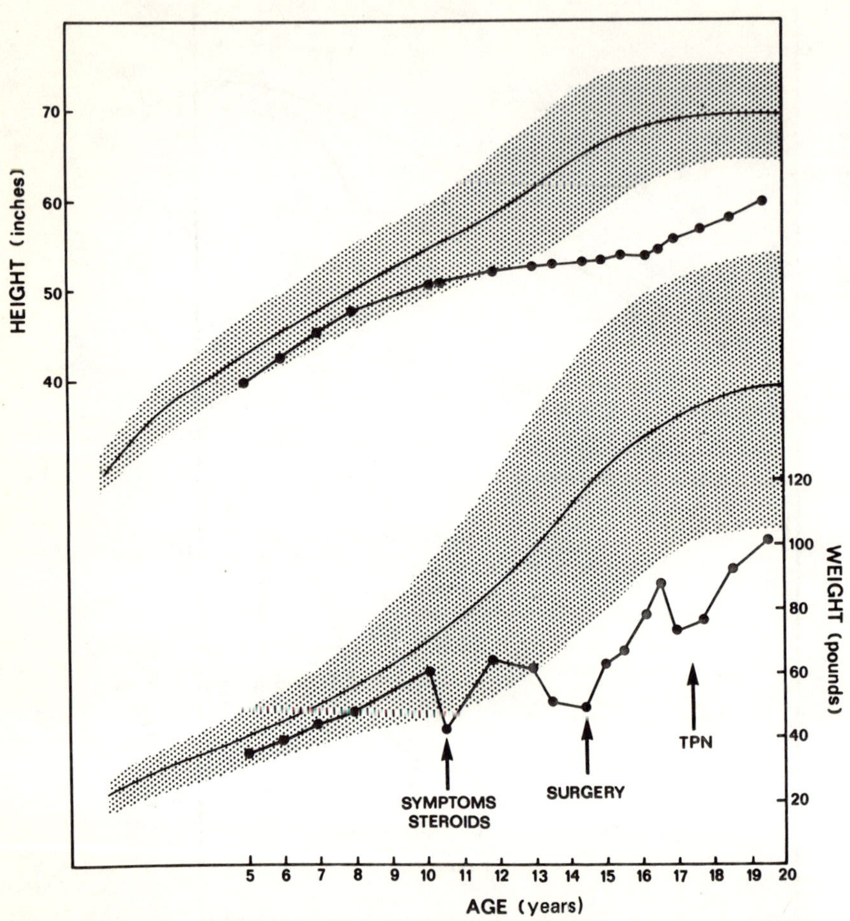

Figure 5 Growth pattern of child with Crohn's disease, demonstrating prolonged and severe growth retardation, despite steroids, surgery, and total parenteral nutrition.

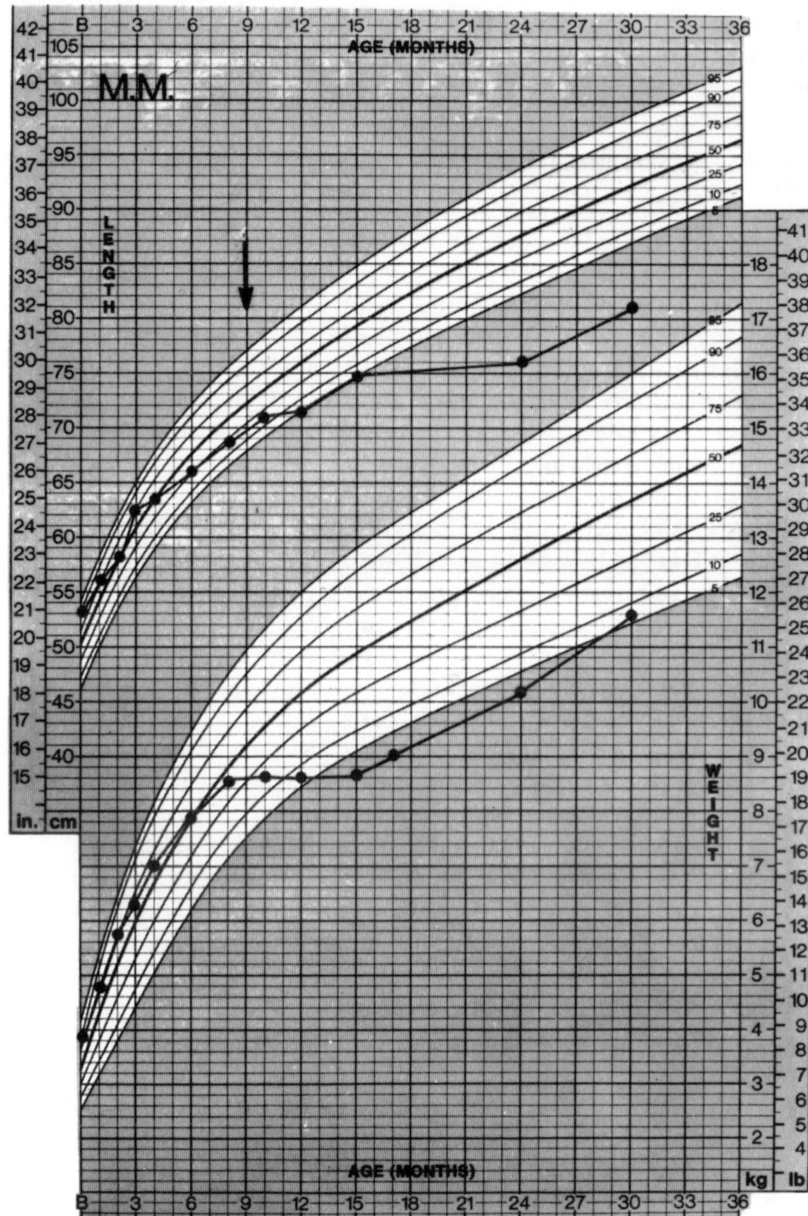

Figure 6 Growth pattern of child with glycogen storage disease (type IV), showing growth retardation beginning before the onset of clinically apparent liver disease (arrow).

syndrome. In addition, chronic diseases of other organ systems may produce similar defects in growth, including chronic congestive heart failure and chronic renal failure.

V. Growth Failure and Inflammatory Bowel Disease

Severe impairment of linear growth in inflammatory bowel disease appears to have been recorded for the first time by Snapper et al. [9] in a 15-year-old boy with Crohn's disease. In 1939, Davidson [10] first reported the association of severe growth failure with ulcerative colitis. These observations have been confirmed over the years by every physician who has ever cared for children with inflammatory bowel disease. Cessation of linear growth, lack of weight gain, retarded bone development, and delayed onset of sexual maturation are seen frequently [11-13], and it is not uncommon to find growth failure preceding clinical evidence of bowel disease—often by years, as demonstrated in the previous figures.

In the series of McCaffery et al. [11], of 130 patients with inflammatory bowel disease and under 21 years of age, 22 patients were found whose growth failure was so severe as to place them more than 2 standard deviations below the mean height for age. Of these patients, 19 had Crohn's disease, 3 had ulcerative colitis. In our own clinic we have had the opportunity to observe 37 children and adolescents with Crohn's disease [13]. These patients were selected from 139 patients with inflammatory bowel disease followed over a 15-year period. The ages of the patients at the time of diagnosis were 8-18 years. Of the 37 patients, 28 had disease involving both colon and terminal ileum; 9 had disease limited to the small intestine or stomach. When first seen, 16 patients were at or below the 3rd percentile for weight, and only 16 of the 37 patients had reached puberty. All of the latter group were older than 14½ years of age. There were 14 of the 37 patients who had severe impairment of linear growth; height was at or below the third percentile, or linear growth had been absent for more than a year. Of these patients 11 were prepubertal, and 3 were pubertal. These 14 patients represented approximately 25% of our population with Crohn's disease (approximately 65 patients in this period of time).

The nutritional classification of some of these patients with growth failure and Crohn's disease is shown in Table 1. These data show that patients with Crohn's disease who fail to grow prior to puberty are indeed "nutritional dwarfs," fitting the criteria of Waterlow [14] for chronic malnutrition. Thus, the majority of the patients, while short for age, are not markedly abnormal for weight, all but three attaining greater than 80% of expected weight for height.

Table 1 Nutritional Classification of Growth Failure in Crohn's Disease

% Expected weight for height	% Expected height for age			
	>95	95-87.5	87.5-80	<80
>90	3	4	3	1
90-80	2	1	0	1
80-70	0	1	1	0
<70	0	1	0	0

Note: Data shown are the numbers of patients in each category.

The etiology of this abnormality in linear growth has not been elucidated. The problem is multifactorial, and in previous studies it has been impossible to assign a single cause in an individual patient—but perhaps because appropriate investigations have not been routinely performed. The factors which are involved are: (1) inadequate intake, (2) excessive losses, (3) malabsorption, (4) possible hormone imbalances, and (5) increased nutritional requirements.

A. Inadequate Intake

Inadequate intake may occur because of anorexia induced by chronic illness. Often, patients may be unwilling to eat because of increases in diarrhea accompanying the ingestion of food or because of exacerbation of abdominal pain following meals. Anorexia is also a common feature of chronic liver disease, celiac sprue, and cystic fibrosis. The anorexia that occurs in cystic fibrosis can be demonstrated to worsen with increasing severity of pulmonary disease. It was previously thought that cystic fibrosis was characterized by a ravenous appetite. However, this appears to be true only for the infancy period. In the first few months of life, the child with untreated cystic fibrosis appears to be able to compensate for the marked losses of fat and nitrogen in the stool by increasing the intake for body size. Once the infant has reached a body size that it can no longer maintain on the basis of appetite alone, growth failure ensues. This appears to be a response of the body to the relatively reduced caloric intake for body mass. It is an estimated observation that children with cystic fibrosis have, as a group, abnormal growth-patterns—particularly in adolescence. Even if intake is not markedly reduced, *defects in intestinal absorption* are common in children and adolescents with Crohn's disease [15-19].

Table 2 reviews data collected from recent studies in adults and children. Approximately one-third of adults and children with Crohn's disease exhibit abnormal xylose absorption tests. This test, therefore, reflects either mucosal

Table 2 Malabsorption in Crohn's Disease

Absorption defect	Frequency of Defect: Adults	Children
Carbohydrate		
Xylose	31/80 (40%)	3/18 (16%)
Lactose	2/23 (10%)	3/17 (17%)
Fat		
Serum carotene	44/47 (94%)	–
Fecal fat	34/79 (43%)	5/17 (29%)
Protein		
Serum albumin <3.3 g%	43/83 (52%)	9/17 (52%)
Protein loss	21/30 (70%)	12/17 (70%)
Bacterial overgrowth	11/36 (30%)	–

Source: From Refs. 15-19, 28.

injury or bacterial overgrowth. Lactose absorption is abnormal in not more than 20% of the patients, reflecting the prevalence of lactose intolerance in the normal mixed white population [20]. Therefore, no specificity can be applied to the abnormality of this test in patients with Crohn's disease, although its presence signifies a need for investigation of mucosal function.

Most of the patients studied for fat malabsorption have shown a quite significant correlation between location of disease and degree of abnormalities in fat metabolism. Those with small-bowel disease tend to have more steatorrhea than those with disease limited to the colon. Interestingly, serum carotene levels are often low in adults, many of whom do not show steatorrhea. Excessive loss of fat in the stools occurs in approximately 40% of adults and children with Crohn's disease. These abnormalities reflect varying combinations of mucosal injury, bacterial overgrowth, bile salt deficiencies, and reduction of the bile salt pool as a consequence of ileal disease. Bacterial overgrowth itself is detected in approximately 30% of patients with Crohn's disease.

In regard to protein abnormalities, hypoalbuminemia occurs in at least 50% of patients with Crohn's disease, and those with active inflammatory states show excessive gastrointestinal protein loss as well. Loss of blood in the stools and fecal losses of cellular constituents as a result of ulceration intensify the nitrogen losses.

Reductions in serum folic acid and iron levels are common, as are aberrations in vitamin B_{12} absorption, signified by low Schilling test results. Hypocalcemia and negative calcium balance are usually a reflection of steatorrhea. Abnormalities in zinc metabolism have been proposed as potential etiologic factors in growth failure in Crohn's disease, but no definitive data are available at present. A small number of patients with Crohn's disease and growth failure have had reduced serum zinc levels [21], but five patients studied by us had normal zinc levels. As for other heavy metals, marked magnesium losses often complicate active Crohn's disease, but the long-range significance of this abnormality is unknown [22, 23].

Defects in intestinal absorption are the basis for the growth failure present in both celiac disease and chronic liver disease. In celiac disease, intestinal mucosal injury leads to reduced surface area, obliteration of absorptive sites, and markedly reduced disaccharidase levels. In chronic liver disease, the major defects in absorption appear to be secondary to a reduced bile acid pool. With reduced intraluminal bile acids, steatorrhea appears, and this complication (including calcium and vitamin D malabsorption and the loss of other fat-soluble vitamins) results in impaired linear growth and weight gain. In cystic fibrosis, both pancreatic insufficiency and increased fecal excretion of bile acids contribute to the steatorrhea and loss of fat-soluble nutrients. Both of these defects can be corrected by exogenous pancreatin, but the degree of correction of the defect depends also on limitation of dietary lipid.

B. Endocrine Function

Many young people with growth failure and Crohn's disease show no measurable defects in absorptive function, although anorexia may persist. As a result, *endocrine failure* has been suggested as a possible contributing factor to poor growth [11]. Such findings as reduced urinary gonadotropins and poor growth hormone release following insulin-induced hypoglycemia have previously been cited as etiologic factors [11]. However, such defects may be related to nutritional status, as they can be seen in children with protein-calorie malnutrition [24]; and recent endocrine studies do not confirm the older data. In fact, children with Crohn's disease and growth failure show elevated levels of growth hormone and exaggerated responses to sleep and to propranolol plus glucagon; these children also have normal thyroid function, thus making primary endocrine abnormalities unlikely as the single explanation for growth failure in this disorder [25]. In addition, exogenously administered growth hormone does not improve growth in such patients [26], suggesting either end-organ resistance to the agent or faulty release of somatomedin. It is of interest that somatomedin levels are depressed in some malnourished children, and rise steadily during the course of nutritional therapy [27]. In three children with Crohn's disease and growth failure studied by us [28], somatomedin levels were normal. Somatostatin levels have not been measured in patients with Crohn's disease.

C. Therapy Effects

In addition to the factors already discussed, certain aspects of therapy for Crohn's disease may contribute to growth failure. For example, large doses of corticosteroids are often used to control inflammatory disease. Ample evidence exists which demonstrates that increased excretion of nitrogen and loss of protein from the carcasses of experimental animals can occur after the administration of pharmacologic doses of corticosteroids [29]. Documentation of abnormalities of linear growth induced by corticosteroids has been provided by the studies of Blodgett et al. [30] in patients with endocrine abnormalities and allergies, without gastrointestinal disease. Nevertheless, it has been observed repeatedly that some patients with inflammatory bowel disease continue to grow despite high-dose steroid therapy, presumably because of suppression of inflammatory activity [12, 13]. The controlling factor for growth in such patients may actually be the caloric intake, but the relative contribution of caloric deprivation to growth failure in children with Crohn's disease has not previously been intensively studied. Indirect evidence for the importance of caloric intake in stimulating growth can be found from the recent data of Layden et al. [31] and Kirschner et al. [32]. These workers have reported the acceleration of linear growth in several children with Crohn's disease—an acceleration initiated by both oral and parenteral nutrition.

For reasons which are still unclear, growth after surgery for both Crohn's disease and ulcerative colitis in childhood and adolescence often remains depressed [12, 13]. In our own series of 37 patients with Crohn's disease (already discussed), of the 11 prepubertal patients with preoperative linear growth failure, only 2 exhibited catch-up growth following surgery. The remaining 9, and all pubertal patients, either failed to grow or maintained their height postoperatively in their preoperative percentile. Thus, growth failure may be considered an important indication for surgery in the prepubertal child with Crohn's disease, but it probably is not an indication after onset of puberty. When growth failure is a major indication for surgery, our experience indicates that the decision to operate should be tempered with the following reservations: (1) all signs of puberty should be absent; (2) radiographically determined bone age should be sufficiently retarded (by at least 2 years) to allow a prediction for future growth; and (3) all tissue showing active disease should be resected at the initial operation. Even under these conditions, an early recurrence will likely retard further linear growth.

VI. Nutritional Studies in Crohn's Disease

In view of the fact that the etiology of growth failure in Crohn's disease is multifactorial, and that comprehensive studies of metabolic abnormalities in

Table 3 Protocol for the Study of Growth Failure in Children with Crohn's Disease

Item of protocol	Period				
	I	II		III	
Weeks	3	5	3	5	3
Hospital	√	√	√	-	√
Studies[a]	A, B, C	-	A	-	A
Oral intake	√	√	√	√	√
Parenteral intake	-	√	√	-	-
Balance studies	√	-	√	-	√

[a]Study A: Complete blood count; serum total protein, albumin, carotene, folic acid, and vitamin B_{12} levels; ^{40}K-counting; basal metabolic rate; creatinine excretion.
Study B: Fecal fat excretion; Schilling test; xylose absorption test; ^{51}Cr-labelled.
Study C: Thyroid and adrenal hormone levels; glucose tolerance test with insulin levels; propranolol and glucagon challenge.

patients with Crohn's disease and growth failure are not available, we have investigated seven patients with Crohn's disease and growth failure, in order to define better the mechanisms of growth disturbance, endocrine dysfunction, malabsorption, and malnutrition in such patients. In addition, using parenteral nutrition as a supplement to oral intake, we have explored the metabolic consequences of this new mode of therapy. Table 3 shows the overall plan of the study, which was divided into three major periods (I, II, III). The table demonstrates duration of hospitalization, oral intake, parenteral intake, and balance studies. The letters (A, B, C) refer to groups of laboratory investigations carried out during each period (see table note). Throughout the entire evaluation, the patients ate a self-chosen, constant, normally balanced diet containing approximately 51% carbohydrate, 35% fat, and 14% protein. Period I consisted of initial metabolic and endocrine studies, with patients on an oral diet only. During period II, patients received a total of 6-8 weeks of central venous hyperalimentation and oral intake, during the last 3 weeks of which they underwent a second metabolic balance study. Both parenteral and oral intake combined were calculated to maintain a total intake of greater than 75 kcal/kg body weight per day for 6-8 weeks. Patients were then sent home during period III for 5 weeks on customary diet and activity. They subsequently returned to the hospital for a final 3-week balance study.

Results of the entire study [28] are summarized here. Seven patients with classic Crohn's disease by the criteria of Schacter and Kirsner [33], and with severe growth failure, were studied in our Clinical Research Center. The patients ranged in age from 9 to 17 years (mean 14 years) and had a height age ranging from 6 to 10 years, a weight age ranging from 6 to 12 years, and a bone age delay of 2-5 years behind chronological age (mean 3 years). Symptoms had been present for an average of 6 years (range 2-8 years) prior to study, and growth failure had been present for an average of 5 years (range 1-8 years) prior to study. Height age and weight age were very close, reflecting the fact that, although short, the patients were of normal proportion (as we have already described above). Six of the seven patients were prepubertal; the other was at Tanner stage III but had amenorrhea. No patient had clinical symptoms of gastrointestinal disease during the study, and four were on stable doses of prednisone not exceeding 20 mg per day throughout the study period.

Included in the baseline observations made in period I were standard evaluations of absorptive function by 72-hr fecal fat excretion, xylose absorption, and serum folic acid, carotene, and vitamin B_{12} levels, all of which were normal in all patients. The only abnormalities which were present at the start of the study, and persisted, were elevated sedimentation rates and mildly abnormal ^{51}Cr-labeled albumin excretion in the stool (not exceeding 3%). Endocrine functions in the patients studied were also normal, including plasma somatomedin levels. Basal metabolic rates when compared to normal values for height age were also normal, strongly suggesting that energy expenditures were not increased by inflammatory disease.

When the daily caloric intake for all of the patients was measured in period I and compared to normal data obtained from the monograph of McCammon [34], it was clear that, in period I, our patients' caloric intake average 82 ± 17% of the normal values for height age; during period II, parenteral nutrition increased the mean intake to 136 ± 21% of caloric requirements; and after cessation of nutritional support in period III, there was a decrease to 78 ± 20% of required calories for height age. The changes in total body weight in seven patients, lean body mass in five patients, and creatinine production in four patients were studied from period I to period III. There was a marked increase in body weight in response to therapy, accompanied by a corresponding increase in total body potassium and creatinine excretion. These data indicate that a significant proportion of total body weight accrued was lean body mass and muscle mass. Data for nitrogen balance indicated that three patients were in nitrogen balance prior to therapy, and their nitrogen retention increased significantly in response to increased nutritional support. One patient (W.T.) was in negative nitrogen balance in period I and had only a small, though statistically significant, increase in nitrogen retention during therapy.

Dramatic and sustained acceleration in growth velocity occurred in response to therapy. Height response data for individaul patients are shown in Table 4. Cumulative growth was from 3 to 22 cm at 1-3 years following

Table 4 Growth Response to Nutritional Support in Crohn's Disease

Patient	Age at onset of treatment (yr)	Cumulative height increase at follow-up (cm)	Time of Follow-up (yr)
E.C.	9.3	6.0	1
W.T.	11.3	7.0	1
K.M.	12.3	6.5	1
R.E.	15.1	13.6	3
A.B.	15.2	22.0	3
G.C.	15.8	3.0	3
D.Z.	17.0	10.0	3

intravenous hyperalimentation. All patients began to grow during therapy. One patient (G.C.), who was the only pubescent patient at the time of the study, grew only 3 cm in 3 years. The most likely explanation for this blunted response was her advanced development. In fact, she had already attained 97% of her projected adult height as estimated from the data of Bayer and Bayley [35]. The other patients all showed a return of growth rate to normal levels. If sustained, these growth patterns would have returned the patients to their premorbid growth channel. However, with cessation of total parenteral nutrition, nutritional intake decreased, and the growth rate fell in parallel. Nevertheless, it was clear that correcting the deficits acquired during the onset of growth failure appeared to have allowed temporary restitution of normal growth rates.

Using supplemental oral nutritional support, Kirschner et al. [32] have reported stimulation of growth in children with Crohn's disease and growth retardation. The difference between those patients and the ones described here are significant. All of Kirschner's patients had active intestinal disease. In addition, growth velocity in three of their seven patients was above 2.5 cm per year and rose to 5-6 cm per year during therapy. The patients we studied had shown long-standing, preexisting growth failure with no intestinal manifestations.

VII. Conclusions

In conclusion, one can state without doubt that:

1. Growth failure in Crohn's disease is usually accompanied by a markedly reduced caloric intake.
2. In our patients, abnormal growth was unrealted to malabsorption, significant intestinal protein loss, steroid effects, or endocrine dysfunction.

3. The normal metabolic rate in the patients studied indicated that the energy cost of disease was not increased.
4. Caloric supplementation begun immediately–at the time growth failure is first noticed–may be adequate to prevent prolonged effects of Crohn's disease on growth.
5. If oral supplementation with an elemental formula fails, central venous parenteral nutrition has been shown by our studies to increase lean body mass and induce linear growth.
6. Dramatic and prolonged increases in linear growth can be achieved by these techniques, and this provides a new approach to the treatment of growth failure in inflammatory bowel disease.
7. It is possible that, to be maximally effective, therapy must be instituted before puberty.

We have successfully applied these principles to the management of patients with other types of gastrointestinal disease and growth failure, namely, eosinophilic gastroenteritis and complicated extrahepatic portal vein obstruction with esophageal resection.

In the clinical management of patients with gastrointestinal disease, the primary goal is to identify the earliest possible stage of nutritional failure and to institute appropriate nutritional support and supplementation before the impact of growth failure becomes manifest. With this approach, it should be possible to prevent in the future the serious complications of growth failure so common in gastrointestinal disease today.

Acknowledgments

Supported in part by Clinical Research Center Grant RR-00128 from the National Institutes of Health, by a grant from the National Foundation for Ileitis and Colitis, and by gifts from the Hazel Dell Foundation, Inc., and the Daughters of Penelope (District 8). Dr. Kelts is a recipient of National Research Service Award AM05594 from the National Institute of Arthritis, Metabolism, and Digestive Diseases, the National Institutes of Health.

Plasma somatedin levels were determined by Dr. Louis Underwood and Mr. Judson VanWyck.

The authors are indebted to many colleagues who have contributed to this study: Dr. Kon-Taik Khaw, Dr. John B. Watkins, Dr. Warren E. Grupe, Dr. John F. Crigler, Dr. Grace Shen, Dr. Steven L. Werlin, Ms. Carol Boehme, Ms. Meryl Adler, and Mr. Ian Barwick.

References

1. D. Smith. *Growth and Its Disorders.* Saunders, Philadelphia, 1977.
2. D. B. Cheek. *Human Growth.* Lea & Febiger, Philadelphia, 1968.
3. R. E. Frisch and R. Revelle. The height and weight of girls and boys at the time of the initiation of the adolescent growth spurt in height and weight and the relationship to menarche. *Hum. Biol. 43,* 140-159 (1971).
4. F. E. Johnston, A. F. Roche, L. M. Schell, et al. Critical Weight at Menarche. *Am. J. Dis. Child. 129,* 19-23 (1975).
5. A. Prader, J. M. Tanner, and G. A. Von Harnack. Catch-up growth following illness or starvation. *J. Pediatr. 62,* 646-659 (1963).
6. G. B. Forbes. A note on the mathematics of catch up growth. *Pediatr. Res. 8,* 929-931 (1974).
7. A. Ashworth. Growth rates in children recovering from protein calorie malnutrition. *Br. J. Nutr. 23,* 835-845 (1969).
8. A. J. Katz, Z. M. Falchuk, and H. Shwachman. The co-existence of cystic fibrosis and celiac disease. *Pediatrics 57,* 715-721 (1976).
9. I. Snapper, J. Groen, and A. Foyer. Observations sur l'ileite regionale. *Proceedings of the Second International Congress of Gastroenterology, Brussels, 1937,* pp. 935-937.
10. S. Davidson. Infantilism in ulcerative colitis. *Arch. Int. Med. 64,* 1187-1196 (1939).
11. T. D. McCaffery, K. Nasr, A. H. Lawrence, and J. B. Kirsner. Severe growth retardation in children with inflammatory bowel disease. *J. Pediat. 45,* 386-393 (1970).
12. M. Berger, D. Gribetz, and B. I. Korelitz. Growth retardation in children with ulcerative colitis: The effect of medical and surgical therapy. *Pediatrics 55,* 459-467 (1975).
13. D. R. Homer, R. J. Grand, and A. H. Colodny. Growth, course and prognosis after surgery for Crohn's disease. *Pediatrics 59,* 717-725 (1977).
14. J. C. Waterlow. Classification and definition of protein calorie malnutrition. *Br. Med. J. 2,* 566-569 (1972).
15. W. Beeken, H. J. Busch, and D. L. Sylvester. Intestinal protein loss in Crohn's disease. *Gastroenterology 62,* 207-215 (1972).
16. W. Beeken. Absorptive defects in young people with regional enteritis. *Pediatrics 52,* 69-74 (1973).
17. C. D. Gerson, N. Cohen, and H. J. Janowitz. Small intestinal absorptive function in regional enteritis. *Gastroenterology 64,* 907-912 (1973).
18. W. L. Beeken and R. E. Kanich. Microbial flora of the upper small bowel in Crohn's disease. *Gastroenterology 65,* 390-397 (1973).
19. E. L. Krawitt, W. L. Beeken, and C. D. Janney. Calcium absorption in Crohn's disease. *Gastroenterology 71,* 251-254 (1976).
20. E. Lebentha, I. Antonowicz, and H. Shwachman. Correlation of lactase activity and lactose tolerance and milk consumption in different age groups. *Am. J. Clin. Nutr. 28,* 595-600 (1975).
21. N. W. Solomons, R. L. Rosenfield, R. A. Jacob, and H. H. Sandstead. Growth retardation and zinc nutrition. *Pediatr. Res. 10,* 923-927 (1976).

22. K. Gerlach, D. A. Morowitz, and J. B. Kirsner. Symptomatic hypomagnesemia complicating regional enteritis. *Gastroenterology 59,* 567-574 (1970).
23. R. J. Grand and A. H. Colodny. Increased requirement of magnesium during parenteral therapy for granulomatous colitis. *J. Pediatr. 8,* 788-791 (1972).
24. D. J. Becker, B. L. Pinstone, and J. D. Hansen. The relation between insulin secretion, glucose tolerance, growth hormone and serum proteins in protein calorie malnutrition. *Pediatr. Res. 9,* 35-39 (1975).
25. A. Tenore, W. F. Berman, J. S. Parks, and A. M. Bongiovanni. Basal and stimulated growth hormone concentrations inflammatory bowel disease. *J. Clin. Endocrinol. Metab. 44,* 622-628 (1977).
26. T. D. McCaffery, K. Nasr, A. M. Lawrence, and J. B. Kirsner. Effect of administered human growth hormone on growth retardation in inflammatory bowel disease. *Am. J. Dig. Dis. 19,* 411-416 (1974).
27. D. B. Grant, J. Hambley, D. J. Becker, and B. L. Pimstone. Reduced sulphation factor in undernourished children. *Arch. Dis. Child. 48,* 596-600 (1973).
28. D. G. Kelts, R. J. Grand, [illegible] Shen, J. B. Watkins, S. L. Werlin, and C. Boehme. Nutritional basis of growth failure in children and adolescent with Crohn's disease. *Gastroenterology 76,* 720-727 (1979).
29. R. W. Wannemacher, Jr. Protein metabolism. In *Total Parenteral Nutrition* (H. Ghadimi, Ed.). John Wiley, New York, 1975, pp. 85-153.
30. F. M. Blodgett, L. Burgin, D. Iezzoni, D. Gribetz, and N. B. Talbot. Effect of prolonged cortisone therapy on the statural growth, skeletal maturation and metabolic status of children. *N. Engl. J. Med. 254,* 636-641 (1956).
31. T. Layden, I. Rosenberg, B. Nemchausky, C. Elson, and I. Rosenberg. Reversal of growth arrest in adolescents with Crohn's disease after parenteral alimentation. *Gastroenterology 70,* 1017-1021 (1976).
32. B. Kirschner, O. Voinchet, and I. H. Rosenberg. Growth retardation in inflammatory bowel disease. *Gastroenterology 75,* 504-511 (1978).
33. H. Schacter and J. B. Kirsner. Definition of inflammatory bowel disease of unknown etiology. *Gastroenterology 68,* 591-600 (1975).
34. R. W. McCammon. *Human Growth and Development.* Chas. C Thomas, Springfield, Ill., 1970, pp. 63-100.
35. L. M. Bayer and N. Bayley. *Growth Diagnosis,* 2d Ed. Univ. of Chicago Press, Chicago, 1976, pp. 214-233.

26 Vitamin and Mineral Deficiencies in Intestinal Malabsorption

HAROLD E. HARRISON / Johns Hopkins University School of Medicine, and Johns Hopkins Hospital, Baltimore, Maryland

I. Fat-Soluble Vitamins

Malabsorption of the fat-soluble vitamins can be seen in all types of steatorrhea. However, there are differences in the degree of malabsorption of the various specific vitamins, depending upon the type of fat malabsorption. Table 1 shows the classification of fat malabsorption which is of interest in this connection.

A. Vitamin A

The major source of vitamin A in food is β-carotene, which is converted to vitamin A chiefly by the intestinal mucosa. In humans β-carotene is also absorbed intact and converted to vitamin A by a cleavage enzyme in the liver. Preformed vitamin A of the diet is present primarily as vitamin A esters of long-chain fatty acids. The retinal esters are hydrolyzed either by a pancreatic hydrolase or a brush border membrane enzyme. Malabsorption of β-carotene and of vitamin A occurs with all types of fat malabsorption, and reduced concentration of β-carotene in plasma is a commonly used index of such malabsorption. Vitamin A deficiency was a major feature of the nutritional deficiency of infants with cystic fibrosis, prior to the use of pancreatic enzyme treatment. Before the development of the sweat chloride test, the vitamin A tolerance test was an important procedure in the diagnosis of cystic fibrosis. Vitamin A deficiency sufficiently severe to produce the characteristic eye lesions, namely, Bitot's spots, xerosis of the conjunctiva, and keratomalacia, is rare. However, milder manifestations with low plasma vitamin A concentrations and night blindness can be seen. Vitamin A preparations in a water-miscible vehicle are

Table 1 Classification of Fat Malabsorption

Defect of lipolysis, secondary to lack of pancreatic lipase
Cystic fibrosis
Abnormality of micelle formation, due to bile salt deficiency
Biliary atresia
Bacterial overgrowth, blind-loop syndrome
Disease of distal small intestine
Congenital defect of bile salt absorption
Cholestyramine administration
Abnormalities of intestinal absorptive surface
Qualitative
Gluten-induced enteropathy
Crohn's disease
Quantitative
Intestinal resection

commonly employed to maintain adequate vitamin A nutrition in patients with fat malabsorption. Huge doses are ordinarily not required, and the dosage can be monitored by serum vitamin A determination.

B. Vitamin D

Skin exposure to the shortwave ultraviolet radiation of sunshine is a natural source of vitamin D for man. However, such exposure can usually not be depended upon for infants and children living in the industrial cities of the temperate zone. Vitamin D, therefore, must be taken orally and absorbed from the small intestine. Absorption of vitamin D is markedly deficient in the absence of bile salts, so that the most severe forms of vitamin D deficiency are seen in children with bile duct obstruction. Vitamin D malabsorption is also seen secondary to bile salt deficiency in patients with ileal disease [1, 2] or as a result of cholestyramine treatment [3]. Pancreatic steatorrhea with failure of lipolysis is less likely to be associated with clinical vitamin D deficiency, although some malabsorption of vitamin D does occur and can be demonstrated with the use of radioactive vitamin D (Fig. 1) [4]. The rarity of clinical rickets in infants and children with cystic fibrosis has often been remarked upon. Poor growth may have been a factor before pancreatic enzyme treatment was employed. Studies of serum 25-hydroxyvitamin D concentrations indicate that vitamin D malabsorption is not severe in cystic fibrosis patients given pancreatic enzyme treatment—which correlates

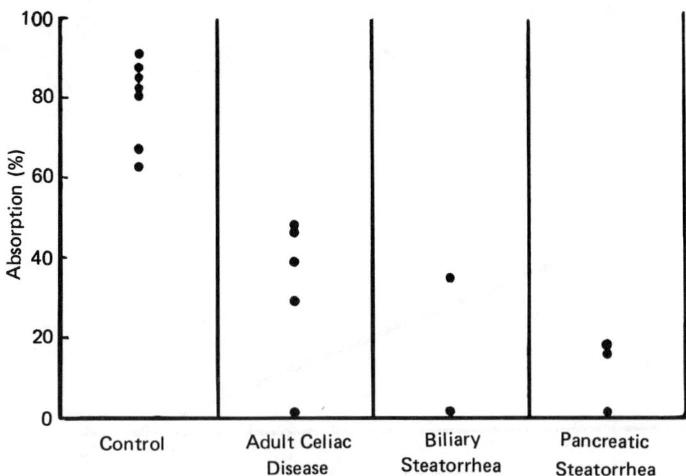

Figure 1 Net absorption of 0.5-1.0 mg [^{3}H] vitamin D_3 in control subjects and patients with intestinal malabsorption. (From Ref. 4.)

with the rarity of vitamin D deficiency and hypocalcemia in patients with cystic fibrosis so treated. Rickets, on the other hand, has been much more commonly seen in association with celiac disease. In the fat malabsorption of intestinal mucosal injury the triglycerides are hydrolyzed, and the free fatty acids combine with calcium to form insoluble calcium soaps. Calcium malabsorption is thus extreme, resulting both from vitamin D deficiency and precipitation of calcium in an unavailable form within the intestinal lumen. In pancreatic steatorrhea the unabsorbed moiety of the unhydrolyzed triglycerides may trap some of the vitamin D, but there is no removal of calcium from solution. The adequacy of vitamin D supplementation can be monitored by serum calcium, phosphate, and alkaline phosphatase measurements. A more precise measurement is that of serum 25-hydroxyvitamin D [1], but this is not yet readily available in most clinical laboratories. An additional measurement of interest is serum immunoreactive parathyroid hormone level, since this should be elevated if calcium malabsorption exists [5]. Patients with steatorrhea do show increased serum 25-hydroxyvitamin D concentrations when exposed to sunshine, and this can be a valid form of treatment.

A special problem of malabsorption of vitamin D or unresponsiveness to pharmacologic doses of vitamin D exists in patients with hypoparathyroidism and steatorrhea. Hypoparathyroid steatorrhea is most commonly found in

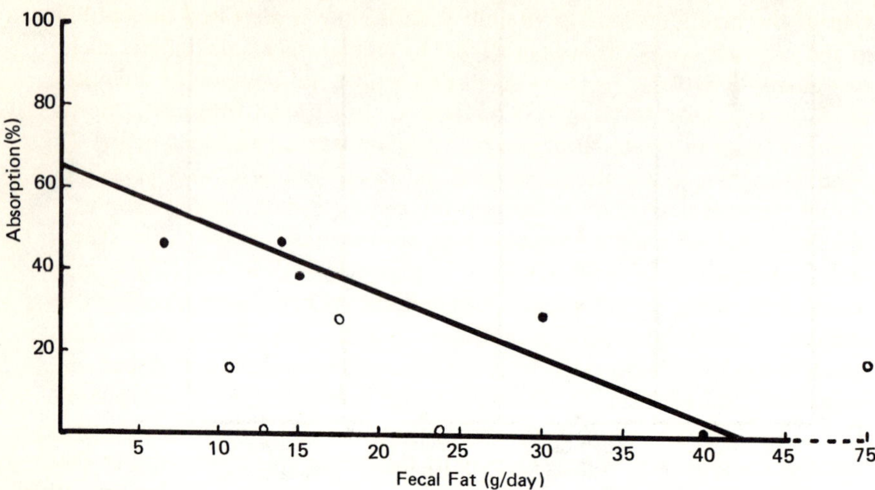

Figure 2 Inverse relationship of percent absorption of oral dose of labeled vitamin D_3 to fecal fat excretion. •, Adult celiac disease; ○, biliary steatorrhea; ⊙, pancreatic steatorrhea. (Taken from Ref. 4.)

patients with autoimmune hypoparathyroidism: i.e., acquired hypoparathyroidism associated with other autoimmune endocrinopathies, particularly adrenal cortical insufficiency, thyroiditis, alopecia, and in some instances intrinsic factor deficiency due to autoimmune injury of the gastric mucosa. The basis of the steatorrhea has been a subject of contention. Reduction of extracellular calcium concentration may be a factor, either through increase of intestinal motility or by inhibition of intestinal absorption of fatty acids. However, it also seems likely that autoimmune injury of intestinal mucosa is an important basis for the fat malabsorption. The possible role of steatorrhea in reducing responsiveness to vitamin D in patients with hypoparathyroidism is suggested by the data in Figure 2, which indicate that the percentage of absorption of fed vitamin D is inversely related to the fecal fat excretion. There is also evidence, however, that unresponsiveness to vitamin D in patients with steatorrhea may, in addition, be due to other factors which interfere with the action of vitamin D, such as unresponsiveness of the target tissues to vitamin D or failure of the metabolic activation of vitamin D. This type of unresponsiveness to vitamin D will be discussed later in connection with mineral deficiencies.

C. Vitamin E

Depletion of α-tocopherol in infants and children with steatorrhea does occur, but the clinical consequences of this depletion have not been clear-cut [6].

One of the manifestations of vitamin E deficiency is increased susceptibility of the red cells to peroxide hemolysis. In prematurely born infants such tocopherol deficiency has been associated with a mild hemolytic anemia which is responsive to vitamin E treatment. In patients with cystic fibrosis or other types of steatorrhea, plasma tocopherol concentrations below 225 μg/dl have been found associated with increased hemolysis with peroxide. Ceroid pigment deposition in smooth muscle, creatinuria and dystrophic lesions of skeletal muscle have also been seen in such patients [7]. The body requirements of tocopherol are increased by high intake of polyunsaturated fatty acid, so that vitamin E requirements have to be considered in relation to unsaturated fatty acid intake. On the other hand, the foods which are rich in unsaturated fatty acids, such as corn oil, cottonseed oil, peanut oil, and soybean oil, also have a high concentration of tocopherol. The tocopherol deficiency of patients with prolonged steatorrhea is presumably the consequence of the trapping of this fat-soluble compound in the unabsorbed fat of the diet. Such patients can be followed by determination of plasma tocopherol and can be treated with additional α-tocopherol if the concentrations of plasma tocopherol are found to be low.

D. Vitamin K

Vitamin K deficiency secondary to bile salt lack is, of course, well known. Hemorrhagic phenomena, resulting from decreased prothrombin activity caused by vitamin K deficiency, were initially detected in patients with failure of delivery of bile salts to the intestinal tract as a result of bile duct obstruction, either intrahepatic or extrahepatic. A deficiency of bile salts in the upper intestine can also result from interruption of the bile salt enterohepatic cycle; the reabsorption of bile salts by the ileal mucosa and reexcretion in the bile. This interruption of the enterohepatic cycle can occur in Crohn's disease with inflammatory lesions of the terminal small bowel, as well as following resection of the terminal small intestine. Recently, specific congenital deficiencies of bile salt absorption by ileum have been reported to result in reduced bile salt concentration of duodenal fluid and in secondary steatorrhea. We have seen two siblings with vitamin D deficiency secondary to steatorrhea of unknown origin, who presented also with reduced prothrombin activity and bleeding, which responded to vitamin K treatment. It is possible that these children represented examples of bile salt deficiency of the type resulting from failure of absorption of bile salts by the distal intestine.

Deficiency of vitamin K is monitored, of course, by determinations of prothrombin time, and in patients with steatorrhea with prolonged prothrombin time the response to injection of vitamin K is perfectly normal.

II. Water-Soluble Vitamins

A. Folic Acid

Dietary folates occur mostly as polyglutamates which are not absorbed intact into the circulation. The orally administered pteroylpolyglutamates are cleaved to pteroylglutamic acid during absorption. The site of cleavage of the polyglutamyl chain seems to be the interior of intestinal epithelial cells. There is no evidence of significant intraluminal conjugase activity nor is the enzyme found in isolated brush border fractions. Malabsorption of dietary folate occurs in gluten-induced enteropathy and tropical sprue. In addition, drugs may interfere with the normal absorption of folate, particularly alcohol and diphenylhydantoin. Folate deficiency, in turn, may also contribute to the abnormality of intestinal mucosal absorptive function. Folate has an essential role in nucleoprotein synthesis, and, since the renewal time of the small-intestinal epithelium is extremely rapid (2-5 days), one would expect a high requirement of folate for mucosal nucleoprotein synthesis, in order to maintain normal villus anatomy and the functional integrity of the mucosal cell [8]. This may explain the therapeutic effect of folate in patients with malabsorption secondary to tropical sprue. Folate is primarily absorbed in the proximal small intestine. When folic acid is administered as the sole form of treatment in tropical sprue, the hematologic lesion, namely the megaloblastic anemia, is usually corrected while the intestinal absorptive defect is only partially improved. It is possible that the intestinal lesion in tropical sprue reflects altered metabolism rather than a simple deficiency of folic acid.

B. Vitamin B_{12}

Vitamin B_{12} and folate play interrelated roles in nucleoprotein synthesis. Deficiency of each is expressed by the same morphologic abnormality of the hematopoietic system, a megaloblastic bone marrow. Vitamin B_{12}, however, is absorbed preferentially in the distal small intestine [9, 10] and, as is known, requires gastric intrinsic factor for its absorption. Vitamin B_{12} malabsorption can be a significant feature in Crohn's disease [9] or following resection of the terminal ileum. In these subjects an inverse relationship between fecal fat and vitamin B_{12} absorption is present (Fig. 3). The vitamin B_{12} deficiency which may occur in patients with autoimmune hypoparathyroidism in association with intestinal malabsorption and steatorrhea has already been mentioned. It is important to distinguish the megaloblastic anemia of this type of vitamin B_{12} deficiency from folate deficiency associated with steatorrhea. In one instance a patient with such steatorrhea was thought to have primary folate deficiency, and treatment with folate did correct the megaloblastic anemia; but serious neurologic manifestations of

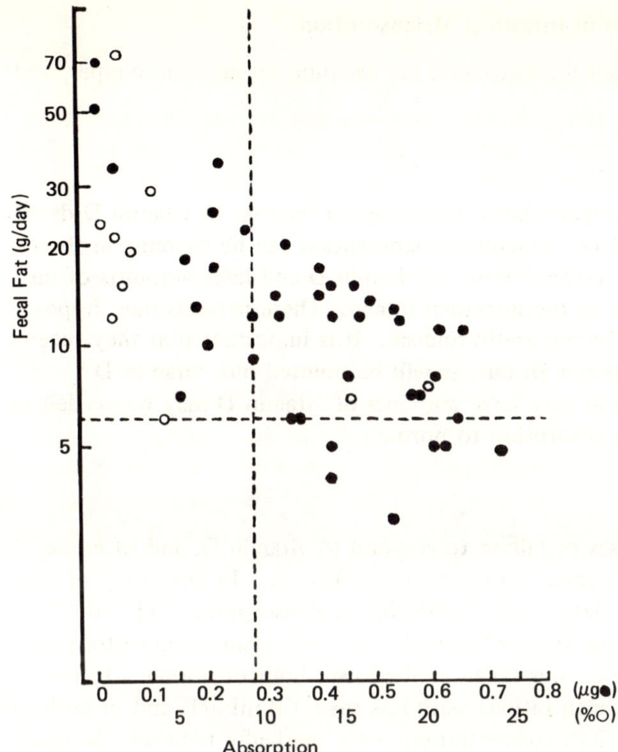

Figure 3 Inverse relationship of vitamin B_{12} absorption and fecal fat excretion. $P < 0.001$; $r = 0.67$. Dashed lines indicate limits of normal values. (Taken from Ref. 10.)

combined system degeneration resulted, which were corrected by the administration of vitamin B_{12}. The deficiency of vitamin B_{12} of the patients with autoimmune hypoparathyroidism is thought to be not simply due to vitamin B_{12} malabsorption resulting from the intestinal disease, but rather to be due to an intrinsic factor deficiency resulting from autoimmune injury to the gastric mucosa. These patients, therefore, must be treated with parenteral vitamin B_{12}, as patients with pernicious anemia are treated. With the availability of serum folate and vitamin B_{12} determinations, the distinction between folate and vitamin B_{12} deficiency can be clearly made. In addition, the Schilling test for absorption of vitamin B_{12} (using radioactive-cobalt-labeled vitamin B_{12}) is of value.

III. Mineral Deficiencies in Intestinal Malabsorption

The four minerals selected for discussion are calcium, magnesium, copper, and zinc.

A. Calcium

Calcium deficiency has already been mentioned in relation to vitamin D deficiency, and, as pointed out, calcium malabsorption can be extreme in those patients who have both reduced levels of vitamin D and large amounts of unabsorbed free fatty acids in the intestinal lumen. These patients have hypocalcemia and secondary hyperparathyroidism. It is important that they receive adequate amounts of vitamin D; but, as will be pointed out, vitamin D resistance can be seen, and very large amounts of vitamin D may be needed in order to restore calcium absorption to normal.

B. Magnesium

One of the possible causes of failure to respond to vitamin D, and of consequent persistent hypocalcemia, is magnesium deficiency. In one study of the incidence of magnesium deficiency in intestinal malabsorption [11], 10 of 24 patients with idiopathic steatorrhea had serum magnesium concentrations less than 1.5 mEq/1, which was taken as the lower limit of normal. In two of these patients, the concentrations were less than 1.0 mEq/1, and in both of these patients serum calcium concentrations were markedly reduced. Serum calcium concentrations were also low in five of the other eight patients. In patients with steatorrhea following partial gastrectomy, only one of the seven patients had a reduced magnesium concentration, and this reduction was slight, to 1.4 mEq/l. Two patients with intestinal resection or blind loops had severe hypomagnesemia as low as 0.3 mEq/l. One patient with marked hypomagnesemia also had hypocalcemia and hypokalemia; the concentration of serum calcium was 7 mg/dl and that of potassium 2.8 mEq/l. A negative correlation was found between serum magnesium and fecal fat, so that patients with the highest fecal fat excretion tended to have the lowest serum magnesium concentrations. In patients with moderate hypomagnesemia, the serum magnesium concentrations returned to normal when the underlying intestinal disorder was treated, or when a low fat diet was given. Patients with severe hypomagnesemia secondary to resection of the distal small bowel required oral magnesium supplements; in this particular study these were given as magnesium chloride 100 mEq/day or 0.5 mEq/kg body weight per day in divided doses.

A considerable amount of interest has developed in the hypocalcemia refractory to vitamin D treatment, a form of hypocalcemia seen in magnesium-deficient subjects. This refractoriness of hypomagnesemic hypocalcemia to

Table 2 Hypocalcemia and Hypomagnesemia in Severe Infection: Role of Gentamicin

	Serum electrolyte concentration							
	Na	Cl	HCO_3	K	Ca	P	Mg	
Date	(mEq/1				(mg/dl)			Remarks
2/10	130	89	32	4.3				Pneumonectomy Gentamicin–I.V. 120 mg Ampicillin I.V.– –6 g
3/7	134	65	46	1.5				
3/10	133	81	37	3.0				Gentamicin D/C
3/11				2.6	6.8	5.0		Tetany
3/12	131			2.6	6.8			Calcium gluconate I.V.
3/14				-	-	-	0.7	M_gSO_4 I.M.
3/16	134	37	36	3.0	8.3		0.7	
3/17					9.2	3.2	1.2	Urine Mg–2.9 mEq/l Urine K–5.5 mEq/l
3/23			32	3.5	8.6	-	0.8	

Note: Patient was an 11-year-old male.

vitamin D does not necessarily involve malabsorption of vitamin D, because it can also be seen in patients with magnesium deficiency due to renal tubular disorders, as shown in Table 2. This patient had aminoglycoside nephropathy resulting from gentamicin treatment of severe infection. One of the manifestations was increased magnesium loss in the urine with hypomagnesemia and hypocalcemia. The hypocalcemia did not respond to injections of calcium gluconate until magnesium sulfate was also given parenterally. There has been conclusive evidence that patients with severe magnesium deficiency have a deficiency of parathyroid hormone output—in other words, a functional hypoparathyroidism. In addition, there is some evidence that magnesium deficiency interferes with the action of parathyroid hormone when parathyroid extract is injected. This target tissue unresponsiveness may be due to an abnormality of vitamin D action.

That magnesium deficiency interferes with response to vitamin D was shown experimentally in rats by Lifshitz [12] in this laboratory. It has also been shown in humans in a study by Medalle et al. [13]. Patients with hypomagnesemia secondary to intestinal disorders had hypocalcemia resistant to vitamin D, with improved responsiveness when magnesium was given orally (Table 3). In one of these patients serum 25-hydroxyvitamin D was quite high, 131 ng/ml, at a time when the serum calcium concentration before magnesium treatment was markedly reduced. The serum calcium concentration rose when the serum nagnesium concentration was increased. In the other patient the serum 25-hydroxyvitamin D was reduced, and the hypocalcemia was extreme. However, treatment with magnesium increased the serum magnesium and simultaneously increased the serum calcium without additional vitamin D therapy. Figure 4 summarizes the studies in several patients. All of these patients had low values for urinary excretion of calcium, serum calcium concentration, urinary magnesium excretion, and serum magnesium concentration, as a result of magnesium depletion due to various forms of intestinal disorders. They had been given vitamin D without response, but, when magnesium hydroxide was added, serum magnesium rose, with a concomitant increase in urine magnesium–indicating increased absorption of magnesium. The serum calcium concentration and urinary calcium excretion also rose into the normal range, with magnesium repletion indicating improved absorption of calcium.

This effect of magnesium deficiency may explain some old studies of ours in patients with disorders of intestinal function. We had found several patients with severe hypokalemia and hypocalcemia who did not respond to vitamin D. The first patient was a Puerto Rican male with tropical sprue. He presented with

Table 3 Magnesium Depletion and Resistance to Vitamin D Treatment

Serum level	Gluten-induced enteropathy	Regional enteritis
25-OH-vitamin D (ng/ml)	131	9
Ca–before Mg[a] (mg/dl)	7.0	5.1
Ca–after Mg (mg/dl)	8.0	8.3
Mg–before Mg (mEq/l)	1.02	0.54
Mg–after Mg (mEq/1)	1.45	1.58

[a]8% Mg $(OH)_2$, 30 ml daily (1.7 g Mg).

Source: Data taken from R. Medalle, C. Waterhouse, and T. J. Hahn. Vitamin D resistance in magnesium deficiency. *Am. J. Clin. Nutr. 29,* 854-858 (1976).

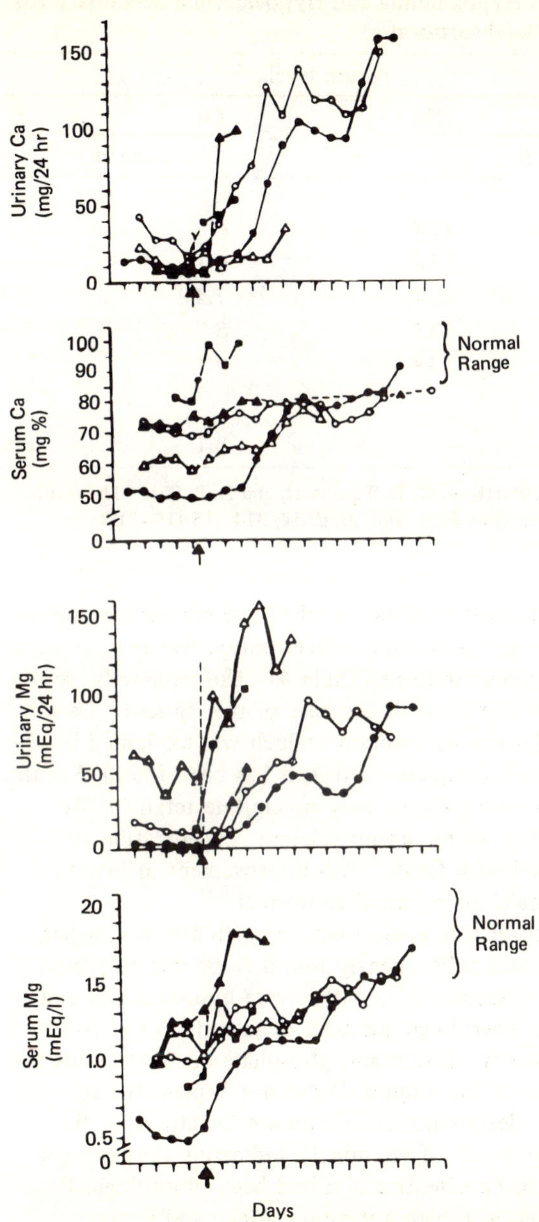

Figure 4 Studies in five patients with magnesium deficiency due to malabsorption. Effect of magnesium repletion on serum concentrations and urinary excretion of calcium, magnesium, and phosphate. Arrow indicates oral administration of 10cc 8% $Mg(OH)_2$ t.i.d. (Taken from Ref. 13.)

Table 4 Studies in Patient with Hypokalemia and Hypocalcemia Secondary to Tropical Sprue with Intestinal Malabsorption

	Serum level			
	K	Na	Ca	P
Date	(mEq/l		(mg/dl)	
1941				
4/1	1.1	138	-	-
4/8	1.6	136	6.1	1.1
4/14	2.6	134	7.2	1.9
4/28	4.2	133	8.7	3.3
5/13	3.4	138	9.1	3.2
1942				
3/38	3.8	-	8.1	3.6

Source: Taken from Ref. 27: H. E. Harrison, R. R. Tompsett, and D. P. Barr. The serum potassium in two cases of sprue. *Proc. Soc. Exp. Biol. Med. 54,* 314-315 (1943).

severe watery diarrhea with increased fecal fat, marked anemia, severe muscle weakness, and hypotension. Serum potassium concentration was low, as were serum calcium and phosphate concentrations (Table 4). Unfortunately, serum magnesium determinations were not done in the case of this patient. Despite the marked hypocalcemia he did not have tetany—which was explained by the severe hypokalemia. (In studies subsequent to this, it has been found that the administration of potassium to such patients may precipitate tetany.) We were puzzled by the refractoriness of his serum calcium concentration to vitamin D. When he was treated with folate, with improvement in intestinal function, both potassium and calcium returned to normal.

An additional patient studied at this time, a woman with severe diarrhea and marked steatorrhea, which was subsequently found to be due to lymphosarcoma of the small intestine, presented also with severe hypocalcemia and hypokalemia. This patient was given huge amounts of vitamin D (up to 2 million units per day) before serum calcium and phosphate concentrations increased (Fig. 5). Malabsorption of the vitamin D did not explain the refractoriness to vitamin D, since determination of vitamin D activity in the plasma by bioassay showed high levels of vitamin D, indicating that enough vitamin D was being absorbed to be effective if it had been physiologically active. When this patient was given a high potassium intake and serum potassium concentration was brought back to normal, serum calcium and phosphate concentrations also rose. There is good evidence to suggest that there is an interrelationship between potassium and magnesium, with

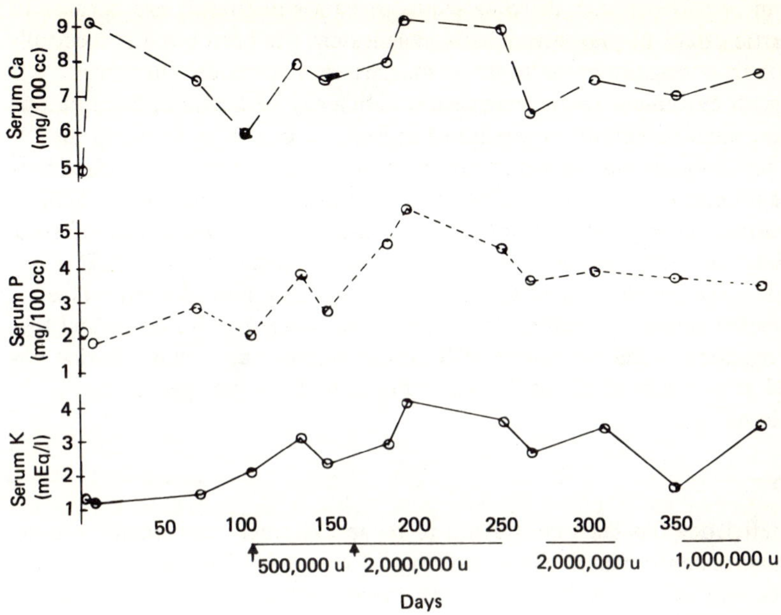

Figure 5 Studies in patient with potassium deficiency and hypocalcemia secondary to intestinal malabsorption. Vitamin D dosage administered as indicated by arrows and units at bottom of diagram. Initial increase of calcium concentration in serum resulted from intravenous injection of calcium gluconate. Subsequent studies on constant intake of calcium with varying daily doses of vitamin D. (Taken from Ref. 28.)

magnesium deficiency often being seen in patients with potassium deficiency [14]. Magnesium concentrations were not determined in this case, but retrospectively we think that these patients with severe potassium deficiency due to severe watery diarrhea may also have had magnesium deficiency, which could explain their poor response to vitamin D. There may be a combined role of potassium and magnesium in the sequence of events responsible for the physiologic activity of vitamin D: either its metabolic activation to the vitamin D hormone, 1,25-dihydroxyvitamin D, or the action of 1,25-dihydroxyvitamin D on intestinal mucosa.

In addition to the secondary magnesium deficiencies due to various forms of loss of small-intestinal function, there is a rare genetic form of hypomagnesemia, primary hypomagnesemia, which is due to an inborn lack of the magnesium transport system in the small bowel. Such patients also present with severe hypocalcemia and tetany, which can be corrected only by the administration of magnesium in adequate amounts. Although the use of magnesium in patients with diarrhea seems to be a paradoxical one because of the cathartic effect of magnesium salts, magnesium has been given successfully orally, either as magnesium chloride or magnesium hydroxide. In some patients with extremely severe magnesium deficiency who cannot tolerate oral magnesium salts, parenteral magnesium has been successful in breaking the chain of unresponsiveness to parathyroid hormone and vitamin D, with subsequent maintenance of the improvement by oral intake of magnesium. Magnesium sulfate can be given intramuscularly, and we have used a dose of 10.0 mg/kg body weight of magnesium (0.2 ml/kg body weight of 50% $MgSO_4 \cdot 7H_2O$ solution), which is slightly less than 1.0 mEq/kg body weight. This dose raises the serum magnesium into the normal range for 6-8 hours and then must be repeated. Oral treatment with magnesium as magnesium chloride has been used at a dosage of about 0.5-1.5 mEq/kg body weight per 24 hr in divided doses.

C. Copper

Copper deficiency has been considered to be an extremely rare manifestation of intestinal malabsorption. Since the original report by Cordano and Graham [15] of copper deficiency in a child with malabsorption, a few other cases have been reported [16-18]. The major incidence of copper deficiency in patients with intestinal disease has been in patients who have been on prolonged parenteral alimentation using fluids deficient in both copper and other trace metals [19, 20]. The chief manifestations of copper deficiency are neutropenia, severe refractory anemia, and osteopenia. Copper deficiency interferes both with intestinal absorption of iron and the incorporation of iron into heme, so that the anemia is a hypochromic microcytic anemia unresponsive to iron. The neutropenia is a very striking manifestation of copper deficiency.

The original patient reported by Graham's group [15] was a child with severe malnutrition secondary to prolonged intestinal malabsorption and dietary restriction, who also had a very severe anemia refractory to treatment with the usual hematinics. The patient had a moderate leukopenia with marked neutropenia (Table 5). When this patient was given a dose of 1 mg copper (as copper sulfate) per day, there was a reticulocytosis, a marked rise of granulocytes, and a return of the hematocrit and red blood count to normal. Similar findings were seen in other patients with copper deficiency. Figure 6 shows the findings in a patient with severe malnutrition and intestinal dysfunction, whose anemia was refractory to iron, and who showed a marked neutropenia. When copper was added, the rise of polymorphonuclear leukocytes and the return of the hematocrit to normal were striking.

The X-ray evidences of the osteopenia of copper deficiency are similar to those of scurvy, namely, a ground-glass appearance of the bones with an increased

Table 5 Copper Deficiency in a Child with Intestinal Malabsorption

Age (hr)	WBC (per mm^3)	PMN[a] (%)	Hct (%)	RBC (10^6/mm^3)	Retic. (%)
6 2/12	5400	30	-	1.63	0
6 3/12	8300	24	8	0.96	0.1
6 4/12	3900	9	10	1.20	0.2
6 4/12: $CuSO_4$, 1 mg/day					
6 5/12	12,400	45	32	1.66	4.5
6 6/12	13,900	71	39	4.10	3.0

[a]Polymorphonuclear cells.

Source: Data taken from A. Cordano and G. G. Graham. Copper deficiency complicating severe chronic intestinal malabsorption. *Pediatrics 38,* 596-604 (1966).

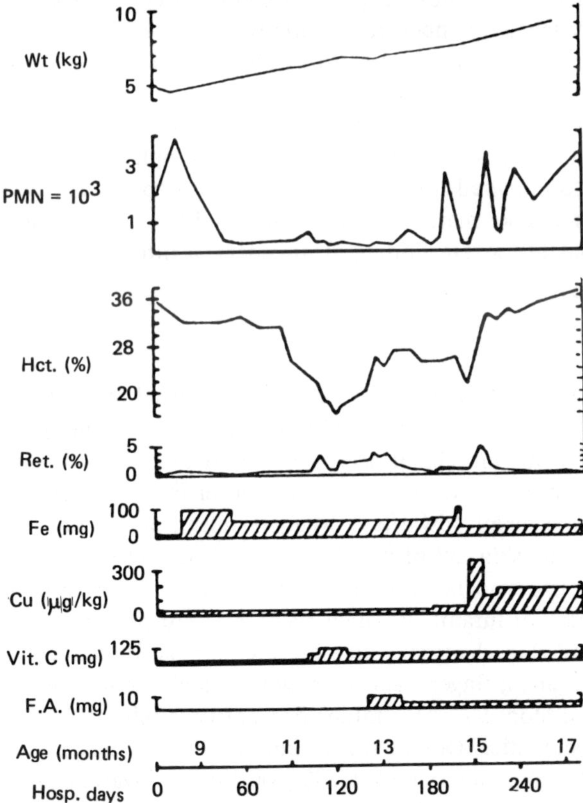

Figure 6 Hematologic findings in patient with copper deficiency. Effect of treatment with copper sulfate. (Taken from Ref. 16.)

density at the periphery of the centers of ossification. This is not surprising because the lesion of copper deficiency is, in part at least, similar to that of scurvy: namely, deficiency of bone matrix formation because of the failure of collagen formation. In the case of scurvy, as in copper deficiency, hydroxylation of the amino acid proline in collagen to hydroxyproline is inadequate, leading to a failure of normal collagen formation. The hemorrhagic manifestations of scurvy are, however, not seen in copper deficiency. The bone lesions of copper deficiency, like the hematologic lesions, are reversed by the administration of copper.

The diagnosis of copper deficiency can be confirmed, once it has been considered, by the determination of serum copper, a procedure which is now available. Total serum copper is reduced, as is serum ceruloplasmin [21], the copper-binding protein which is formed in response to absorption of copper. Total serum copper concentrations of less than 90 μg/dl or ceruloplasmin concentrations of less than 20 mg/dl are characteristic features of copper deficiency. Sternlieb and Janowitz [22] have studied copper absorption by means of radioactively labeled copper in patients with a wide variety of malabsorption syndromes and varying degrees of steatorrhea. They found reduced concentrations of ceruloplasmin, particularly in patients with gluten-induced enteropathy, but also in patients with lymphosarcoma of the small bowel, scleroderma, and tropical sprue. The low serum ceruloplasmin concentrations were secondary to impaired intestinal absorption of copper, as studied by the radioactive copper uptake method. They concluded from their studies that copper deficiency was not a rare finding in disorders of intestinal absorption.

D. Zinc

Various clinical syndromes of zinc deficiency have been reported in humans. The first was a dietary deficiency of zinc, possibly aggravated by reduced absorption due to a high phytate and clay intake in the particular children involved. This deficiency syndrome was found in children in Iran and Egypt, and the manifestations were mainly dwarfism, hypogonadism, poor hair growth, and roughness of the skin, all of which responded to zinc supplementation. The next disease entity associated with zinc was acrodermatitis enteropathica, a hereditary disease of infants in which there is severe persistent diarrhea with malnutrition and skin changes, which are predominantly vesicobullous lesions around the mouth, anus, fingers, and toes, with pustular and eczematoid skin lesions elsewhere, and alopecia. This rather rare entity is inherited as an autosomal recessive characteristic. One of the striking findings in this disorder was the improvement following human-milk feeding and its aggravation or initial development when there was a change from breast milk to cow's milk. Several years ago, Moynahan, studying synthetic diets in this disorder, found that the addition of zinc caused remission of symptoms [23]. This has been confirmed, and there is evidence that acrodermatitis enteropathica is a conditioned zinc deficiency due to failure of absorption of zinc. The mechanism has not been entirely elucidated; the effect of human milk seems to be the improvement of zinc absorption, perhaps by the chelation of zinc with some component of human milk. Zinc deficiency, as manifested by reduced serum zinc concentrations, may be seen in other forms of malabsorption syndromes. A chemical entity resembling acrodermatitis enteropathica has been produced in infants given prolonged parenteral alimentation [24].

Since both copper and zinc deficiency may be complications of prolonged parenteral alimentation [19, 20] unless these trace metals are supplied in the intravenous fluids, it is incumbent upon those using this form of treatment to determine the copper and zinc concentrations in plasma [25, 26]. Techniques are now available for such studies. It is also worth looking at plasma zinc values in children with chronic intestinal disorders, particularly those with persistent growth retardation. Growth retardation is, of course, a major manifestation of Crohn's disease. There are obviously many other reasons for the growth retardation, but in patients who are not showing good growth response with traditional treatment, particularly those who have had major resection of the bowel, the study of trace metal metabolism may be of help in deciding whether zinc deficiency is a factor in the poor growth.

IV. Conclusions

In conclusion, techniques are now available for measuring the concentrations of vitamins or vitamin metabolites in plasma, as well as the important trace metals, for the study of patients with chronic malabsorption syndromes. In such patients, and particularly in patients who have had major loss of intestinal absorptive surface and are being maintained on parenteral alimentation, measurements of vitamin and trace metal concentrations in blood plasma are of importance, in order to ensure that the diet of these patients or the parenteral fluid administered contains adequate amounts of the necessary vitamins and minerals to maintain normal plasma concentrations.

References

1. J. E. Compston and B. Creamer. Plasma levels and intestinal absorption of 25-hydroxyvitamin D in patients with small bowel obstruction. *Gut 17,* 171-175 (1977).
2. J. E. Compston and B. Creamer. The consequences of small intestinal resection. *Q. J. Med. N. S. 46,* 485-497 (1977).
3. J. E. Compston and R. P. H. Thompson. Intestinal absorption of 25-hydroxyvitamin D and osteomalacia in primary biliary cirrhosis. *Lancet 1,* 721-724 (1977).

4. G. R. Thompson, B. Lewis, and C. C. Booth. Absorption of vitamin D_3-^3H in control subjects and patients with intestinal malabsorption. *J. Clin. Invest. 45,* 94-102 (1966).
5. J. A. Fischer, U. Binswanger, R. Schenk, W. Merz, and H. J. Kistler. Normocalcemic secondary hyperparathyroidism and malabsorption. *Helvet. Med. Acta 35,* 30-42 (1969, 1970).
6. J. G. Bieri. Vitamin E. *Nutr. Rev. 33,* 161-167 (1975).
7. H. J. Binder, D. C. Herting, V. Hurst, S. C. Finch, and H. M. Spiro. Tocopherol deficiency in man. *N. Engl. J. Med. 273,* 1289-1297 (1965).
8. C. H. Halsted. The small intestine in vitamin B_{12} and folate deficiency. *Nutr. Rev. 33,* 33-37 (1975).
9. K. Lenz. The effect of the site of lesion and extent of resection on duodenal bile acid concentration and vitamin B_{12} absorption in Crohn's disease. *Scand. J. Gastroenterol. 10,* 241-248 (1975).
10. J. S. Stewart, D. J. Pollock, A. V. Hoffbrand, D. L. Mollin, and C. C. Booth. A study of proximal and distal intestinal structure and absorptive function in idiopathic steatorrhea. *Q. J. Med. N. S. 36,* 425-444 (1967).
11. C. C. Booth, S. Hanna, N. Babouris, and I. MacIntyre. Incidence of hypomagnesemia in intestinal malabsorption. *Br. Med. J. 2,* 141-144 (1963).
12. F. Lifshitz, H. C. Harrison, and H. E. Harrison. Response to vitamin D of magnesium deficient rats. *Proc. Soc. Exp. Biol. Med. 125,* 472-476 (1967).
13. R. Medalle, C. Waterhouse, and T. J. Hahn. Vitamin D resistance in magnesium deficiency. *Am. J. Clin. Nutr. 29,* 854-858 (1976).
14. V. P. Peterson. Potassium and magnesium turnover in magnesium deficiency. *Acta Med. Scand. 174,* 595-604 (1963).
15. A. Cordano and G. G. Graham. Copper deficiency complicating severe chronic intestinal malabsorption. *Pediatrics 38,* 596-604 (1966).
16. A. Cordano, J. M. Baertl, and G. G. Graham. Copper deficiency in infancy. *Pediatrics 34,* 324-336 (1964).
17. G. G. Graham and A. Cordano. Copper depletion and deficiency in the malnourished infant. *Johns Hopkins Med. J. 124,* 139-150 (1969).
18. G. G. Graham and A. Cordano. Copper deficiency in human subjects. In *Trace Elements in Human Health and Disease,* Vol. 1, Zinc and Copper. Academic Press, New York, 1976.
19. C. R. Fleming, R. E. Hodges, and L. S. Hurley. A prospective study of serum copper and zinc levels in patients receiving total parenteral nutrition. *Am. J. Clin. Nutr. 29,* 70-77 (1976).
20. E. C. Hauer and M. V. Kaminski, Jr. Trace metal profile of parenteral nutrition solutions. *Am. J. Clin. Nutr. 31,* 264-268 (1978).
21. N. A. Holtzman, P. Charache, A. Cordano, and G. G. Graham. Distribution of serum copper in copper deficiency. *Johns Hopkins Med. J. 126,* 34-42 (1970).
22. I. Sternlieb and H. D. Janowitz. Absorption of copper in malabsorption syndromes. *J. Clin. Invest. 43,* 1049-1055 (1964).

23. (Editorial). Zinc in human medicine. *Lancet 2,* 351-352 (1975).
24. T. Arakawa, T. Tamura, Y. Igarashi, H. Suzuki, and H. H. Sandstead. Zinc deficiency in two infants during total parenteral alimentation for diarrhea. *Am. J. Clin. Nutr. 29,* 197-204 (1976).
25. K. N. Jeejeebhoy, B. Lauger, G. Tsallas, R. C. Chu, A. Kuksis, and G. H. Anderson. Total parenteral nutrition at home: Studies in patients surviving 4 months to 5 years. *Gastroenterology* 943-953 (1976).
26. N. W. Solomons, T. J. Layden, I. H. Rosenberg, K. Vo-Khactu, and H. H. Sandstead. Plasma trace metals during total parenteral alimentation. *Gastroenterology* 1022-1025 (1976).
27. H. E. Harrison, R. R. Tompsett, and D. P. Barr. The serum potassium in two cases of sprue. *Proc. Soc. Exp. Biol. Med. 54,* 314-315 (1943).
28. H. E. Harrison, H. C. Harrison, R. R. Tompsett, and D. P. Barr. Potassium deficiency in a case of lymphosarcoma with the sprue syndrome. *Am. J. Med. 2,* 131-143 (1947).

27 Nutritional and Economic Implications of Soil-Transmitted Helminths with Special Reference to Ascariasis

LANI S. STEPHENSON / Cornell University, Ithaca, New York

> It is difficult for those living in temperate climates with good standards of public health and medical care to realize the impact of disease on rural communities in the tropics. For example, if you happen to be born and grow up in rural Africa, you are liable to harbor four or more different disease-producing organisms simultaneously. And yet as a parent, you must be fit enough to work, or your family will starve. In your village every child at times suffers the paroxysms of malaria fever and you and your wife will mourn the death of one or two children from this disease . . . . But lacking effective remedies, you tend to philosophize in the face of sickness. You make the effort to walk the ten miles to the nearest dispensary when you or your child is ill, but there may be no remedies, and it may be too late . . . . [1]

I. To Treat or Not to Treat

There has long been a controversy in the medical literature over whether or not a clinician should provide treatment for common intestinal helminthic infections, particularly when they appear to be light or asymptomatic. A recent statement by Gilles [2] illustrates what is probably the most commonly held viewpoint: "In nonendemic areas it is justifiable to treat all [intestinal worm] infections however light, while in areas where reinfection is likely to occur, only heavy or moderate infections are worth treating unless simultaneous attempts are made to improve environmental hygiene." On the other hand, Pawlowski [3] recently stated, with reference to infection by *Ascaris*, that "intestinal ascariasis should always be treated when diagnosed because it is potentially a very serious infection.

The treatment of suspected cases is also recommended . . . ." In the past, when drugs available—particularly for hookworm and trichuris infections—were somewhat toxic, difficult to administer, and/or not particularly efficacious, it may have been justified to discourage treatment. However, recent developments seriously place in doubt former conservative viewpoints. These developments include: the appearance of broad-spectrum anthelmintic drugs which are relatively safe and inexpensive; the fact that prevalence of soil-transmitted helminths is not rapidly decreasing [4]; and a realization that hoped-for large improvements in environmental hygiene have not occurred for a majority of poor families in many developing countries.

II. Prevalence and Epidemiology

Four common soil-transmitted helminths, roundworm (*Ascaris lumbricoides*), hookworms (*Ancylostoma duodenale* and *Necator americanus*), and whipworm (*Trichuris trichiura*), constitute public health problems from the point of view of prevalence. Recent global estimates indicate that ascariasis is one of the most common parasitic infections in the world, with an estimated 986 million persons or one-quarter of the world's population infected [5]. Hookworms are estimated to infect about 716 million persons, while *Trichuris* is thought to infect 536 million persons [5].

Transmission of all four parasites is through improper disposal of feces from infected persons; the feces contain potentially infective ova or larvae which require relatively warm temperatures and moisture for development. Once at the infective stage, eggs of *Ascaris* and *Trichuris* are capable of surviving considerable cold and dehydration. This means that infections tend to be endemic in poverty areas, anywhere that sanitation is poor, especially in the warm, humid areas of the tropics and subtropics. It may be improbable that light intestinal worm infections cause serious disease in otherwise healthy well-nourished persons. However, the vast majority of people infected with intestinal helminths live in developing countries or areas where various forms of malnutrition and other diseases are common. There is increasing evidence of synergistic relationships not only between malnutrition and infections but also between one infection and another. In the case of *Ascaris,* infections are most common and heaviest in children of preschool age, who are also most likely to suffer from or succumb to protein-energy malnutrition, gastroenteritis, respiratory infections, malaria, and a variety of other nutritional, infectious, and parasitic diseases [6].

III. Nutrition-Helminth Interactions: Possible Mechanisms

The helminths discussed here are in excellent physiologic positions to be able to interact with the nutritional status of their hosts. The adult forms of

Ascaris and the hookworms are commonly located in the jejunum of the small intestine, where most nutrient digestion and absorption take place, and where antigenic components and toxic or bioactive compounds produced by the worms can be easily absorbed. In addition, hookworms suck blood from the mucosal surface, causing blood loss and tissue destruction. *Trichuris,* although located primarily in the colon, where they often bury their heads deeply into the colonic mucosa, are in a position to interfere with water and electrolyte absorption.

Intestinal parasites may directly affect the nutritional status of a child by causing either a decrease in nutrient consumption or a functional increase in the body's nutrient requirements. Any condition causing anorexia, such as general malaise due to larval migration through the tissues or intestinal upset due to the presence of adult parasites in the small intestine, would decrease total nutrient consumption. Increases in nutrient requirements may arise from a number of factors, including: (1) interference with absorption at the brush border because of diffuse mucosal damage, physical obstruction by worms, or production of antiproteolytic substances by worms; (2) loss of macronutrients, fluid, and electrolytes through diarrhea and vomiting; and (3) consumption by the worms of nutrients which are needed by the host [7, 8]. These effects would be much more likely to achieve clinical significance when a child is heavily infected with parasites, has a marginal nutrient intake, and/or already has other debilitating infections. While the above interactions may be logical from a physiologic standpoint, it is complicated and ethically difficult to confirm their occurrence in human clinical studies. Layrisse and Vargas [4] have described the dilemma faced by researchers in this way:

> Much has been written on the synergistic interaction between parasitic infection and malnutrition in which malnutrition decreases the capacity of the host to invasion of parasites and, vice versa, the effect of parasitic infection influences the host's nutrition. But although this concept of mutual effect seems very logical, it has not as yet received substantial support due in part to the fact that human parasitic infection flourishes mostly in areas where malnourishment exists since early life and partly because the experimental studies carried out so far have not been entirely satisfactory.
>
> The difficulties confronted for a perusal study of a single parasitic infection in man should also be taken into account. There are environmental influences which can affect either host or parasites, or both, and which vary according to the ecological area under study. It is also important to bear in mind the difficulty in finding populations infected with a single parasite. In many instances, students are forced to work in multiparasitized areas and make a decision which infection is paramount in inducing malnourishment and rule out other less harmful

> infections. The literature on this topic reflects pathetically all these inconveniences. Controversial results, such as ascribing to a parasite a detrimental nutritional effect by a group of investigators and a nondetrimental effect by others, are not unusual. In other cases, malnourishment effects ascribed to a parasite have been denied after more careful studies.

Well-controlled animal studies can provide clear-cut evidence of parasitic effects, but it is difficult for the clinician to extrapolate these results for use in the clinical setting.

IV. Nutrient-Parasite Interactions

A. Ascaris lumbricoides

1. Life Cycle. Adult *Ascaris lumbricoides* normally live in the small intestine and are most often found in the proximal jejunum and mid jejunum at autopsy. The female worms are from 20 to more than 35 cm in length and about 4-6 mm in diameter, while the males are 15-30 cm long and more slender [9].

The female worms produce ova which are passed in the feces of the host. *Ascaris* are much more prolific in terms of potential ova production than are the other intestinal helminths. One female worm can contain 27,000,000 ova, and may pass as many as 200,000 ova per day into the feces [10].

Humans contract ascariasis by ingestion of embryonated ova. The ova are passed unembryonated in the feces. In the presence of sufficient oxygen, moisture, and warmth, larvae develop in about 2-3 weeks and become infective about 1 week later. The ova have a tough protein coat and, prior to embryonation, are extremely resistant to drying or to destruction by various chemicals. They have been known to remain viable in the soil for over 10 years. Development generally ceases above 100°F and below 60°F. Tropical temperatures of about 85°F are ideal for embryonation, although prolonged direct sunlight is said to kill embryos.

Ova ingested by the host hatch in the small intestine and liberate larvae, which pass through the mucosa and are carried to the liver in the enterohepatic circulation. The larvae develop further and roam about in the liver for about 4-5 days, then proceed via the bloodstream to the heart, and on to the lungs. In the lungs they continue growth, finally break out into the alveoli, pass up the trachea, and are either swallowed or spit out by the host. The swallowed larvae develop in the small intestine where they grow into juvenile and then adult worms of both sexes, which mate to produce fertilized ova. Many of the larvae that originally hatched are destroyed or lost and do not become adult *Ascaris.*

The entire process, from ingestion of ova to production of fertilized ova by gravid *Ascaris,* takes about 2 months. Adult *Ascaris* continue to grow in width and length throughout their normal 1-2 year lifespan. More detailed information on the life cycle of *A. lumbricoides* is available [9, 11].

2. General Pathology and Morbidity of Ascaris Infection. The evidence for pathologic effects of *A. lumbricoides* in humans comes mainly from the clinical and surgical experiences of practicing physicians in many countries (Table 1). In general the pathologic processes have been little studied under controlled conditions. Symptoms reported to occur in ascariasis include digestive disorders, colic, nausea, vomiting, respiratory disorders and pneumonitis, restless sleep, and teethgrinding during the night [12]. Neurologic disorders, including convulsions, and serious allergic manifestations are also reported in the medical literature [13].

Adult *A. lumbricoides* are thought to live peacefully in the lumen of the small intestine, indiscriminately ingesting food particles and other substances,

Table 1 Manifestations of Ascariasis

Allergic action of the adult and larva
- Substances from adult
  - Allergic phenomena among laboratory workers
- Substances from larva
  - Cutaneous signs: urticaria, erythematous lesions
  - Blood eosinophilia
  - Loffler's syndrome
- Associated infections
  - Complications due to *Strongyloides stercoralis* and *Escherichia coli*
  - Cryptogenetic and malignant eosinophilia
  - Cutaneous, ophthalmic, and visceral larva migrans due to the migration of the larvae

Action of the adult on the intestinal tract
- Nutritional disorders and enterocolitis of the diarrheal type
- Surgical forms
  - Intestinal subocclusions and occlusions caused by mass of *Ascaris*
  - Intussusception (in children), volvulus, and hernial strangulation (penetration of *Ascaris* into the loop involved)
  - Acute mesenteric adenitis
  - Penetration into the appendiceal lumen or into an intestinal diverticulum
  - Postoperative troubles due to movement of *Ascaris* (colic, peritonitis, fistula)

Wandering of the adult
- From mouth, nose, lacrimal fossa, or through eustachian tube to the middle ear
- Through glottis (glottal edema) to trachea or bronchi
- Into bile ducts: obstructive jaundice, gallstones, cholangitis, liver abscess
- Into pancreatic duct: acute hemorrhagic or purulent pancreatitis
- Migration across tissue walls from intestine to peritoneal cavity and elsewhere

Source: Taken from *Control of Ascariasis* [13].

such as barium sulfate from a barium meal, that pass through the gastrointestinal tract [14]. However, it seems likely that adult *Ascaris* cause a variety of digestive disturbances. To substantiate this view, Lagundoye [15] found that 92% of 53 adult Nigerian hospital outpatients infected with adult *Ascaris* exhibited a disordered small-bowel pattern when a plain abdominal X-ray film was taken. The most common abnormality seen was coarsening of the mucosal folds, although flocculation and dilution of barium, segmentation, bowel dilatation, and nonobstructive localized intussusception were also seen.

But most published reports on the effects of adult worms deal with surgical or other complications, due to wandering of the adults to abnormal sites such as the liver or pancreas [16, 17]. These complications include, among others, intestinal obstruction, obstructive jaundice, cholangitis, liver abscesses, acute pancreatitis, peritonitis, and appendicitis (Table 1). These are discussed in detail by Pawlowski [3].

Ascariasis in humans is generally thought to cause few if any symptoms in most infected perons [13] and to be rarely fatal. However, in Sri Lanka in 1954, one large hospital reported that ascariasis was *the* most common cause for admission of inpatients. In 12.8% of cases admitted for ascariasis, the disease was fatal [18]. This fatality rate was halved in the following year, in response to the introduction of piperazine compounds. This mortality rate seems unusually high; the author did not report whether deaths were due primarily to ascariasis or to other causes.

Complications due to ascariasis in the United States are relatively rare, but are still encountered, particularly in the southern states. In 1975, Blumenthal and Schultz [19] observed, in three rural Louisiana public hospitals, that 21 patients had been hospitalized with intestinal obstruction secondary to ascariasis over a 3-year period. They estimated that this incidence approximated two cases of obstruction per thousand infected children.

Regarding symptomatology, it is pertinent to point out that tolerance to and admission of pain are often determined by culture and previous experience. Also, full medical histories are difficult to obtain, and may even be dispensed with, in overcrowded outpatient clinics where the patrons are mostly illiterate parents with 2- or 3-year-old children who, at best, have difficulty explaining their symptoms. In any case the idea that ascariasis is either harmless or symptomless may be only medical folklore.

3. Nutritional Effects. The report of a World Health Organization Expert Committee on control of ascariasis [13] cites relationships between ascariasis and stunting, general undernutrition, avitaminosis, decreased protein absorption, xerophthalmia, and ascorbic acid deficiency. There is a huge literature available on various aspects of ascariasis, but very few well-controlled studies deal with the nutritional effects of *Ascaris* on the human host. Those studies that have been conducted involved the selection of children who were mostly of school age, and therefore less vulnerable to malnutrition than preschool children. Also, many of the children studied harbored a number of other gastrointestinal parasites—making assessment of the effects of ascariasis itself difficult.

A few clinical studies of *A. lumbricoides* infection in children indicate lower apparent absorption and retention of protein and lower apparent absorption of fat and carbohydrate in infected children *prior to,* as opposed to *after,* deworming. In the first of these studies, Venkatachalam and Patwardhan [20] found that deworming of nine hospitalized infected children, who harbored a mean of 26 adult parasites each, caused the mean fecal nitrogen excretion per day to decrease from 1.32 to 0.76 g ($P < 0.01$). The authors also showed experimentally that neither the improved hospital diet fed, nor the ova excreted by *Ascaris,* nor the effects of the drugs used in deworming could have accounted for this change in nitrogen excretion. They concluded that even moderate burdens of *Ascaris* could be responsible for nutritionally significant losses of dietary protein in children receiving diets marginal in protein content.

Improvement in protein nutrition after deworming was also noted by Tripathy et al. [21] in five hospitalized children harboring a mean of 30 adult *Ascaris* and receiving relatively low levels of protein in the diet (1.0-1.5 g/kg body weight per day). Fecal nitrogen after deworming decreased by a mean of 6.5 percentage points of dietary nitrogen: 33.5% before and 27% after deworming ($P < 0.01$). The same authors [22] also found, in three other *Ascaris*-infected children harboring more than 48 worms each, that the decrease in nitrogen excretion after deworming was accompanied by an increase in nitrogen retention.

More important from the standpoint of energy balance, Tripathy et al. [21] found that four of five infected children exhibited mild to moderate steatorrhea. Fecal fat excretion decreased in all five children after deworming (9.9 versus 2.3% of dietary fat, $P < 0.001$). They also found impaired D-xylose absorption in three of the five children prior to treatment; the absorption improved slightly in two of their cases immediately after deworming. They reported generalized mucosal damage in small-intestinal biopsy specimens taken prior to deworming and postulated that mucosal damage was responsible for the defects in absorption. The degree of mucosal damage showed a decrease in biopsy specimens taken after deworming.

On the other hand, Teotia et al. [23] found that only one of five *Ascaris*-infected children exhibited fat malabsorption, but severity of the infections was not measured. Also, Bray [24], in a nitrogen balance study in four children (ages 7-10 yr), found no consistent differences in nitrogen absorption or utilization prior to and after deworming. The children studied exhibited wide variations in severity of ascariasis and in clinical signs of malnutrition, and one subject also harbored *Ancylostoma.*

Recently two clinical studies in India have indicated that ascariasis may interfere with vitamin A absorption. Mahalanabis et al. [25] determined vitamin A absorption in *Ascaris*-infected adults and 12 healthy controls. More than 70% of infected patients had malabsorption of vitamin A, as indicated by serum levels after a radioactive dose. In addition, 7 of 23 infected patients who receive a D-xylose absorption test had abnormally low values (below 20% of dose excreted in urine in 5 hr). Immediately after deworming, vitamin A absorption improved in 13 of the 14 patients retested, and D-xylose absorption increased in all 5 patients retested.

Sivakumar and Reddy [26] demonstrated that six *Ascaris*-infected children absorbed less of a test dose of vitamin A from the gut than did five control children (80 versus 99%, $P < 0.01$). The percentage of the radioactive label excreted in the urine did not vary between groups; hence the infected children retained less vitamin A than did controls (68 versus 82%, $P < 0.01$). None of the children had steatorrhea, since stool fat content was less than 5 g per 24 hr. Two of the infected children were retested 2 months after deworming; vitamin A absorption improved from 83-86% to 95-96%. Only trace amounts of the vitamin A label were found in excreted worms, indicating that sequestering of the vitamin by the worms could not have caused the defect in absorption. The authors concluded that ascariasis may be aggravating vitamin A deficiency in areas where xerophthalmia is common.

In one of the few published studies relating ascariasis to preschool child growth, Gupta and co-workers [27] reported from India that the deworming of malnourished preschool children every 3 months in villages where *Ascaris* was common resulted in increased weight for age after 8 months of study, in comparison with nontreated controls. Children 6-48 months old in two villages were given tetramisole every 3 months for a year, and control children in two other villages received a placebo; children in all four villages received food supplements, immunizations, and simple medical care.

When children whose stools had been positive for ascaris ova were considered, 13 treated children gained over one percentage point in weight for age during the year, and only 2 lost over 1 percentage point. In the placebo group, 16 children gained, but 27 children lost over one percentage point (chi-square $P < 0.01$). The authors concluded that periodic deworming should be an integral part of a supplementary feeding program or a child health care package where roundworm is a severe problem. They also pointed out that the six tablets of tetramisole needed per child per year cost only about 4% as much as a year's supply of supplementary food the the same child.

In 1975-1976, an investigation was undertaken in Kenya to measure the effects of ascariasis on growth, nutritional stutus, and health of preschool-age children [28, 29]. The study was conducted in two Kenyan villages where 186 children, aged 12-72 months, were examined three times at 14-week intervals, and anthropometric, clinical, and stool examinations were performed. At visit I, 85% of the children were below 90% weight for age by the Harvard standard, and 27% had ova of *Ascaris* in their stools; mean anthropometric measurements between infected and control children did not differ significantly. All children received an anthelmintic (levamisole) at visit II; the mean number of worms collected was approximately 7 per infected child.

In the 14 weeks between visits I and II (before deworming) children infected by *Ascaris* (n = 61) did not differ from controls (n = 125) in weight gain or percent expected weight gain. In the 14 weeks after deworming (II-III) previously infected children showed higher weight gain (0.7 versus 0.5 kg, $P < 0.05$) and percent expected weight gain (130 versus 98%, $P < 0.025$) than controls. Before deworming, triceps skinfold thickness decreased in *Ascaris*-infected children as compared with controls (−1.6 versus 0.3 mm, $P < 0.0005$). After deworming, skinfold thickness increased markedly in previously infected children as compared with controls (2.0 versus −1.1 mm, $P < 0.0005$). Multiple regression analysis showed that ascariasis was by far the most important variable of 37 possible health, nutritional, and socioeconomic variables explaining decrease in skinfold thickness before, and increase after, deworming. Thus it was concluded that even light infections of *Ascaris* adversely influence nutritional status, and deworming enhanced growth.

Cross-sectional nutrition-parasite surveys in the United States have recently found ascariasis in children from Louisiana to be associated with low serum albumin and plasma ascorbic acid levels and to be weekly associated with low weight for height and with signs of riboflavin deficiency [30]. Also, *Ascaris*-infected preschoolers on Hilton Head Island, South Carolina, more frequently had serum vitamin A levels below 20 μg/dl than did noninfected children (43 versus 21%), but the association was not statistically significant [31].

In short, ascariasis has been linked to deficiencies or malabsorption of calories, protein, fat, carbohydrate (D-xylose), vitamin A, riboflavin, and ascorbic acid. These findings deserve further study, particularly in preschool-age children in areas where poor growth and development are common.

B. Hookworms

"Hookworm is never spectacular like some other diseases, but is essentially insidious; year after year, generation after generation, it saps the vitality and undermines the health and efficiency of whole communities"—thus write Chandler and Read [9]. The life cycles of the human hookworms are grossly similar to the life cycle of *Ascaris* except that one contracts the infection from infective larvae which penetrate the skin or oral cacity, rather than from ingestion of ova. Details of the life cycles, epidemiology, diagnosis, and drug treatment are well described elsewhere [9, 32]. The adult parasites live mainly in the upper small intestine and are 7-12 mm in length; their life-span may be 5 years or longer. An individual can harbor more than a thousand adult hookworms at once.

The relationships between hookworm and human nutritional status have been more thoroughly studied than such relationships for the other soil-transmitted helminths–and are discussed in detail by Roche and Layrisse [33], Layrisse and Vargas [4], and Banwell and Shad [32]. The worms feed by biting off pieces of the mucosal surface (a process which causes bleeding into the gut) and also by actively sucking the host's blood. Daily blood loss due to hookworm infection has been estimated to vary from 2-3 ml in light infections to about 100 ml in heavy infections. Studies with infected humans have determined, by means of radioisotopic techniques, that *Necator* causes a blood loss of approximately 0.03 ml per day per worm, or 2 ml per day per 1000 necator ova found per gram of feces. The daily blood loss is generally greater per worm with *Ancylostoma,* being approximately 0.20 ml per worm or 4 ml per 1000 ova per gram of feces.

Perhaps 40-60% of the hemoglobin iron lost into the gut lumen is reabsorbed farther down the gastrointestinal tract [4], but iron losses can be considerable, and hookworms are an important cause of iron deficiency anemia in humans when the dietary iron absorption is not sufficient to replace both iron lost through normal iron losses and iron losses due to the parasites. Layrisse and Roche, in a classic field study among more than 1100 rural Venezuelans, demonstrated that hemoglobin level correlated inversely with number of hookworm ova per gram of feces [33, 34].

Human hookworm infection may also be responsible for severe hypoproteinemia due to serum albumin loss and a protein-losing enteropathy [32]. In *uncomplicated* hookworm infection, macro- and micronutrient absorption for those nutrients studied is said to be adequate, except for an impairment of folic acid absorption [4]. Some workers have reported malabsorption and mucosal injury in infected subjects, but others have not, and have suggested that the mucosal changes seen were actually caused by factors other than hookworms: e.g., poor diet or tropical sprue [4, 35-37].

When considering treatment of hookworm infection, one must realize that a majority of patients, and particularly children, living in tropical and subtropical areas where hookworm is endemic, are likely to be presently or potentially malnourished to some degree, are likely to be exposed to many other infections, and are likely to have infrequent access to medical care. Provided that the drugs are available, it may be wiser, even in presumably light infections, to treat rather than to assume that the infection is harmless.

C. Trichuris trichiura

Trichuriasis is contracted by ingestion of infective ova, as is ascariasis, and causes blood loss from the gut, as do the hookworm infections. The adult

Trichuris trichiura worms are 30-50 mm in length and live for up to 3-5 years or perhaps longer. They attach themselves to the mucosa in the colon, usually in the cecum and appendix. Infections can range from only a few to more than a thousand worms. Signs and symptoms of heavy infections may resemble those of hookworm infection and may include loss of appetite, abdominal discomfort, nausea, diarrhea, blood-streaked stools, weakness, weight loss, eosinophilia, and anemia [9]. Rectal prolapse can occur in severe or chronic cases [9]. Further details of interest to physicians and other researchers are available elsewhere [4, 9, 38].

Recent reviews indicate the role of *Trichuris* in causing blood loss, but it appears that other possible relationships between the worms and malnutrition have not been extensively studied in humans. Layrisse et al. [39] determined blood loss in nine *Trichuris*-infected children by means of a ^{51}Cr tracer and reported that the children lost about 0.005 ml of blood per worm per day, or about 0.25 ml per 1000 ova per gram of feces. They estimated that infections of more than 800 worms can induce iron-deficiency anemia in children. While *Trichuris* do not cause the degree of blood loss that hookworms do, the symptoms attributed to them (loss of appetite, diarrhea, weight loss) suggest that they may negatively influence the nutritional status of malnourished children through a number of mechanisms, even when infections are light. Previously, the most effective treatment for trichuriasis was the difficult and time-consuming hexylresorcinol retention enema. Under these conditions, it was not surprising that light infections were not treated. An effective and reportedly safe drug, mebendazole, is now available [38], and perhaps it is time to reconsider treatment of lighter infections and to continue research on interactions between *Trichuris* and malnutrition in children.

V. Economics of Ascariasis

From the foregoing discussion one can see that some relationships between human malnutrition and intestinal helminths have been studied. However, with the possible exception of hookworm anemia, very little of a quantitative cause-and-effect nature is actually known. The economic implications of intestinal parasites on the family and society have been studied much less, with a few notable exceptions [40]. Yet the cost of a disease—relative to other diseases and to available financial resources—is important in determining whether or not the medical care system chooses to prevent and control the disease.

In the past, treatment of lighter infections of *Ascaris*, hookworm, and *Trichuris* has been discouraged, with the following justifications:

1. Light loads are "asymptomatic" (and therefore presumably harmless).
2. The children will just get reinfected anyway.

3. Environmental hygiene and health education are the true answers to control.
4. It costs nothing, economically speaking, to ignore light infections.
5. To treat light, presumably harmless, infections uses scarce health resources that are better spent on diseases with higher mortality rates.

In view of recent research into the nutritional and economic implications of ascariasis in particular, a review of these arguments is now in order. It may be true that light infections of *Ascaris* are asymptomatic, though this depends upon the amount of discomfort a person is used to experiencing; but field studies have now shown that deworming of infected malnourished children improves weight gain [27-29]. While it is true that treated children often become reinfected in endemic areas, the fact that treatment may improve growth, even if only for a short period, justifies treatment, particularly in preschool children, who are most vulnerable to growth failure and protein-energy malnutrition.

It is true that a general rise in the standard of living and significant improvements in environmental hygiene should prevent transmission of soil-transmitted helminths. This has been the gospel put forth for decades. But for millions of people in rural areas, environmental sanitation has not improved markedly, and the prevalence of intestinal parasites in many communities has hardly decreased. A recent study in Iran [41] illustrated that improved sanitation by itself may be unlikely to lower drastically the prevalence of ascariasis and hookworm infections. Three villages in Iran were supplied with either improved sanitation alone (one latrine per family plus a clean village water supply), treatment alone (piperazine for ascariasis and bephenium for hookworm infection, these drugs being given alternately every 3 months), or both. Four years later, the reduction in rates of ascariasis for the different methods were: sanitation, infection reduced by 28%; treatment, 84%; and both, 79%. For hookworm, reduction rates were: sanitation, 4%; treatment, 73%; and both, 69%. Thus even after a 4-year period, sanitation alone did little to decrease prevalence of both parasites, while treatment decreased prevalence by 70% or more.

Provision and usage of latrines and safe water supplies and health education are, of course, essential parts of community development and can drastically reduce transmission of many diseases, particularly those due to certain bacteria and viruses. However, in the short term, it is questionable whether the increased usage of latrines alone can be expected to greatly lower the prevalence of ascariasis. Recent village studies in Kenya showed that most older children and adults used latrines, but that some young preschool children did not, partly because they could not use a pit latrine properly, and partly because they were too young to understand the need for proper feces disposal [29].

Mothers can encourage their children to use a latrine as early as possible. But the average rural Kenyan mother may have two or three preschool children to care for and is responsible for cultivation of all food crops, food preparation, and fetching the entire family's supply of water and firewood on foot. Thus it is unrealistic to expect her to ensure that every stool passed by all of her children ends up in a latrine. Fecal contamination of the environment by young children cannot help but continue.

Spread of ascariasis is further complicated by the prolific ova production of the female worms. Only one contaminated stool that is passed in the yard contains enough ova to theoretically infect an entire village for years.

One adult female *Ascaris* may produce about 200,000 ova per day, and each ovum, if embryonated and swallowed by a human, can produce one adult worm. Ova are extremely hardy and can survive for more than a year in the soil, if not destroyed by sunlight, radiation, or desiccation. If one young child harbors only 10 adult worms, 5 of which are female, the number of ova passed in the child's stools per day is on the order of 1,000,000, and the yearly ova output is about 365,000,000. Thus even if all older family members religiously use a latrine, and the youngest preschool child uses the latrine at least 90% of the time, that one child, if only lightly infected, can deposit up to 36,500,000 ascaris ova per year in the soil around the family dwelling. These ova can obviously be spread from dwelling to dwelling by movement of animals or people, or possibly by wind and rain, or on contaminated food. So even if the availability and use of latrines becomes near-perfect, ascaris ova will remain in large numbers in the environment. This is also true for the other soil-transmitted helminths, although their reproductive capacities are much lower per worm than is that of *Ascaris.*

The other health education technique that can be used to prevent ascariasis is to promote thorough hand-washing before eating. This of course is already being done, but large quantities of clean water are simply not available to many rural families. And even when access to water is not a problem, it is at best difficult to convince very young children that they should not put unwashed hands into their mouths.

The fourth assumption about nontreatment of mild infections is that lack of treatment involves no economic costs. But there clearly are costs attached to the mere existence and persistence of a disease. In Kenya in 1976, the minimal economic costs incurred due to ascariasis were estimated for the entire country [29]. These computations included costs to the medical care system and to private citizens. Health care costs were estimated from inpatient and outpatient statistics from government hospitals where a primary diagnosis of ascariasis was made. These costs were extrapolated to include mission hospitals (but not rural health centers or dispensaries). From this the cost of health care was estimated to be $180,000 in 1976, excluding anthelmintic drugs. Figures were obtained on anthelmintic drugs purchased by the government, and the cost of these was estimated to be $160,000. The general public, it was estimated, purchased $195,000 worth of anthelmintic drugs from retail stores in 1976. *Ascaris*-infected Kenyans seeking treatment in hospitals were estimated to have spent $199,000 because of lost work time and transportation costs resulting from their trips to the hospital. Based on the assumption that absorption and utilization of calories in food in those infected with *Ascaris* is reduced by only 2.8% of total calories, then the retail value of this food lost to Kenyans was estimated to be $4,400,000 in 1976. The total of these economic costs of *Ascaris* is over $5,000,000 in a single year for a country with 10 million persons, and these estimates are quite conservative.

The fifth and strongest argument against treating light intestinal worm infections is that to do so would use up scarce health care funds which should be used to prevent and treat diseases with higher child mortality rates, such as protein-energy malnutrition (PEM), gastroenteritis, and malaria. Since Gish and Walker [42] have estimated that many developing countries spend only $2 per capita per year on health care, this point is well taken. On the other hand, diseases such as PEM and gastroenteritis are much more complicated and expensive to treat and control than ascariasis. And, since ascariasis may inhibit growth in malnourished children, the treatment and prevention of ascariasis may very well have a beneficial effect on the prevalence of PEM and its associated diseases.

VI. Drug Treatment Programs

Thus, despite efforts to improve health knowledge, sanitation, and health care, *Ascaris*, hookworms, and *Trichuris* are still very prevalent and, because of their ubiquitous natures, very likely to persist or even increase in prevalence. Substantial improvements in education, housing, sanitation, and the economic situation are being made in many areas, but these improvements are unlikely to occur fast enough to stay or decrease the prevalence of soil-transmitted helminths in general, and *Ascaris* in particular, in the next 10 years. This is especially true if the only weapons used are health education and symptomatic treatment after diagnosis in hospitals.

Given that significant fecal contamination of the environment is destined to continue, the remaining approach to decrease ascariasis is to decrease the likelihood that those feces contain helminth ova. For *Ascaris* in particular, this can be done by periodic mass anthelmintic treatment of persons in areas where *Ascaris* is prevalent. In the past, anthelmintic drugs, especially the more toxic ones, have been given to a person only after a stool examination has shown which parasites the person has. The development of less toxic drugs, coupled with the realization that most *Ascaris*-infected persons never get a stool examination and hence never receive drug treatment, has caused a number of physicians to suggest mass treatment programs as an alternative [43]. In mass treatment, an anthelmintic is periodically given to all persons in a vulnerable group in an area where certain parasites are known to be common. This approach has important medical and economic advantages over other methods of control:

1. Time and cost of stool examinations are saved.
2. For the same amount of money, many more persons can be treated than is possible in conventional health care facilities.
3. The person administering the drug needs very little if any genuine medical training.
4. Prevention and cure are combined, in one delivery system in that present effects of the disease are temporarily arrested, and fecal contamination is temporarily halted in all infected persons.

This mass treatment approach is likely to be the only way–significantly and economically–to decrease ascariasis and the prevalence of three other soil-transmitted helminths within the next 10 years.

The three main components of a mass treatment program are: (1) choice of target groups, (2) choice of drug, and (3) choice of delivery system.

Regarding target groups, it seems that preschool children are the most likely to suffer from the effects of ascariasis and are also most likely to promote transmission of the disease to others. Hence they probably require frequent deworming, perhaps 2-3 times per year at the outset. Prevalence surveys in some areas also show that *Ascaris* and other soil-transmitted helminths are extremely prevalent in school-age children and adults. If cost permits, they too should receive routine anthelmintic therapy, although less often than preschoolers: e.g., once per year or every 2 years.

Regarding choice of drug, one can either opt for the traditional, less expensive piperazine compounds, or one can choose the more expensive, broad-spectrum anthelmintics. The author feels that the preferable choice, for Kenya in particular, is a broad-spectrum-type drug–for a number of reasons:

1. Prevalence studies show that the soil-transmitted helminths tend to coexist. Cases of multiple parasites are often common. If one is going to treat and help prevent infections by *Ascaris,* one might as well also be treating and helping to prevent infections by hookworm, *Trichuris,* and *Strongyloides* at the same time. This cannot be done using piperazine compounds alone.

2. The major difficulty and a significant proportion of the cost of a mass treatment program is likely to be the choice and development of the delivery system, rather than the choice and purchase of drugs. It is sensible to combat all four soil-transmitted helminths with a single delivery system.

3. Although the cost per dose of the borad-spectrum anthelmintics is greater than the cost of piperazine compounds, the cost per dose of bephenium, used in the treatment of hookworm, is greater than the cost per dose of levamisole, a broad-spectrum drug that reportedly lowers individual worm burdens of hookworm, *Trichuris,* and *Strongyloides,* as well as virtually eliminating *Ascaris.* In the long run, it is probably cheaper to treat and prevent all four diseases at once than to deal with them separately.

VII. Conclusions

There is a great need for more applied research to determine the relationships between nutrition, particularly childhood malnutrition, and intestinal parasitic infections. Nevertheless, it is clear that hookworm infection can cause iron-deficiency anemia and that infection by *Ascaris* is associated with poor growth in malnourished children. Periodic deworming of children, using a mass treatment approach, is highly recommended to control soil-transmitted helminths in areas where parasites and protein-energy malnutrition are highly prevalent. The main aims of treatment should be to reduce parasite loads below the level of clinical significance for the individual child [2] and to reduce future environmental contamination with infective feces for the sake of the community.

Acknowledgments

The studies on the nutritional and economic aspects of ascariasis quoted here were supported in part by a grant from the World Bank, Washington, D.C.

These studies were made possible by the assistance and advice of many persons, including Dr. M. C. Latham and Dr. M. C. Nesheim in the United States; Dr. D. W. T. Crompton, Ms. S. Arnold, and Mr. D. Barnard in England; and Dr. T. Schulpen, Dr. A. A. J. Jansen, Dr. M. L. Oduori, Mr. H. Kinyanjui, Ms. B. Maina, Dr. D. Wijers, Dr. T. Hanegraaf, Dr. A. Voorhoeve, Ms. W. van Steenbergen, Dr. A. Muller, Ms. M. van Rens, Ms. S. Lakhani, Mr. J. Mbuvi, Mr. S. Nzomo, Dr. A. Cross, and Dr. C. Forbes in Kenya. The author is indebted to Dr. M. C. Latham, Dr. J. R. Georgi, and Dr. M. C. Nesheim for reviewing the manuscript and to Ms. D. Doty for typing the manuscript.

References

1. D. Rowe. *Tropical Diseases.* WHO Pamphlet, Geneva, 1976, pp. 4-7.
2. H. M. Gilles. Diseases of the alimentary system. Treatment of intestinal worms. *Br. Med. J. 2,* 1314-1316 (1976).
3. Z. S. Pawlowski. Ascariasis. *Clin. Gastroenterol. 7,* 157-178 (1978).
4. R. Layrisse and A. Vargas. Nutrition and intestinal parasitic infection. *Prog. Food Nutr. Sci. 1,* 645-667 (1975).

5. W. Peters and H. M. Gilles. *A Color Atlas of Tropical Medicine and Parasitology*. Wolfe Medical, London, 1977.
6. World Health Organization Expert Committee. *Nutrition and Infection.* WHO Technical Report Series No. 314, Geneva, 1965.
7. D. B. Jelliffe. *Ascaris lumbricoides* and malnutrition in tropical children. *Doc. Med. Geogr. Trop. 5,* 314-320 (1953).
8. A. W. Woodruff. Pathogenicity of intestinal helminthic infections. *Trans. R. Soc. Trop. Med. Hyg. 59,* 585-606 (1978).
9. A. C. Chandler and C. P. Read. *Introduction to Parasitology,* John Wiley, New York, 1961.
10. E. B. Cram. Ascariasis in preventive medicine. *Am. J. Trop. Med. Hyg. 6,* 91-114 (1926).
11. H. C. Jeffrey and R. M. Leach. *Atlas of Medical Helminthology and Protozoology*. Williams & Wilkins, Baltimore, Md., 1966.
12. A. E. Keller, H. Casparis, and W. S. Leathers. A clinical study of ascariasis. *JAMA 97,* 302-306 (1931).
13. World Health Organization Expert Committee. *Control of Ascariasis.* WHO Technical Report Series No. 379, Geneva, 1967.
14. V. W. Archer and C. H. Patterson. Roentgen diagnosis of ascariasis. *JAMA 95,* 1819-1821 (1930).
15. S. B. Lagundoye. Disordered small bowel pattern in ascariasis. *Trop. Geogr. Med. 24,* 226-313 (1972).
16. M. P. Moore. The pathological aspects of ascariasis. *South. Med. J. 47,* 825-831 (1954).
17. J. Piggot, E. A. Hansbarger, and R. C. Neafie. Human ascariasis. *Am. J. Clin. Pathol. 53,* 223-234 (1970).
18. C. C. de Silva. Tropical ascariasis. *J. Trop. Pediatr. 3,* 62-73 (1957).
19. D. S. Blumenthal and M. G. Schultz. Incidence of intestinal obstruction in children infected with *Ascaris lumbricoides. Am. J. Trop. Med. Hyg. 24,* 801-805 (1975).
20. P. S. Venkatachalam and V. N. Patwardhan. The role of *Ascaris lumbricoides* in the nutrition of the host: Effects of ascariasis on digestion of protein. *Trans. R. Soc. Trop. Med. Hyg. 47,* 169-175 (1953).
21. K. Tripathy, E. Duque, O. Bolaños, H. Lotero, and L. G. Mayoral. Malabsorption syndrome in ascariasis. *Am. J. Clin. Nutr. 25,* 1276-1281 (1972).
22. K. Tripathy, F. Gonzalez, H. Lotero, and O. Bolaños. Effects of *Ascaris* infection on human nutrition. *Am. J. Trop. Med. Hyg. 20,* 212-218 (1971).
23. S. P. S. Teotia, M. Teotia, K. B. Kunwar, and S. S. Misra. Fat malabsorption in intestinal parasitic infections. *J. Indian Med. Assoc. 53,* 577-582 (1969).
24. B. Bray. Nitrogen metabolism in West African children. *Proc. Nutr. Soc. 7,* 3-13 (1953).
25. D. Mahalanabis, K. N. Jalan, T. K. Maitra, and S. K. Agarwal. Vitamin A absorption in ascariasis. *Am. J. Clin. Nutr. 29,* 1372-1375 (1976).

26. B. Sivakumar and V. Reddy. Absorption of vitamin A in children with ascariasis. *J. Trop. Med. Hyg. 78,* 114-115 (1975).
27. M. G. Gupta, S. Mithal, K. L. Arara, and B. N. Tandon. Effects of periodic deworming on nutritional stauts of *Ascaris*-infested preschool children receiving supplementary food. *Lancet 3,* 108-110 (1977).
28. L. S. Stephenson, D. W. T. Crompton, M. C. Latham, M. C. Nesheim, and T. W. J. Schulpen. The influence of *Ascaris* infection on growth of malnourished preschool children. *Fed. Proc. 37,* 264 (1978).
29. L. S. Stephenson (Latham), M. C. Latham, and S. Basta. The nutritional and economic implications of *Ascaris* infection in Kenya. *World Bank Staff Working Paper No. 271.* World Bank, Washington, D.C., Sept. 1977.
30. D. S. Blumenthal and M. G. Schultz. Effects of *Ascaris* infection on nutritional status. *Am. J. Trop. Med. Hyg. 25*, 682-690 (1976).
31. J. P. Carter, R. Vanderzwaag, W. J. Darby, E. J. Lease, F. H. Lauter, B. W. Dudley, E. G. High, D. J. Wright, and T. Murphree. Nutrition and parasitism among rural pre-school children in South Carolina. *J. Natl. Med. Assoc. 62,* 181-191 (1970).
32. J. G. Banwell and G. A. Shad. Hookworm. *Clin. Gastroenterol. 7,* 129-156 (1978).
33. M. Roche and M. Layrisse. The nature and causes of "hookworm anemia." *Am. J. Trop. Med. Hyg. 15,* 1032-1100 (1966).
34. M. Layrisse and M. Roche. The relationship between anemia and hookworm infection. Results of surveys of rural Venezuelan populations. *Am. J. Hyg. 79,* 279-301 (1964).
35. J. M. Falaiye, J. M. Oladapo, and S. C. Wali. Hookworm enteropathy. *J. Trop. Med. Hyg. 77,* 211-214 (1974).
36. B. W. Tandon, R. K. Kohle, A. K. Saraya, K. Ramachandra, and O. M. Prakash. Role of parasites in the pathogenesis of intestinal malabsorption in hookworm disease. *Gut 10,* 293-298 (1969).
37. J. G. Banwell, P. D. Marsden, V. Blackman, P. J. Leonard, and M. S. R. Hutt. Hookworm infection and intestinal absorption amongst Africans in Uganda. *Am. J. Trop. Med. Hyg. 16,* 304-308 (1967).
38. M. S. Wolfe. *Oxyuris, Trichostrongylus,* and *Trichuris. Clin. Gastroenterol.* 7, 201-217 (1978).
39. M. Layrisse, L. Aparcedo, C. Martinez-Torres, and M. Roche. Blood loss due to infection with *Trichuris trichiura. Am. J. Trop. Med. Hyg. 16,* 613-619 (1967).
40. S. S. Basta and A. Churchill. Iron deficiency anemia and the productivity of adult males in Indonesia. *World Bank Staff Working Paper No. 175.* World Bank, Washington, D.C., April 1974.
41. F. Arfaa, G. H. Sahba, I. Farahmandian, and H. Jalali. Evaluation of the effect of different methods of control of soil-transmitted helminths in Khuzestan, Southwest Iran. *Am. J. Trop. Med. Hyg. 26,* 230-233 (1977).

42. O. Gish and G. Walker. Transport and communication systems in health services. *Trop. Doc. 7,* 119-122 (1977).
43. R. E. Brown. Some nutritional considerations in times of major catastrophe. *Clin. Pediatr. 11,* 334-342 (1972).

Author Index

Numbers in brackets are reference numbers and indicate that an author's work is referred to although the name is not cited in the text. Italic numbers give the page on which the complete reference is listed.

B

C

D

E

F

G

H

I

J

K

O

P

Q

R

S

T

W

Y

Z

Subject Index

Acknowledgement is given to the valuable assistance of Ms. Mary Ann Bayne, with the subject index and bibliography; Ms. Jean Burton and Ms. Jan Coyle for their secretarial support.

F

I

L

M

V

W

X

Y

Z